MEDICAL MASTERCLASS

EDITOR-IN-CHIEF

JOHN D FIRTH DM FRCP

Consultant Physician and Nephrologist
Addenbrooke's Hospital
Cambridge

CARDIOLOGY AND RESPIRATORY MEDICINE

EDITORS

PAUL R ROBERTS MD FRCP

Consultant Cardiologist
Southampton General Hospital
Southampton

STEPHEN J FOWLER MD MRCP(UK)

Lecturer and Honorary Consultant in Respiratory Medicine
University of Manchester and Lancashire Teaching Hospitals NHS Trust
Royal Preston Hospital
Preston

Second Edition

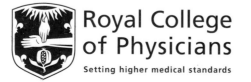
Royal College
of Physicians
Setting higher medical standards

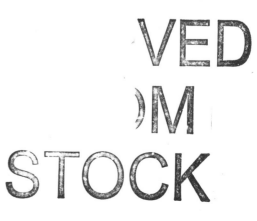

Disclaimer

LIST OF CONTRIBUTORS

Dr P Bhatia MBBS MRCP(Ireland)
Consultant Physician Respiratory and
Internal Medicine
Tameside General Hospital
Ashton-Under-Lyne

Dr B Chandrasekaran MRCP(UK)
Clinical Research Fellow
The Royal Brompton Hospital
London

Dr PWX Foley MRCP(UK)
Specialist Registrar in Cardiology
and Honorary Research Fellow
(University of Birmingham)
Cardiology Department
Portsmouth Hospitals NHS Trust
St Mary's Hospital
Portsmouth

Dr SJ Fowler MD MRCP(UK)
Lecturer and Honorary Consultant
in Respiratory Medicine
University of Manchester and Lancashire
Teaching Hospitals NHS Trust
Royal Preston Hospital
Preston

Dr PR Kalra MRCP(UK)
Consultant Cardiologist
Cardiology Department
Portsmouth Hospitals NHS Trust
St Mary's Hospital
Portsmouth

Dr S Kaul MRCP(UK)
Specialist Registrar in Respiratory
and Intensive Care Medicine
Department of Respiratory Medicine
King's College Hospital
London

Dr DKC Lee MRCP(UK)
Specialist Registrar
Department of Respiratory Medicine
Papworth Hospital
Cambridge

Dr N Melikian BSc (Hons) MBBS MRCP(UK)
British Cardiac Society
John Parker Research Fellow
Cardiology Department
King's College Hospital
London

Dr A Pawlowicz PhD FRCP
Consultant Physician in General
and Respiractory Medicine
Department of Respiratory Medicine
The Queen Elizabeth Hospital
King's Lynn

Dr PR Roberts MD FRCP
Consultant Cardiologist
Southampton General Hospital
Southampton

Dr R Sharma MRCP(UK)
Consultant Cardiologist
Ealing Hospital NHS Trust
London

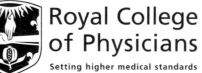

Royal College
of Physicians
Setting higher medical standards

© 2008 Royal College of Physicians of London

Published by:
Royal College of Physicians of London
11 St. Andrews Place
Regent's Park
London NW1 4LE
United Kingdom

Set and printed by Graphicraft Limited, Hong Kong

First edition published 2001
Reprinted 2004
Second edition published 2008

ISBN: 978-1-86016-270-1 (this book)
ISBN: 978-1-86016-260-2 (set)

Distribution Information:
Jerwood Medical Education Resource Centre
Royal College of Physicians of London
11 St. Andrews Place
Regent's Park
London NW1 4LE
United Kingdom
Tel: +44 (0)207 935 1174 ext 422/490
Fax: +44 (0)207 486 6653
Email: merc@rcplondon.ac.uk
Web: http://www.rcplondon.ac.uk/

CONTENTS

CARDIOLOGY

PACES Stations and Acute Scenarios 3

Diseases and Treatments 69

CONTENTS

FOREWORD

Since its initial publication in 2001, *Medical Masterclass* has been regarded as a key learning and teaching resource for physicians around the world. The resource was produced in part to meet the vision of the Royal College of Physicians: *'Doctors of the highest quality, serving patients well'*. This vision continues and, along with advances in clinical practice and changes in the format of the MRCP(UK) exam, has justified the publication of this second edition.

The MRCP(UK) is an international examination that seeks to advance the learning of and enhance the training process for physicians worldwide. On passing the exam physicians are recognised as having attained the required knowledge, skills and manner appropriate for training at a specialist level. However, passing the exam is a challenge. The pass rate at each sitting of the written papers is about 40%. Even the most prominent consultants have had to sit each part of the exam more than once in order to pass. With this challenge in mind, the College has produced *Medical Masterclass*, a comprehensive learning resource to help candidates with the preparation that is key to making the grade.

Medical Masterclass has been produced by the Education Department of the College. A work of this size represents a formidable amount of effort by the Editor-in-Chief – Dr John Firth – and his team of editors and authors. I would like to thank our colleagues for this wonderful educational product and wholeheartedly recommend it as an invaluable learning resource for all physicians preparing for their MRCP(UK) examination.

Professor Ian Gilmore MD PRCP
President of the Royal College of Physicians

PREFACE

The second edition of *Medical Masterclass* is produced and published by the Education Department of the Royal College of Physicians of London. It comprises 12 textbooks, a companion interactive website and two CD-ROMs. Its aim is to help doctors in their first few years of training to improve their medical knowledge and skills; and in particular to (a) learn how to deal with patients who are acutely ill, and (b) pass postgraduate examinations, such as the MRCP(UK) or European Diploma in Internal Medicine.

The 12 textbooks are divided as follows: two cover the scientific background to medicine, one is devoted to general clinical skills [including specific guidance on exam technique for PACES, the practical assessment of clinical examination skills that is the final part of the MRCP(UK) exam], one deals with acute medicine and the other eight cover the range of medical specialties.

The core material of each of the medical specialties is dealt with in seven sections:

- Case histories – you are presented with letters of referral commonly received in each specialty and led through the ways in which the patients' histories should be explored, and what should then follow in the way of investigation and/or treatment.

- Physical examination scenarios – these emphasise the logical analysis of physical signs and sensible clinical reasoning: 'having found this, what would you do?'

- Communication and ethical scenarios – what are the difficult issues that commonly arise in each specialty? What do you actually say to the 'frequently asked (but still very difficult) questions?'

- Acute presentations – what are the priorities if you are the doctor seeing the patient in the Emergency Department or the Medical Admissions Unit?

- Diseases and treatments – structured concise notes.

- Investigations and practical procedures – more short and to-the-point notes.

- Self assessment questions – in the form used in the MRCP(UK) Part 1 and Part 2 exams.

The companion website – which is continually updated – enables you to take mock MRCP(UK) Part 1 or Part 2 exams, or to be selective in the questions you tackle (if you want to do ten questions on cardiology, or any other specialty, you can do). For every question you complete you can see how your score compares with that of others who have logged onto the site and attempted it. The two CD-ROMs each contain 30 interactive cases requiring diagnosis and treatment.

I hope that you enjoy using *Medical Masterclass* to learn more about medicine, which – whatever is happening politically to primary care, hospitals and medical career structures – remains a wonderful occupation. It is sometimes intellectually and/or emotionally very challenging, and also sometimes extremely rewarding, particularly when reduced to the essential of a doctor trying to provide best care for a patient.

John Firth DM FRCP
Editor-in-Chief

ACKNOWLEDGEMENTS

Medical Masterclass has been produced by a team. The names of those who have written or edited material are clearly indicated elsewhere, but without the support of many other people it would not exist. Naming names is risky, but those worthy of particular note include: Sir Richard Thompson (College Treasurer) and Mrs Winnie Wade (Director of Education), who steered the project through committees that are traditionally described as labyrinthine, and which certainly seem so to me; and also Arthur Wadsworth (Project Co-ordinator) and Don Liu in the College Education Department office. Don is a veteran of the first edition of *Medical Masterclass*, and it would be fair to say that without his great efforts a second edition might not have seen the light of day.

John Firth DM FRCP
Editor-in-Chief

KEY FEATURES

We have created a range of icon boxes that sit among the text of the various *Medical Masterclass* modules. They are there to help you identify key information and to make learning easier and more enjoyable. Here is a brief explanation:

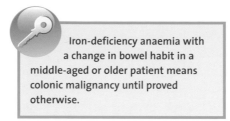

Iron-deficiency anaemia with a change in bowel habit in a middle-aged or older patient means colonic malignancy until proved otherwise.

This icon is used to highlight points of particular importance.

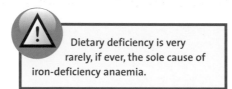

Dietary deficiency is very rarely, if ever, the sole cause of iron-deficiency anaemia.

This icon is used to indicate common or important drug interactions, pitfalls of practical procedures, or when to take symptoms or signs particularly seriously.

CARDIOLOGY

Authors:

B Chandrasekaran, PWX Foley, PR Kalra, N Melikian, PR Roberts and R Sharma

Editor:

PR Roberts

Editor-in-Chief:

JD Firth

CARDIOLOGY: SECTION 1
PACES STATIONS AND ACUTE SCENARIOS

1.1 History-taking

1.1.1 Paroxysmal palpitations

Introduction

The symptom of palpitations (abnormal awareness of the heart beat) can be caused by a range of clinical conditions, from the very benign to the potentially life-threatening. Approach the patient with this in mind. It is unusual to see someone during a symptomatic episode, so as much information as possible should be gained from the history, with the main aim being to assess the patient's potential risk from life-threatening ventricular arrhythmias. You should always have in mind a list of the possible causes of palpitations (Table 1). In most situations it will be essential to perform investigations during a symptomatic episode. Remember that the severity of symptoms does not always reflect the seriousness of the underlying problem: some patients in sinus rhythm may experience severe palpitations, whereas others may be asymptomatic when in ventricular tachycardia (VT). In this case the family history should make you particularly keen to exclude significant inherited conditions that may predispose to arrhythmias, eg hypertrophic cardiomyopathy.

> Severe symptoms do not necessarily mean a dangerous arrhythmia and minor symptoms do not necessarily mean a benign arrhythmia.

History of the presenting problem

What are the palpitations like?

The characteristics of the palpitations can provide valuable clues in making the diagnosis. Question the patient about the following.

- Ask her to 'tap out' the rhythm of her palpitations. Note how fast this is and whether it is regular or irregular. Irregular means that AF or frequent extrasystoles (ectopics) are most likely. A 'missed beat' is typically caused by an extrasystole: after the compensatory pause the next sinus beat is felt with extra force. These missed beats are almost always of no pathological significance. However, they can cause worry that is likely to be reinforced because anxiety is the most common cause of awareness of extrasystoles. They are likely to have been long-standing and previously asymptomatic.

TABLE 1 POTENTIAL CAUSES OF PALPITATIONS	
Type of palpitation	**Cause**
No arrhythmia	Anaemia Anxiety Panic attacks Depression
Extrasystoles	Atrial Ventricular
Bradyarrhythmia	Atrioventricular block Sinus node disease
Tachyarrhythmia	VT Atrial fibrillation (AF)/flutter Atrioventricular nodal re-entry tachycardia Atrioventricular re-entry tachycardia Sinus tachycardia
VT, ventricular tachycardia.	

- Does she feel the palpitations in the neck? These are suggestive of cannon waves, indicating simultaneous atrial and ventricular contraction. This can occur in atrioventricular (AV) block, AV dissociation associated with VT or atrioventricular nodal re-entry tachycardia (AVNRT).

- How do the palpitations start, what brings them on and how do they stop? Does she get any warning at all? Do attacks come on gradually or suddenly? Palpitations that come on and go away gradually are most likely due to sinus tachycardia.

- Are there accompanying symptoms? Does she feel faint or dizzy when these occur? Has she ever collapsed? Arrhythmias causing these symptoms are more likely to be serious (potentially life-threatening) and clearly mandate thorough investigation. Some patients with supraventricular tachycardia (SVT) develop polyuria as a result of atrial stretch causing the release of atrial natriuretic peptide.

- How frequent are the palpitations? Palpitations that occur infrequently are likely to be difficult to catch on simple ambulatory monitoring.

- What treatments have been tried already? An SVT may be terminated by a Valsalva manoeuvre.

Other relevant history

- General health: is there anything to suggest thyrotoxicosis? (See *Endocrinology*, Section 1.1.3.)

- Smoking, alcohol, tea and coffee consumption: acute excess of these can trigger arrhythmia in those predisposed to it.

- Drugs (prescribed and non-prescribed): a range of these can cause arrhythmia. Always consult the drug datasheet or the *British National Formulary*.

- Family history is clearly an important element in this case, so it is important to obtain as much information as possible, eg which particular relatives were involved, what were the surroundings of their deaths and at what ages did they die? It is often helpful to draw a simple family tree. A patient is much more likely to be concerned about palpitations, even if of benign cause, if a relative has died at a young age of heart disease. Check if there is any post-mortem information available for any members of the patient's family who have died from heart disease.

- Is the patient prone to anxiety? Does she ever have anxiety attacks? Has she a history of recurrent presentation to doctors with medically unexplained symptoms? This aspect of the history needs to be explored sensitively. It is unhelpful if the patient thinks that this line of questioning infers that you do not believe her. If there is a high degree of anxiety, it may be the cause of her symptoms, although other pathological substrates may be present.

Plan for investigation and management

After examining the patient and confirming no abnormalities, you would plan as follows.

ECG

In most situations only a 12-lead ECG in sinus rhythm is available. When assessing the 12-lead ECG of a patient with palpitations:

- look for sinus bradycardia or tachycardia;

- check if there are features suggestive of a cardiac structural abnormality, eg P mitrale or left ventricular hypertrophy (LVH) (Fig. 1);

- measure the PR interval;

- check if there is AV block;

- check for delta waves (Fig. 2);

- ask the patient if she has had a previous myocardial infarction (Q-wave or T-wave changes);

- measure the QT interval and calculate the QT correction (QTc, QT adjusted for rate);

- check for any atrial or ventricular extrasystoles.

However, if an ECG has been recorded during symptoms and documents an arrhythmia, it may not be necessary to investigate further because this alone may enable a precise diagnosis to be made.

Chest radiograph

This is likely to be normal, although an increased cardiothoracic ratio or abnormal cardiac outline may suggest significant pathology.

Ambulatory monitoring

See Section 3.3. An example of an arrhythmia captured on an ambulatory monitor record is shown in Fig. 3.

Echocardiography

This is an important test that helps stratify the patient's risk. If this shows the patient to have a structurally and functionally normal heart, it puts her into a very low-risk group. However, it is important not to discount the possibility of significant arrhythmia just because

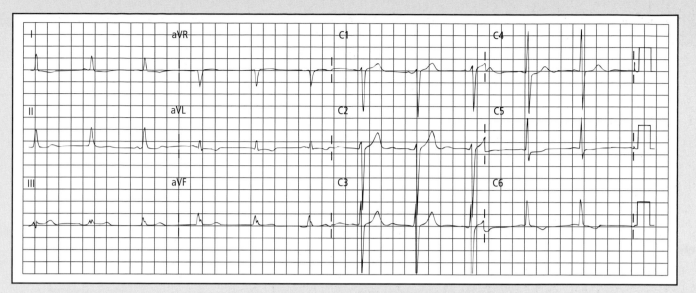

▲ **Fig. 1** ECG showing LVH with strain (lateral ST/T changes) in a patient with previously undiagnosed aortic stenosis.

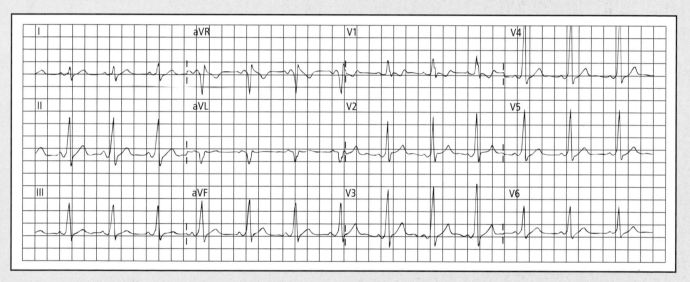

▲ **Fig. 2** Twelve-lead ECG of patient with Wolff–Parkinson–White syndrome. Note the short PR interval and delta waves.

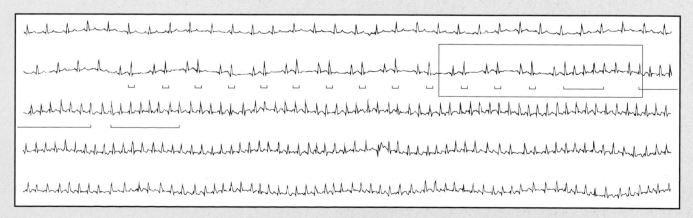

▲ **Fig. 3** Ambulatory monitor of a patient with SVT. Sinus tachycardia is followed by ventricular bigeminy before the sudden onset of SVT.

the echocardiogram is normal, particularly in a patient with a potentially significant family history.

> A patient with a normal physical examination, normal ECG and normal echocardiogram is at very low risk of life-threatening arrhythmia.

Blood tests

- Abnormal electrolytes, particularly hypokalaemia, may predispose to arrhythmias.

- Hyperthyroidism may cause AF or sinus tachycardia and hypothyroidism sinus bradycardia.

Review in clinic with results of investigations when available.

Further discussion

In many cases a benign arrhythmia is detected, such as ventricular or atrial ectopy, and occasionally symptoms are clearly associated with sinus rhythm. In most cases explanation and positive reassurance to the patient are all that is required. Only in rare instances, where the patient is very debilitated, should a beta-blocker be prescribed.

Significant symptoms can occasionally be associated with sinus tachycardia. In these circumstances it is important to exclude causes of sinus tachycardia, the most common being anxiety, before attributing the arrhythmia to inappropriate sinus node function.

If an arrhythmia has been found to be associated with symptoms, management will be tailored to the individual and the specific arrhythmia. In different situations this may require reassurance,

antiarrhythmic medication or referral to a specialist electrophysiologist for consideration of catheter ablation (see Section 3.4).

1.1.2 Palpitations with dizziness

Letter of referral for urgent assessment in the cardiology clinic

Dear Doctor,

Re: Mr Matthew Carney, aged 57 years

Please assess this retired policeman who has a 2-month history of rapid palpitations. Initially he was well during the episodes, but more recently he has noticed that he is dizzy when they go on for more than 20 seconds. He came to see me today as he nearly blacked out this morning. He has previously been very well and this is the first time he has asked to see a doctor. Examination today was unremarkable but I am quite concerned about the presyncopal episode today and would value your opinion. Does he require detailed cardiac investigation?

Yours sincerely,

Introduction

Your main concern is that this patient gives a history of presyncope, which places him in a higher risk category for life-threatening arrhythmia. The main objective must be to exclude a significant ventricular arrhythmia. With the little information available, it is apparent that the palpitations are directly related to the presyncope,

which would be consistent with the diagnosis of ventricular tachycardia (VT).

It is vital to ensure that the patient is safe while a diagnosis is being established. He should thus be admitted from clinic for investigation and monitoring. It is essential to document his heart rhythm during an episode. Some patients with VT are asymptomatic, whereas others are extremely symptomatic from only short runs of VT. Both groups are at risk of cardiac arrest as a result of VT or the VT degenerating into ventricular fibrillation.

History of the presenting problem

What is the relationship of the presyncope and palpitations?

It is important to determine the order of symptoms; many patients with presyncope or syncope will have a reactive sinus tachycardia after the event that might cause a feeling of palpitation. In this case it is clear that the presyncope is occurring with more prolonged episodes of palpitation.

Aside from ventricular arrhythmia, consider other causes of palpitations and syncope:

- bradyarrhythmias;

- atrial flutter with 1:1 conduction;

- atrial fibrillation (AF) and Wolff–Parkinson–White syndrome;

- aortic stenosis.

And do not forget the following.

- Vasovagal syncope: the most common cause of presyncope and syncope.

- Epilepsy: a common cause of syncope, but there seem to be no features here to support this diagnosis.

- Acute blood loss: this will usually be obvious, but it is a mistake to miss the fact that the patient has had melaena.

> **Cardiac arrhythmias that can cause syncope:**
>
> - VT/ventricular fibrillation;
> - bradyarrhythmias;
> - atrial flutter with 1:1 conduction;
> - AF and Wolff–Parkinson–White syndrome.

Other relevant history

Ischaemic heart disease

This is a common cause of VT. In this situation there appears to be no previous history, but it is important to clarify whether there is a previous history of angina or myocardial infarction. If not, then specific symptons of angina should be sought: 'What is the most exercise that you do? Have you had any tightness in your chest when you've been doing that recently?' It will also be appropriate to ask about risk factors for ischaemic heart disease.

Cardiomyopathy

Most forms can cause VT. It is important to find out whether there is a history of breathlessness, lethargy or recent viral illness. An alcohol history should be taken, both for the current time and for the past.

Drugs (prescribed and non-prescribed)

Drug toxicity can provoke VT, eg digoxin, quinidine and catecholamines. Check the datasheet or *British National Formulary* for details of any drug that the patient is taking. Is arrhythmia reported as a side effect? Recreational drugs such as cocaine and ecstasy are associated with arrhythmias.

Family history

This is particularly pertinent in young patients presenting with arrhythmias. Always enquire if anyone in the family has had a similar problem, or if anyone has died suddenly and unexpectedly. VT may be part of a primary electrophysiological disturbance or secondary to any pathology that produces structural changes in the ventricles. Any 'cardiac history' could therefore be relevant, eg valvular heart disease, congenital heart disease, right ventricular dysplasia or previous cardiac surgery.

Epilepsy

The history in this case points very clearly to a cardiac arrhythmia, but it would be sensible to enquire briefly to ensure that the patient does not have epilepsy and confirm that there are no features to suggest that this might be responsible for the current episodes (eg aura, tongue biting or urinary incontinence).

Plan for investigation and management

In this case examination of the patient was normal. You would plan as follows.

ECG

Obtaining an ECG during an episode is a key objective in establishing a diagnosis (Fig. 4). Beware of confusing VT and supraventricular tachycardia with aberrant conduction (see Section 3.1).

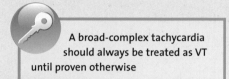

> A broad-complex tachycardia should always be treated as VT until proven otherwise

Ambulatory monitoring

If the diagnosis is not apparent, monitoring for longer periods may be necessary (see Section 3.3).

Electrophysiology study

If symptoms are infrequent or doubt exists as to the diagnosis, then provocation of the rhythm during an electrophysiological study will provide definitive evidence (see Section 3.2).

Other

If VT is suspected, investigations to identify possible causes should be considered. Specifically, investigations should be concerned with identifying any structural cardiac abnormality (Table 2).

TABLE 2 INVESTIGATIONS FOR IDENTIFYING A CARDIAC ABNORMALITY THAT MAY PROVOKE VENTRICULAR ARRHYTHMIAS	
Investigation	**Looking for:**
CXR	Cardiomegaly, cardiac silhouette and pulmonary oedema (Fig. 5)
Electrolytes	Abnormalities of potassium or magnesium can be associated with arrhythmia
Echocardiogram	Cardiac function, valve structure/function and intracardiac masses (Fig. 6)
Exercise ECG	Ischaemia and exercise-induced arrhythmias
Coronary angiography	Coronary atherosclerosis and valvular function
CT or MRI	Mediastinal pathology and pericardial/myocardial disease

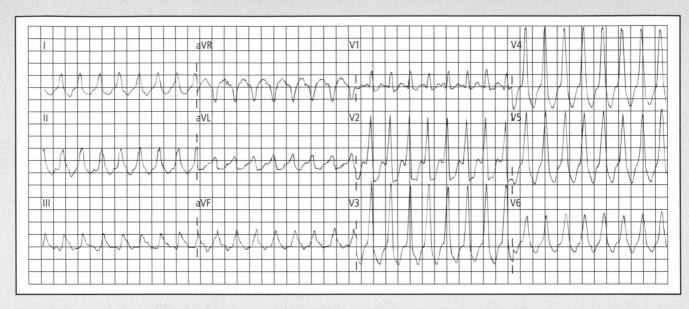

▲**Fig. 4** Twelve-lead ECG of VT. Note broad complexes and concordance across chest leads. Right bundle-branch block morphology suggests left ventricular origin.

Further discussion

The patient is likely to be having presyncope associated with VT. Management will consist of treating any immediate episodes of VT (DC shock/pharmacological cardioversion) and identification of the cause of the arrhythmia (see Section 2.2.2). If possible, the underlying cause should be corrected and the risk of arrhythmia then reassessed. In this case it may turn out that the patient has significant coronary artery disease that warrants revascularisation, either with percutaneous intervention or coronary artery bypass grafting. Following this it would be important to reassess left ventricular function and consider an electrophysiological study to determine whether recurrent VT was likely (see Section 3.2). All patients with VT should be assessed as to whether they would benefit from an implantable cardioverter defibrillator (ICD) (see Section 3.4).

In those patients who do not have an indication for an ICD, either catheter ablation or pharmacological therapy may be considered. It is essential to monitor the patient to ensure suppression of the arrhythmia; symptomatology is not always adequate because the drugs may slow but not prevent the VT, thus making it better tolerated or unnoticed. Monitoring will usually be by ambulatory ECG recording, but exercise testing if the arrhythmia is induced by exercise or provocation during electrophysiological study may be appropriate in some cases.

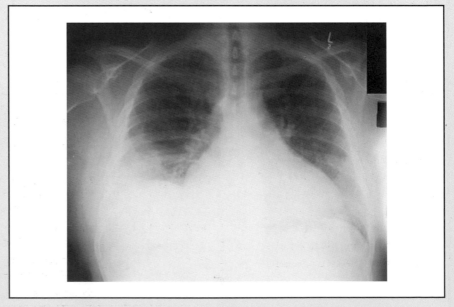

▲**Fig. 5** Chest radiograph of patient with dilated cardiomyopathy. The cardiothoracic ratio is increased. There is a pleural effusion at the right base.

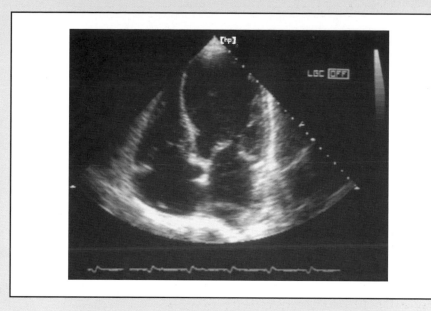

▲ **Fig. 6** Echocardiogram demonstrating dilated cardiomyopathy. This is a 'four-chamber' view with both ventricles dilated, particularly the left ventricle (seen in the centre at the top).

1.1.3 Breathlessness and ankle swelling

Letter of referral to cardiology outpatient clinic

Dear Doctor,

Re: Professor Freddie Walsh, aged 48 years

Thank you for seeing this professor of mathematics who has a 3-month history of progressive exertional dyspnoea, fatigue and peripheral oedema. He has generally been fit and well without prior history. His father died in his forties of a 'large heart'. He is not taking routine medication, although I have started him today on furosemide 40 mg once a day. Please assess the cause of his symptoms.

Yours sincerely,

Introduction

These symptoms are most commonly caused by cardiac or pulmonary disease. The cause usually becomes apparent early in the history: subsequent questions, examination and investigation should be directed to providing confirmatory details. The common differential diagnoses are given in Table 3. Consider the main causes of chronic heart failure when taking the history. It is important to assess the impact of symptoms on general daily activities, including work.

History of the presenting problem

If the following do not emerge spontaneously, make specific enquiry about them.

- Chest pain: if present, does this sound like ischaemic cardiac pain or like pleurisy?

- Cough/sputum: has it been present and has there been haemoptysis?

- Wheeze: note that this is not synonymous with airway disease. It may occur in pulmonary oedema when it is known as 'cardiac asthma'.

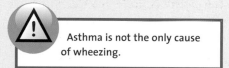

Asthma is not the only cause of wheezing.

Cardiovascular system

Progressive breathlessness associated with orthopnoea,

System	Condition
Cardiac	**Left ventricular dysfunction** **Valvular heart disease** Pericardial effusion/constriction Cyanotic congenital heart disease High-output cardiac failure secondary to anaemia
Pulmonary	**Chronic airway or parenchymal lung disease (cor pulmonale)** Chronic, repeated pulmonary embolism (PE) Primary pulmonary hypertension
Gastrointestinal	Liver failure Protein-losing enteropathy
Renal	Nephrotic syndrome Chronic renal failure
Endocrine	Hypothyroidism

TABLE 3 DIFFERENTIAL DIAGNOSIS OF ANKLE SWELLING AND BREATHLESSNESS

Notes – most common causes in bold.

paroxysmal nocturnal dyspnoea and cough productive of clear frothy sputum would suggest a cardiac cause. The ankle swelling in cardiac failure is usually bilateral and symmetrical, but it is not uncommon for one ankle to swell initially.

A preceding episode of severe central chest pain at rest, particularly if occurring against a background of stable angina, would suggest a precipitating myocardial infarction (MI). A 'really bad episode of indigestion' may have been something different.

Has the patient been started on diuretic therapy? Has this helped? A good response would support but not prove a cardiac cause for the symptoms.

Respiratory system

The development of increasing breathlessness and ankle swelling may indicate the development of cor pulmonale in a man with long-standing respiratory disorder. His symptoms are said to have started only 3 months ago, but what was he like before then? What is the most vigorous exercise he ever took? Three months ago was his breathing more laboured than that of his wife, family or friends?

Stepwise progression (sudden deterioration followed by periods of stability) should raise the suspicion of multiple recurrent PE, even in the absence of pleuritic chest pain or haemoptysis.

Other relevant history

It is clearly important to establish any history of cardiovascular or respiratory disease. Ask about the following.

- Rheumatic fever or history of a cardiac murmur.

- Recurrent asthma/bronchitis or any other respiratory problem.

- Smoking, which is obviously a substantial risk factor for both chronic airway disease and ischaemic heart disease.

- Alcohol intake, which is a risk factor for cardiomyopathy. Ask: 'How much alcohol do you drink now? Have you ever been a heavy drinker in the past?'

- Previous BP measurements: untreated hypertension can lead to left ventricular failure.

- Previous cardiac surgery might be suggestive of impaired left ventricular function or constrictive pericarditis.

Whilst the GP's letter has stated that the patient is not taking any regular medication, it is essential to confirm this and ensure that he has not been taking non-prescribed treatment that may be causing or exacerbating his symptoms, eg NSAIDs.

A detailed family history is particularly important in this case. His father died at a young age of presumed cardiomyopathy ('a large heart'). This might reflect a familial dilated cardiomyopathy or premature coronary artery disease.

Plan for investigation and management

After explaining to the patient that you would normally complete a full examination, plan the following baseline investigations.

ECG

A routine ECG is very helpful. If it is completely normal, then a diagnosis of chronic heart failure is unlikely. Other abnormalities may help elucidate the aetiology of the patient's symptoms.

- A dominantly negative P wave in lead V1, reflecting left atrial hypertrophy, is an indirect sign of left heart dysfunction (Fig. 7).

- Right ventricular hypertrophy (right bundle-branch block with dominant R waves in V1) secondary to any cause of pulmonary hypertension.

- Low voltages and electrical alternans, which occur with a large pericardial effusion.

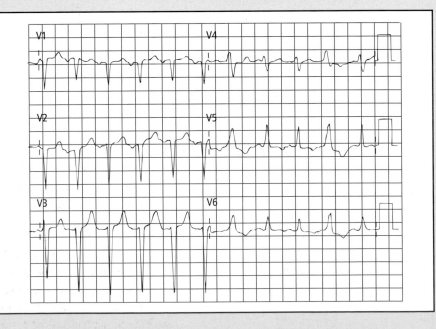

▲**Fig. 7** ECG showing left atrial strain (inverted P wave in V1) and partial left bundle-branch block in a patient with severe congestive cardiac failure secondary to alcoholic cardiomyopathy.

requires cardiac catheterisation for confirmation.

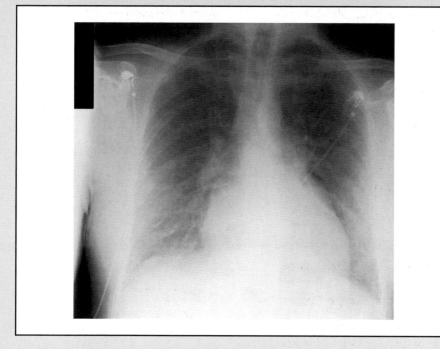

▲**Fig. 8** Chest radiograph showing cardiomegaly and pulmonary oedema in a patient with congestive cardiac failure caused by severe mitral regurgitation. Note cardiomegaly and enlarged left atrium.

- Atrial arrhythmias: common in both cardiac and pulmonary disease.

- Previous MI, left bundle-branch block or poor R-wave progression indicating left ventricular disease.

Chest radiograph

In the context of an elevated JVP:

- a large heart should prompt echocardiography (Fig. 8);

- check for signs of pulmonary oedema;

- if heart size is normal, inspect the lung fields closely for evidence of chronic obstructive airway disease or parenchymal lung disease;

- if the heart size and lung fields are both normal, consider PE or pericardial constriction.

Blood tests

Check FBC, electrolytes and renal, liver and thyroid function tests.

Urinalysis

Do not forget this simple test. If there is significant proteinuria on dipstick testing (>2+), then nephrotic syndrome is possible. In this case check serum albumin and urinary albumin/creatinine ratio or 24-hour urinary protein excretion. Remember that proteinuria of up to 1 g/day (occasionally more) can be caused by severe cardiac failure.

Echocardiography

This is most useful for excluding significant valvular or left ventricular disease. If a pericardial effusion is found, then careful clinical and echocardiographic assessment is required to judge whether this is contributing to his symptoms. Assessment of right heart function is largely subjective, but reasonably accurate indirect measurements of pulmonary artery systolic pressure can be obtained. Echocardiography may suggest pericardial constriction or restrictive cardiomyopathy, which

Other tests

Other more specialist investigations may be required and will be directed by the clinical features and initial investigations. These include cardiac catheterisation (for coronary artery anatomy and valvular dysfunction) and spiral CT (for PE).

Management

If chronic heart failure is suspected and supported by initial investigations, eg abnormal ECG and CXR, then initial management might include the adjustment of diuretic dose and commencement of an angiotensin-converting enzyme (ACE) inhibitor. The patient should be reviewed with results in due course, but remember that renal function should be monitored in the interim. This should occur approximatey 1–2 weeks after starting ACE inhibitor treatment (see Section 2.3), with advice given to the GP to stop the ACE inhibitor if serum creatinine rises by more than 20%.

Further discussion

The impact of symptoms on daily living are very important. Recommendations regarding work and exercise should all be discussed. Education, with particular emphasis on the rationale for treatment, may help compliance. Involvement of a specialist heart failure nurse is extremely helpful.

If the patient were to deteriorate despite full medical therapy, then cardiac resynchronisation therapy, with or without implantable cardioverter defibrillator (see Section 3.4), or referral for transplant assessment might be required (see Section 2.3).

1.1.4 Breathlessness and exertional presyncope

Letter of referral to cardiology outpatient clinic

Dear Doctor,

Re: Miss Susan Ward, aged 38 years

Thank you for seeing this accountant who is currently out of work. Over the last few months she has complained of gradually worsening fatigue and exertional dyspnoea. A year ago she was fit and active but is now unable to jog or attend her usual exercise classes. There has been no improvement with bronchodilator therapy. She is extremely anxious about an episode last week when she nearly fainted while hurrying for a train to a job interview. Please advise on further management.

Yours sincerely,

Introduction

There are suggestions in this history that stress or anxiety may be contributing to this patient's symptoms, but your primary concern should be to exclude the significant organic conditions that can present insidiously in this way (Table 4).

 Exertional syncope or presyncope is a symptom to be taken seriously. It usually indicates an inability to increase the cardiac output appropriately as a result of a fixed obstruction or ventricular dysfunction.

Although not usually associated with exertional dyspnoea, other causes of syncope and sudden cardiac death in young subjects such as arrhythmogenic RV dysplasia and QT prolongation should also be considered. An accurate and detailed family history is imperative.

Fatigue is a non-specific symptom of multifactorial aetiology, but is a common limiting symptom in patients with heart failure and valvular disease.

History of the presenting problem

- Is the patient limited by fatigue (may indicate low cardiac output), breathlessness or by something else? If so, what?

- How far can she walk/run? How many flights of stairs can she climb? Be specific about this, and try to get a feeling for the pace of progression by asking: 'How does this compare with last Christmas or during your summer holidays?'

- Have there been any other instances of syncope/presyncope, and exactly what were the circumstances? It is important to establish the environment in which these episodes occurred (eg warm and not having eaten, or following alcohol consumption might suggest a vagal component) and if there was any warning.

Ask specifically about the following associated symptoms.

- Chest pain: if present, is this pleuritic or anginal? This woman is young for ischaemic heart disease, but anginal pain can be associated with pulmonary hypertension. This is thought to originate from the hypertrophied (and therefore relatively hypoxic) RV. Rare other causes include anomolous origins of coronary arteries.

- Haemoptysis: a feature of pulmonary hypertension, but could also indicate PE.

- Cough/wheeze/sputum: features that would suggest chronic lung disease.

- Orthopnoea/paroxysmal nocturnal dyspnoea: suggests incipient pulmonary oedema.

- Palpitations (see Sections 1.1.1 and 1.1.2).

TABLE 4 DIFFERENTIAL DIAGNOSIS OF EXERTIONAL DYSPNOEA AND PRESYNCOPE

Pathophysiology	Specific conditions
Left ventricular outflow tract obstruction	Hypertrophic cardiomyopathy (HCM) Aortic subvalvular/valvular/supravalvular stenosis
Pulmonary hypertension	Primary pulmonary hypertension Secondary, eg to respiratory disease, pulmonary thromboembolism or mitral valve disease (see Section 2.12.2)
Right ventricular (RV) outflow tract obstruction	Infundibular/pulmonary stenosis
Left ventricular dysfunction	See Section 2.3
Pericardial compromise of cardiac filling	Effusion Constriction
Anaemia	–
Sustained arrhythmia	Atrial fibrillation Complete heart block

- Ankle oedema/calf swelling or tenderness: unilateral problems raise the possibility of venous thromboembolism; bilateral swelling suggests RV failure.

- Raynaud's phenomenon: this may be present in autoimmune rheumatic disease and also in 10% of women with primary pulmonary hypertension (PPH).

- Any features that would suggest autoimmune rheumatic disease, eg joint pains and rashes.

Other relevant history

Enquire specifically about a history of the following:

- venous thromboembolism;

- rheumatic fever or 'heart murmur';

- any problems during a previous pregnancy (if relevant, see below);

- chest trauma or tuberculosis (may lead to pericardial problems);

- respiratory disease.

Also ask about the following.

- Smoking.

- Alcohol.

- Pregnancy: many previously silent cardiorespiratory conditions manifest themselves in pregnancy because of the physiological changes it engenders.

- Other risk factors for ischaemic heart disease (eg hypertension, smoking, hypercholesterolaemia, family history and diabetes).

- Other risk factors for PE (eg immobility and clotting abnormalities).

Drug history

Ask directly about the use of the following.

- Oral contraceptive: this carries a risk factor for thromboembolism.

- Appetite suppressants: these have been implicated in valve disease and pulmonary hypertension.

- Cardiotoxic chemotherapy.

- Cocaine: this can cause left ventricular dysfunction and pulmonary hypertension.

Family history

A detailed family history is important. Ask broad questions such as 'Has anyone in your family died suddenly at a young age?' Specifically consider:

- premature ischaemic heart disease;

- PE;

- HCM;

- pulmonary hypertension.

Social history

Stress may be a contributary factor. Ask questions regarding work (financial consequences of currently being unemployed), the implications of looking for a new job and her general home circumstances.

Plan for investigation and management

> The echocardiogram is the key investigation in the patient with dyspnoea and syncope on exertion.

Explain that you will carry out a full clinical examination before conducting the following investigations.

ECG

Note the rhythm, axis, and any atrial or ventricular hypertrophy

(see Section 3.1). Left bundle-branch block is commonly associated with a dilated left ventricle (LV).

Chest radiograph

Note heart size and shape, pulmonary arteries, lung fields and any valve calcification or pleural effusions.

Echocardiography

Enables visualisation of ventricular dimensions, hypertrophy and function, together with outflow tracts and valves (with gradients) and any intracardiac shunt or pericardial effusion. If there is significant pulmonary hypertension, a dilated hypertrophied RV that compresses the LV into a 'D' shape (Fig. 9) can usually be seen, and the presence of tricuspid regurgitation enables the estimation of pulmonary artery pressure.

Ambulatory monitoring

To exclude tachyarrhythmias, particularly if structural abnormalities are found on echocardiography.

Oxygen saturation

Check pulse oximetry. Perform arterial blood gases if oxygen saturation is below 95% or the patient looks cyanosed.

Blood tests

Check FBC, electrolytes, renal and liver function, glucose, cholesterol and inflammatory markers (C-reactive protein and erythrocyte sedimentation rate). Other tests for autoimmune rheumatic disease may be indicated (see *Rheumatology and Clinical Immunology*, Section 3.2).

Urinalysis

Look specifically for protein, blood and glucose. Could there be a multisystem inflammatory condition?

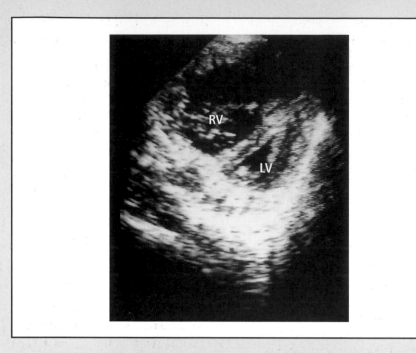

▲**Fig. 9** Short-axis echocardiographic view of a patient with PPH showing the high-pressure, dilated right ventricle (RV) compressing the left ventricle (LV) into a characteristic 'D' shape. (Courtesy of Dr L.M. Shapiro.)

Other tests

If the echocardiogram suggests pulmonary hypertension but no cause is apparent, further investigations are needed (see Section 2.12.1). These should initially be directed towards excluding secondary causes of pulmonary hypertension. If a cause is not discovered and the diagnosis of PPH is made, other investigations (eg right heart catheterisation) are used to determine prognosis and optimise treatment. Consider pulmonary function tests.

Management

Further management will depend on the specific diagnosis. Urgent referral for specialist care is required if a structural cardiac abnormality is found, eg HCM or pulmonary hypertension. In contrast, if examination and investigations are normal, provide reassurance and encourage the patient to maintain activity. Make sure you retain an open mind and keep her under review on at least one further

occasion. If exercise limitation persists, then an exercise test (with monitoring of arterial oxygen saturation) can be valuable in providing reassurance that it is safe to resume previous levels of activity.

Further discussion

Exertional breathlessness is a common reason for referral to cardiology clinics. Identifying patients with significant pathology can sometimes be difficult, and even if patients do have genuine pathology, anxiety may influence how their symptoms are manifested. Exertional syncope should be taken seriously even in a young, apparently fit individual; in rare cases it can precede sudden cardiac death. Initial investigations should be ordered on an urgent basis, particularly if the ECG is abnormal.

If HCM is diagnosed, it will be important to ask about children and other family members because issues of screening will need to be considered and discussed. This is

generally best performed via a specialist service with trained counsellors.

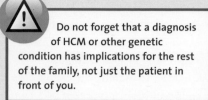 Do not forget that a diagnosis of HCM or other genetic condition has implications for the rest of the family, not just the patient in front of you.

1.1.5 Dyspnoea, ankle oedema and cyanosis

Letter of referral to cardiology outpatient clinic

Dear Doctor,

Re: Mr Rob Owen, aged 45 years

Many thanks for assessing this reclusive 45-year-old man. Despite having been registered at the practice for over 10 years he has recently presented for the first time. His major complaint was ankle swelling that has prevented him from putting on his shoes. I was, however, surprised to find that he was centrally cyanosed and moderately dyspnoeic. Many thanks for your urgent help in investigating his symptoms.

Yours sincerely,

Introduction

Cyanosis can be of cardiac (right-to-left shunting) or respiratory origin or (very rarely) associated with abnormal haemoglobin. If cyanosis develops over a long period it can be reasonably well tolerated, but may lead to other complications (see Section 2.7). The list of differential diagnoses for this patient includes:

- respiratory failure and cor pulmonale secondary to chronic obstructive pulmonary disease (COPD), but also bronchiectasis, pulmonary fibrosis or hypoventilation syndromes;

- Eisenmenger's syndrome (see Section 2.7.3);

- primary pulmonary hypertension (not likely in a middle-aged man, see Section 1.1.4);

- secondary pulmonary hypertension of another cause (see Section 2.12);

- other congenital heart disease (patients with Ebstein's anomaly or mild cases of tetralogy of Fallot may survive to middle age).

You need to determine the cause of his cyanosis by looking for evidence of respiratory disease, pulmonary hypertension and intracardiac shunts.

Causes of cyanosis in an adult:

- respiratory failure and cor pulmonale;
- Eisenmenger's syndrome;
- pulmonary hypertension (primary or secondary);
- other congenital heart disease;
- abnormal haemoglobin (very rare).

History of the presenting problem
Enquire about the duration and severity of the presenting symptoms, remembering that some patients, perhaps such as this man, may not be reliable witnesses, tending to deny ill-health and generally playing down the issues. Ask specifically about the following.

- How long has his ankle swelling been going on for?

- Has he noticed that he has become blue and, if so, when? Has he been a 'funny colour' for as long as he can remember? If this has been very long-standing, it suggests a cardiac rather than a respiratory explanation.

- Is he limited by breathlessness? Quantify his functional status. How far can he go on the flat? Can he go up stairs? How many times does he have to stop?

Also ask about the following:

- Has he suffered from dizziness, headache, visual disturbance or paraesthesiae? These could be symptoms of hyperviscosity, probably indicating secondary polycythaemia in this case.

- Has he had any episodes of syncope or presyncope? These are worrying signs in patients with pulmonary hypertension.

- Does he find it difficult to stay awake sometimes? Has he ever fallen asleep during the day when he was not trying to, eg when driving a car? Has anyone ever complained that he snores excessively when he sleeps? Does he wake up with headaches in the mornings? Any of these features would suggest obstructive sleep apnoea.

- Does he smoke? Does he have chronic cough, sputum or wheeze? Is there any history of asbestos exposure? These may suggest chronic lung disease.

Ask about features that would suggest thromboembolic disease:

- asymmetrical calf swelling or tenderness;

- pleuritic chest pain;

- haemoptysis.

Other relevant history
Ask specifically about the following.

- Does he know if he was a blue baby? Did he have a heart murmur? Did he have rheumatic fever (try St Vitus' dance) as a child or as a young man?

- Tuberculosis and whooping cough: these would put him at risk of bronchiectasis.

- Did any siblings die young? If so, consider cystic fibrosis.

Also ask about the following:

- Symptoms of autoimmune rheumatic disease, which can be associated with interstitial lung disease.

- Use of prescribed medications and other drugs: are any associated with chronic lung disease or pulmonary hypertension?

- History of stroke or transient ischaemic attack. These would be uncommon in a patient aged 45 years, but may be attributable to paradoxical embolism from right-to-left shunting in this case.

Plan for investigation and management

Cardiac cyanosis will not improve with maximal inspired oxygen, whereas respiratory cyanosis generally will.

Explain that after examining him you would want to organise the following tests.

Oxygen saturation
Check pulse oximetry. Also check arterial blood gases for Po_2 and Pco_2

when he is breathing air and (monitoring him continuously in case he retains CO_2 and is dependent on hypoxic drive) after 10 minutes on high-flow oxygen (see *Respiratory Medicine*, Section 2.11.1).

ECG

Look for evidence of right ventricular hypertrophy (RVH; see Section 3.1).

Chest radiograph

Look for signs of pulmonary hypertension and chronic lung disease, particularly the hyperexpansion of COPD and the interstitial shadowing of parenchymal lung disease.

Blood tests

Check his FBC: is the patient polycythaemic? Check electrolytes, and renal and liver function. Other tests, eg for autoimmune rheumatic disorders, may be indicated in some cases.

Echocardiography

This is a key investigation for assessing right ventricular (RV) function, RVH and pulmonary pressures. Examine the heart valves and look for septal defects and shunts.

Pulmonary function tests

Does the patient have severe obstructive or restrictive lung disease? Check spirometry, lung volumes and gas transfer. Depending on the initial results consider the following:

- high-resolution CT scan of the chest (see Section 3.8);

- transoesophageal echocardiography for atrial septal defect if there is pulmonary hypertension and a shunt is suspected but not seen on

transthoracic echocardiography (see Section 3.10);

- ventilation–perfusion scan or spiral CT scan if pulmonary thromboembolism is considered possible (see Section 3.11);

- MRI of the heart to define anatomy more clearly (see Section 3.8).

Management

Management depends on the underlying condition. Note that in all patients with pulmonary hypertension, great care must be taken with the use of diuretics for oedema: the risk is that overzealous fluid removal can lead to reduction in RV filling pressure, thereby causing circulatory collapse.

- Swollen ankles do not mean diuretic deficiency.
- Be very careful with diuretics in patients with pulmonary hypertension: overzealous fluid removal can cause circulatory collapse.

Further discussion

The optimal management of severe pulmonary hypertension requires early referral to a specialist clinic. Patients with Eisenmenger's syndrome should be referred to a cardiologist with an interest in adult congenital heart disease; other patients may benefit from referral to a specialist pulmonary hypertension service. If anticoagulation is required, it will be important to ensure that the patient will be compliant with monitoring and understand the key importance of this.

1.1.6 Chest pain and recurrent syncope

Letter of referral to cardiology outpatient clinic

Dear Doctor,

Re: Mr John Morris, aged 65 years

This man works as a farmer and presents with a 3-month history of syncopal episodes and exertional chest pain. He has been seen in the practice over the last few years with a number of minor ailments, but has no significant past medical history. I would be grateful if you would see him and advise on further investigation and management.

Yours sincerely,

Introduction

The history of syncope and exertional chest pain strongly suggests a cardiac problem, with syncope due to outflow tract obstruction or arrhythmia and pain due to cardiac ischaemia. Severe pain can sometimes cause vasovagal syncope, and patients on vasodilatory medications can develop orthostatic syncope. However, neither of these would seem likely from the history given.

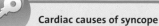

Cardiac causes of syncope

- Vasovagal.
- Arrhythmia.
- Aortic stenosis.
- Hypertrophic cardiomyopathy.
- Orthostatic hypotension.

History of the presenting problem

Syncope

Ask the patient to provide as detailed an account of the syncopal episodes as they can.

- Outflow tract obstruction resulting from vasodilatation and reflex bradycardia usually occurs on exertion.

- Arrhythmias can occur at any time, although some may be provoked by exertion due to ischaemia or increased release of catecholamines. Was the patient aware of his heart beating in an unusual way at any time?

- Orthostatic hypotension can occur after variable periods of standing and may be prominent after exertion.

- Vasovagal syncope is typically preceded by a definite prodrome of worsening nausea and sweating.

Chest pain

Confirm the nature of the pain: it is important to be clear that he is experiencing angina rather than any other pain. Establish quickly its character, radiation, etc.

Other features

Ask directly if any witnesses have told the patient what happened when he collapsed. Did he change colour? If so, this suggests a cardiac cause. Did anyone check his pulse? This may firmly establish the diagnosis if done by a reliable witness. And were there any features to suggest epilepsy (aura, limb shaking, tongue biting and urinary incontinence)? However, remember that seizures can occasionally be secondary to a cardiac cause of collapse.

Other relevant history

Does the patient have a history of ischaemic heart disease, valvular heart disease or arrhythmia? Has he ever had a heart attack? Has he ever seen a specialist for his heart? Has he ever been aware of his heart beating fast or abnormally?

Does he have any risk factors for ischaemic heart disease? Does he smoke? Is there a family history of this condition? Does he have diabetes or high blood cholesterol?

Ask specifically about rheumatic fever. This usually occurs in childhood and may have involved a sore throat, prolonged bed-rest and aching joints. Also, although clearly not relevant in this case, note if a patient has congenital heart disease such as tetralogy of Fallot, which can be associated with exertional syncope.

At the age of 65 years and with the history of chest pain, the following conditions are not likely but check if there is any family history of sudden death, especially at a young age. If there is, this may suggest hypertrophic cardiomyopathy, long QT syndrome with associated arrhythmias, Brugada syndrome or arrhythmogenic right ventricular dysplasia.

Plan for investigation and management

The diagnosis will be aided by the examination and confirmed by the following investigations.

ECG

Is it normal? Is there any evidence of heart block or other arrhythmia? Measure the PR interval and QRS duration. Is there evidence of left ventricular hypertrophy (LVH) (Fig. 10a)? This could suggest aortic stenosis, hypertrophic cardiomyopathy or dilated cardiomyopathy, or a previous myocardial infarct, which may predispose to ventricular arrhythmia (Fig. 10b). Are there other abnormalities such as delta waves or long QT interval (Fig. 10c)?

Chest radiograph

Look for LVH and for evidence of aortic valve calcification.

Echocardiography

This will determine the presence of aortic valve stenosis and left ventricular outflow obstruction and allow measurement of left ventricular function, which if poor may predispose to ventricular arrhythmias (Fig. 11).

Ambulatory ECG monitoring

Prolonged monitoring, initially with a 24-hour tape, may pick up ventricular or other arrhythmias, which can sometimes be revealed on standard 12-lead recordings (Fig. 12).

Blood tests

These are not likely to be critical investigations in this case, but anaemia may worsen the symptoms of ischaemic heart disease or aortic valve disease, and assessment of cardiovascular risk factors (glucose and cholesterol) would be appropriate.

If doubt about the diagnosis remains, then further tests to be considered would including tilt-table testing (vasovagal syncope may be provoked, with either bradycardia or hypotension initiating the event) and coronary angiography.

If you consider that the patient may be at risk of ventricular arrhythmias, then consider admitting him for further investigation and management (see Section 1.1.2).

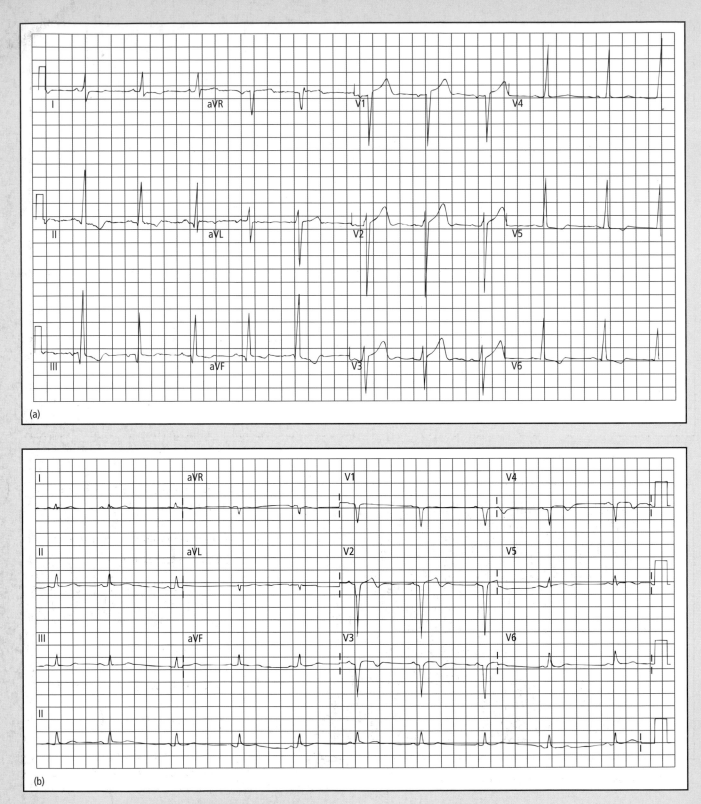

▲ **Fig. 10** Twelve-lead ECGs: (**a**) LVH; (**b**) old anterior myocardial infarction.

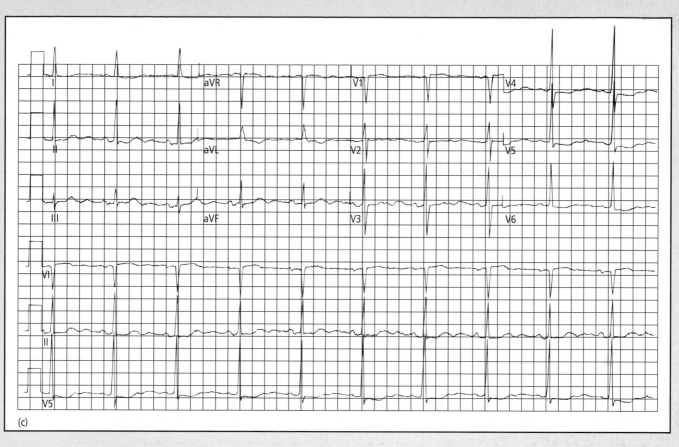

▲**Fig. 10** Twelve-lead ECGs: **(c)** long QT.

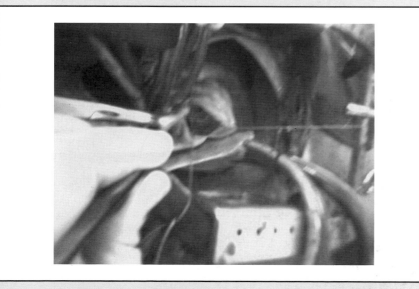

▲**Fig. 11** Stenotic aortic valve seen at operation prior to replacement.

Further discussion

Driving
Patients with syncope cannot drive until they satisfy the Driver and Vehicle Licensing Agency

(DVLA) that recurrence is unlikely (see Section 2.19).

General advice
Advise the patient to avoid heavy lifting and vigorous exercise until a

diagnosis is made and treatment established.

1.1.7 Hypertension found at routine screening

Letter of referral to medical outpatient clinic

Dear Doctor,

Re: Mrs Joy King, aged 30 years

This Afro-Caribbean woman attended the family planning clinic to obtain a prescription for the oral contraceptive pill (OCP). However, her BP on numerous occasions is typically around 180/100 mmHg. She smokes between 10 and 20 cigarettes a day but drinks minimal amounts of alcohol. She has no other known medical problems, but

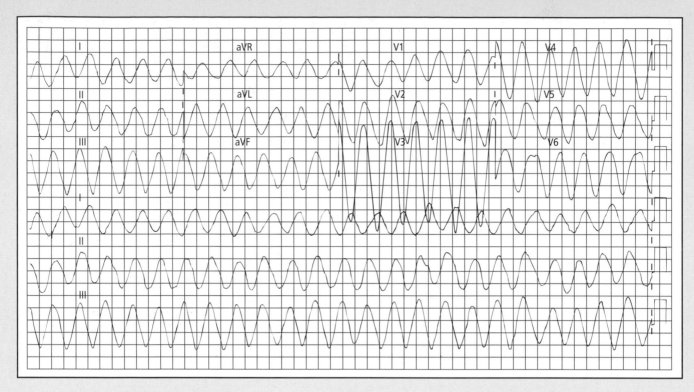

▲ **Fig. 12** Twelve-lead ECG showing ventricular tachycardia.

there is strong family history of high BP with her mother, older sister and one maternal aunt all being treated for the condition. Her father died from a haemorrhagic stroke when she was a child. On examination she is overweight with a BMI of 28. Please can you advise on further investigation and management?

Yours sincerely,

Introduction

Hypertension is a common problem, especially in black people. Although there may be multiple causes for her father's death from a haemorrhagic stroke, uncontrolled and unrecognised hypertension is certainly a possibility. The initial approach in managing this patient should be directed towards confirming the diagnosis of hypertension (ie to ensure there

is no element of 'white coat' hypertension) and, if hypertension is confirmed, treating the blood presssure. This should then be followed by an assessment of whether there are secondary causes for her hypertension, followed by advice and management of her other vascular risk factors (her weight and

smoking) and a decision regarding prescription of the OCP.

The differential diagnosis of this woman's high BP reading is summarised in Table 5.

History of the presenting problem

Hypertension is usually asymptomatic until there is

TABLE 5 DIFFERENTIAL DIAGNOSIS OF HYPERTENSION	
Comment	**Diagnosis**
Common	Essential hypertension
	False elevation as a result of inadequate BP cuff size
	Isolated clinic ('white coat') hypertension
Must consider	Renal hypertension
	Renovascular hypertension
	Primary hyperaldosteronism (Conn's syndrome)[1]
	Phaeochromocytoma[1]
	Coarctation of the aorta[1]
Other causes[2]	Cushing's syndrome
	Acromegaly
	Polycystic ovarian syndrome

1. Rare or very rare.
2. Hypertension not likely to be the dominant feature of these conditions.

progression to end-organ damage. Some patients, on being given a diagnosis of hypertension, will ascribe many different and varied complaints to it. A multitude of symptoms, eg headache, epistaxis, tinnitus, dizziness and fainting, are often blamed on an elevated BP, but probably occur with similar frequency in those whose BP is normal. It is important to elicit any potential complications of untreated hypertension, as detailed below.

Cardiovascular system

Hypertension initially results in left ventricular hypertrophy (LVH), followed by diastolic and finally systolic left ventricular dysfunction. Pursue a history of shortness of breath on exertion or at rest, as well as one of pulmonary oedema. Enquire about swelling of ankles. Other non-specific symptoms can include palpitations and potentially chest pain (if associated with ischaemic heart disease, although this is unlikely in this patient).

Neurological system

Ask about any transient or prolonged episodes of weakness in any of her limbs, or problems with her speech or eyesight. The answers to these questions can rule out transient ischaemic attacks or a stroke. Ask whether the patient has had any episodes of loss of vision or blurred vision that may have been caused by retinal bleeds.

Peripheral vascular system

Ask about symptoms that might indicate intermittent claudication, although this would be extremely unlikely in a 30-year-old woman.

Other relevant history

Could there be a secondary cause of hypertension?

It is important to address specific symptoms that may point towards

TABLE 6 POSSIBLE SECONDARY CAUSES OF HYPERTENSION AND RELEVANT QUESTIONS TO BE ASKED IN THE HISTORY	
Cause of hypertension	**History to be elicited**
Atheromatous renovascular disease	The presence of other atheromatous complications such as peripheral vascular disease and cerebrovascular disease increase the likelihood of renovascular hypertension Does she get pain in the legs on walking? Has she had any neurological symptoms?
Renal parenchymal disease	Has she ever had tests on her urine or kidneys (eg during pregnancy or for insurance purposes)? Has she ever been told that she had a problem with her kidneys? Is there any family history of kidney disease? Has she noticed any blood in her urine, or ever had bad swelling in her legs?
Phaeochromcytoma	Ask about intermittent episodes of panic attacks (anxiety), sweating, tremors, palpitations and chest pain
Primary hyperaldosteronism (Conn's syndrome)	There are no specific symptoms, but a history of muscle cramps secondary to low potassium levels, and possibly polyuria and polydipsia, may be relevant
Cushing's syndrome	Has she gained weight? Has she noticed striae, or thinning of her hair or skin? Does she bruise easily? Any changes in menstrual cycle? Has she been prescribed steroids?
Acromegaly	Any change in her hand or foot size? Has anyone commented on changes in her facial appearance? Has she noticed any change in vision? Does she have any joint problems?
Drugs	Has she taken any prescribed or non-prescribed medication? Has she been eating lots of liquorice?

Note: it is very rare for a secondary cause of hypertension to be diagnosed from history alone, but the history can provide useful clues to follow.

a secondary cause of high BP (Table 6). In most cases, however, a secondary cause is not found and hypertension is classified as primary or 'essential'. A strong family history of hypertension would support the diagnosis of essential hypertension and hence a detailed family history must always be pursued, or confirmed when it is stated (as in this case).

Cardiovascular risk factors

In any patient presenting with hypertension it is very important to assess other cardiovascular risk factors, including the following:

- smoking;

- diabetes;

- hyperlipidaemia;

- family history of cardiovascular events;

- alcohol consumption.

Plan for investigation and management

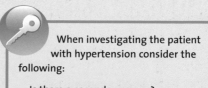

When investigating the patient with hypertension consider the following:

- Is there a secondary cause?
- Is there evidence of end-organ damage?

After examining her your strategy for investigation should be directed towards detecting secondary causes and identifying evidence of end-organ complications (see Section 2.17).

ECG

Look particularly for evidence of LVH (see Fig. 10a).

Urine

Check for proteinuria and haematuria using dipsticks. If positive for protein, quantification of albumin/creatinine ratio with a spot urine or 24-hour collection is required. The presence of proteinuria and/or haematuria would be consistent with the patient having a renal disorder with secondary hypertension, or with renal damage caused by hypertension.

Blood tests

Check FBC, electrolytes, renal and liver function, uric acid, fasting glucose and lipid profile. The most common cause of hypokalaemia is diuretic treatment, but low values are often found in untreated accelerated-phase hypertension and in primary hyperaldosteronism (suspect only if patients are not on diurectic treatment). Is her renal function normal? Does she have glucose intolerance or diabetes? Is her cholesterol elevated?

Chest radiograph

Assess heart size and look for pulmonary oedema and possible (but very unlikely) radiographic signs of coarctation (Fig. 13).

Echocardiography

This is more sensitive than ECG at detecting LVH, especially if patients are of Afro-Caribbean descent (Fig. 14). Look for evidence of diastolic and systolic left ventricular impairment.

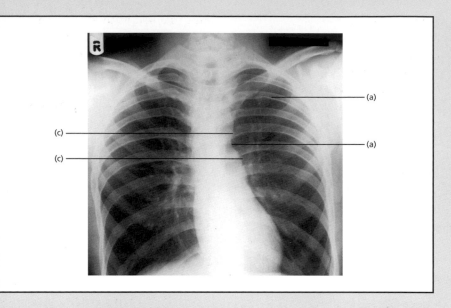

▲ **Fig. 13** CXR of patient with coarctation of the aorta, showing (**a**) rib notching, (**b**) site of coarctation and (**c**) prestenotic and poststenotic dilatation. (Reproduced with permission from Ray KK, Ryder REJ and Wellings RM, *An Aid to Radiology for the MRCP*. Oxford: Blackwell Science, 1999).

Other tests

Other tests may be appropriate depending on the findings of those detailed above. Ambulatory blood pressure monitoring may be needed to confirm the diagnosis and exclude 'white coat' hypertension, the latter being suspected particularly in cases where BP recorded in clinic is very high but there seems to be no evidence of end-organ damage.

Other specific tests may be required as dictated by the clinical setting to diagnose primary renal disease (serological tests or renal biopsy),

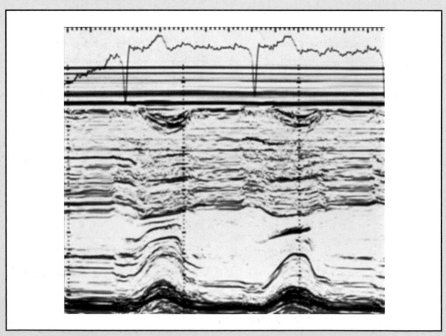

▲ **Fig. 14** LVH: compared with the normal parasternal M-mode (see Fig. 121), it is evident that the interventricular septum is grossly thickened in this patient. (Courtesy of Dr J. Chambers.)

renovascular disease (renal ultrasound and Doppler examination, or MRI angiography), Conn's syndrome (plasma renin and aldosterone levels) or phaeochromocytoma (24-hour urinary and blood catecholamine levels). (See Section 2.17.)

Management

Management consists of treating any underlying secondary cause of hypertension if present. Otherwise, a stepwise approach to antihypertensive medication is most likely.

Further discussion

Do not forget to offer advice and treatment (where possible) to reduce other cardiovascular risk factors. Decisions regarding the treatment of hypertension (or hypercholesterolaemia) should never be taken in isolation. For example, in this patient it is important that any treatment for high BP is combined with general lifestyle measures (stop smoking, increase physical activity and try to lose weight). Should she have an abnormal lipid profile this should also be actively managed with dietary advice (and possibly review by a dietitian) and statin therapy. It is only after addressing these issues that the choice of OCP or other method of contraception should be made on the basis of overall cardiovascular risk and benefits.

1.1.8 Murmur in pregnancy

Letter of referral to cardiology outpatient clinic

Dear Doctor,

Re: Mrs Rose Berry, aged 23

Thank you for seeing this woman who is 29 weeks pregnant and was noted to have a systolic murmur at one of her routine antenatal visits. This is her first pregnancy and there have been no other problems. The rest of her history and examination are unremarkable and I would be grateful for your opinion as to the significance of her murmur.

Yours sincerely,

Introduction

Your major concern will be to differentiate an innocent murmur from one that suggests underlying pathology (Table 7). Can you reassure the patient or, if there is a structural cardiac lesion, can you predict and prevent problems that might arise during the pregnancy? The most common diagnosis will be an innocent systolic murmur due to the hyperdynamic circulation of pregnancy, requiring no further intervention. Mitral or aortic valve disease, hypertrophic cardiomyopathy (HCM) and congenital abnormalities such as a ventricular septal defect may require careful monitoring; at the very least they require antibiotic prophylaxis during vaginal delivery. Occasionally, rare and severe conditions such as cardiomyopathy of pregnancy can present in the third trimester.

History of the presenting problem

Most patients who present in this way will be asymptomatic. The presence of symptoms should raise the suspicion of significant pathology. However, bear in mind that a degree of weakness, exertional dyspnoea, dizziness and peripheral oedema are quite common during pregnancy and are a result of physiological adaptation rather than intrinsic cardiac disease. Be sure to gauge the precise severity of the symptoms and relate it to the stage of the pregnancy.

Ask some general questions.

- Have you been getting out of breath more easily?

- How far can you walk?

- Have you woken up breathless at night?

- Have you had any chest pains?

- Have you had any palpitations, when your heart seems to beat with an unusual rhythm?

- When do you get them?

- Have you experienced any blackouts? What were you doing at the time?

TABLE 7 DIFFERENTIAL DIAGNOSIS OF A SYSTOLIC MURMUR DURING PREGNANCY	
Comment	**Diagnosis**
Common	Innocent systolic murmur Mitral valve prolapse
Must consider	Mitral valve disease (regurgitation/mixed/stenosis with tricuspid regurgitation) Aortic valve disease (stenosis/mixed/regurgitation with flow murmur) HCM Atrial or ventricular septal defect
Other causes	Peripartum cardiomyopathy

HCM, hypertrophic cardiomyopathy.

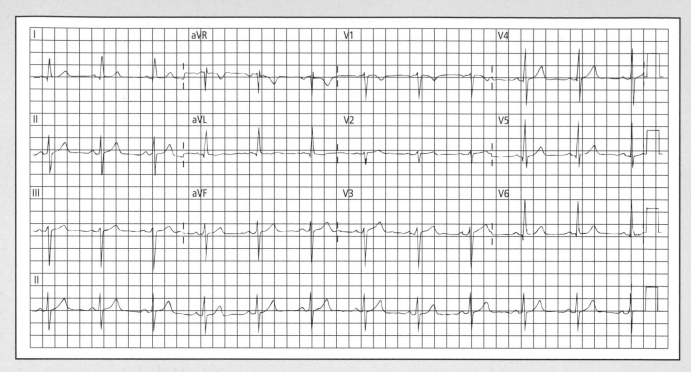

▲ **Fig. 15** ECG: axis shift in pregnant woman.

- Do you ever feel as if you are going to pass out?

Other relevant history

Enquire about any previous cardiac history. Occasionally, a minor abnormality will have been documented in infancy or childhood, and the patient may have been told that she has a murmur, 'hole' or 'sound' in her heart. Ask about any difficulties before the pregnancy that might also suggest a congenital abnormality. Also ask about any heart problems in other family members: a history of sudden death at a young age might raise the possibility of a hereditary cardiomyopathy or Marfan's syndrome.

Plan for investigation and management

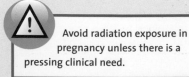 Avoid radiation exposure in pregnancy unless there is a pressing clinical need.

After explaining to the patient that under normal clinical circumstances you would examine her to confirm the clinical findings as stated on the referral letter, you would plan as follows.

ECG

Minor flattening of T waves or axis shift (Fig. 15) are common in normal pregnancy, as are sinus tachycardia and ectopic beats. Look for evidence of atrial enlargement, left or right ventricular hypertrophy, or conduction abnormalities.

Chest radiograph

This is best avoided (because of the radiation dose) unless there are clear clinical indications.

Echocardiography

This is the investigation of choice to confirm or rule out cardiac pathology (Fig. 16).

Management

Management will depend on the diagnosis. Most patients will have

an innocent murmur: they, and other doctors involved in their care, can be reassured. For information regarding other conditions, see the relevant sections in Part 2 of this module.

Further review for innocent murmurs is not usually required. Patients with structural heart disease will need further input in liaison with the obstetric team. The timing and frequency of follow-up will depend on the nature and severity of the structural abnormality.

Further discussion

Congenital heart disease in pregnancy is the third commonest cause of maternal death. It will become an increasing problem as more patients survive with complex congenital cardiac abnormalities: the recurrence rate for most (non-syndromic) congenital abnormalities in the offspring is 5%.

Mild lesions may get worse or ventricular function may deteriorate

prevent endocarditis. Warfarin is teratogenic; hence special arrangements (usually conversion to low-molecular-weight heparin) are required for those who need anticoagulation during pregnancy.

1.2 Clinical examination

1.2.1 Irregular pulse

Instruction
This woman has had palpitations. Please examine her heart.

General features

Your approach to this case will be aimed at identifying any systemic condition that may cause palpitations and identifying whether there is any specific cardiovascular abnormality present.

Look for thyrotoxicosis or anaemia. Consider the conditions associated with atrial fibrillation (AF) (Table 9). Are there any general features that would support one of these diagnoses? Look for surgical scars (eg thoracotomy or pacemaker/implantable

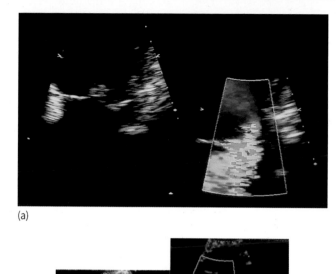

(a)

(b)

▲ **Fig. 16** (a) Mitral valve prolapse: in the two-dimensional image on the left, the anterior mitral valve leaflet is seen to bow into the left atrium. The effect of this can be seen in the colour-flow mapping in the image on the right: a broad regurgitant jet can be seen. (b) Ventricular septal defect: in these parasternal long- and short-axis views, a small jet of orange colour represents the abnormal blood flow across the septum from the left to right ventricle. LA, left atrium; LV, left ventricle; RV, right ventricle; Ao, aorta. (Courtesy of Dr J. Chambers.)

as pregnancy progresses, and hence careful monitoring with specialist input is necessary. In some patients careful consideration will need to be given to advising termination of pregnancy on medical grounds; when the current pregnancy is over, patients with high-risk and intermediate cardiac lesions should be offered advice about contraception (Table 8).

Patients with significant cardiac lesions undergoing vaginal delivery require antibiotic prophylaxis to

TABLE 8 RISKS OF PRE-EXISTING HEART DISEASE IN PREGNANCY

Level of Risk	Condition
High	Pulmonary hypertension Mitral stenosis Aortic and pulmonary stenosis Marfan's syndrome
Intermediate	Coarctation of aorta HCM Cyanotic congenital heart disease without pulmonary hypertension
Low	Well-tolerated valvular regurgitation Septal defects without pulmonary hypertension Totally corrected congenital heart disease Prosthetic valves

HCM, hypertrophic cardiomyopathy.

TABLE 9 CAUSES OF AF

System	Cause
Cardiac	**Hypertension**
	Ischaemic heart disease
	Non-ischaemic cardiomyopathy
	MV disease
	Pericardial disease
	Endocarditis
	Atrial myxoma
Respiratory	**Chest infection**[1]
	Pulmonary infarction
	Bronchial carcinoma
Other	Hyperthyroidism
	Alcohol
	Haemochromatosis
	Sarcoidosis
	Recreational drug use

Notes: common causes in bold; [1]common in routine clinical practice but not in PACES.
AF, atrial fibrillation; MV, mitral value.

cardioverter defibrillator), evidence of hypercholesterolaemia (xanthelasma or tendon xanthomata) and the characteristic skin colour of chronic amiodarone use (Fig. 17).

Cardiovascular examination

Key points to look for include the following.

Pulse

Check rate and rhythm. Is there an arrhythmia now? Is the pulse small volume suggestive of low cardiac output? Are there alternate large- and small-amplitude beats (alternans) suggestive of impaired left ventricular (LV) function? Is the radial pulse absent? This may be the case with congenital abnormalities, arterial embolism, and Blalock shunt or those used as surgical conduits.

Signs of heart failure

Look for evidence of congestive heart failure or tricuspid regurgitation by examining the JVP. Is the apex beat displaced? What is the character of the apex beat? Is there evidence of pulmonary oedema or right-sided heart failure?

Heart sounds

Careful auscultation should reveal any valve abnormalities. Particular focus should be on the mitral valve as there is an increased incidence of AF with mitral stenosis or regurgitation. Mitral regurgitation is common in patients with impaired dilated left ventricles. Is there an ejection systolic murmur that might suggest hypertrophic cardiomyopathy (HCM) (Table 10)?

Further discussion

An irregular pulse may obviously be the cause of her symptoms, and

to confirm the diagnosis of an arrhythmia an ECG will clearly be the first investigation to perform. If the pulse is rapid and regular, then it suggests sinus tachycardia, supraventricular tachycardia (SVT) or ventricular tachycardia (VT). In a formal examination such as PACES it is highly improbable that the patient will be in VT, although SVT is possible, eg atrial flutter with a pulse of 150 bpm. If the pulse is irregularly irregular, then it is either AF or sinus rhythm with frequent ectopics. A regularly irregular rhythm will either be sinus rhythm with regular ectopic beats (eg ventricular trigeminy) or heart block (eg Wenckebach).

Patients with structural cardiac abnormalities are more likely to have arrhythmias: specific conditions to look for are impaired LV function, valvular abnormalities and cardiomyopathies. Many cardiomyopathies may just have features of impaired left or right ventricular function, but some may have very specific findings, eg HCM (Table 10). A CXR and echocardiogram would clearly be the first-line investigations to look for structural cardiac lesions.

Remember that in routine clinical practice many patients who complain of palpitations do

TABLE 10 CLINICAL FEATURES OF HCM

Pulse	'Jerky': brisk rising and declines in mid-systole (as gradient develops)
JVP	Prominent *a* wave (reduced right ventricular compliance due to massive hypertrophy of septum)
Apex beat	May be displaced laterally and often forceful. Presystolic impulse may produce a 'double' apical beat
Heart sounds	Fourth heart sound precedes first sound (corresponds to presystolic impulse)
Murmurs	Harsh crescendo–decrescendo murmur heard after the first heart sound at the left sternal edge (flow over obstructed outflow tract). Tends to radiate to axilla rather than the carotids. With severe gradients there may be an associated murmur of mitral regurgitation. Approximately 10% of cases will also have aortic regurgitation

HCM, hypertrophic cardiomyopathy

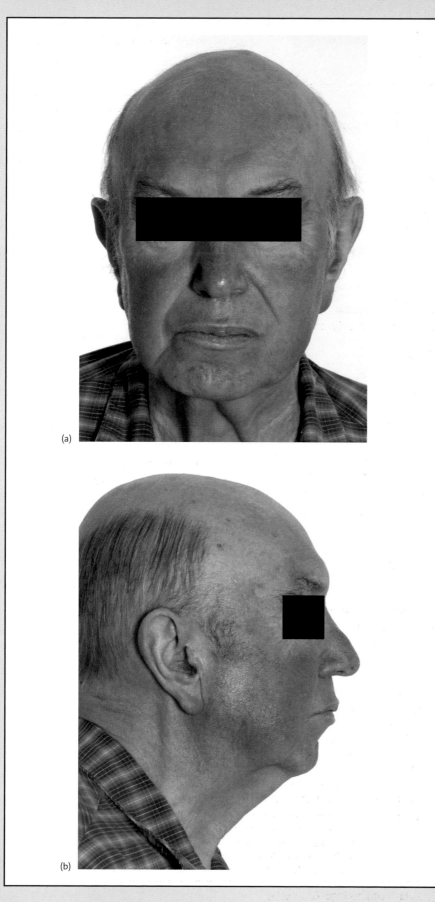

(a)

(b)

▲ **Fig. 17** Typical slate-grey skin coloration associated with long-term amiodarone treatment.

not have a pathological arrhythmia: anxiety can lead to an increased awareness of sinus rhythm or normal ectopic beats.

1.2.2 Congestive heart failure

Instruction

This 78-year-old man has a 6-week history of progressive breathlessness, orthopnoea and swollen ankles. Please examine his cardiovascular system.

General features

Look for cyanosis, anaemia, stigmata of chronic liver disease or nicotine-stained fingers.

Are there any features to suggest previous cardiac interventions, such as a sternotomy scar or presence of pacemaker?

Although this is not a respiratory station, note the shape of the chest and whether it seems to expand normally as the patient breathes. Do appearances suggest chronic airways disease? If they do, and particularly if you find signs other than basal crackles when you listen to the patient's lungs, then a respiratory cause of breathlessness and oedema is likely (consider right heart failure of cor pulmonale).

Expose both arms fully to ensure that there are no fistulae present.

⚠ Oedema of the hands and face is a feature of hypoalbuminaemia and very rarely the result of congestive cardiac failure (Fig. 18).

Cardiovascular examination

Key points to look for during the cardiovascular examination include the following.

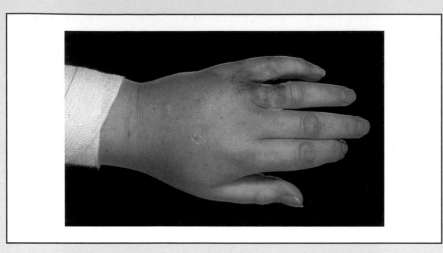

▲ **Fig. 18** Hand oedema in a patient with hypoalbuminaemia.

Signs of cardiac dysfunction

- Pulse: rate, rhythm, volume and character. A sinus tachycardia may be caused by anxiety or cardiac failure; consider specifically atrial fibrillation (AF). A low-volume pulse might indicate cardiac failure or alternatively severe mitral regurgitation, but is there anything about the character to suggest either aortic stenosis or incompetence?

- BP, including pulsus paradoxus, which suggests pericardial effusion/tamponade.

- JVP: is this raised? Check for the features of JVP, including the effect of respiration (eg increasing with inspiration in constrictive pericarditis and *cv* waves in tricuspid regurgitation).

- Apex beat: is this displaced? Is it hyperdynamic, in keeping with a volume-overloaded left ventricle (eg mitral or aortic incompetence)?

- Heart sounds: is there an S3 gallop? Are there murmurs (especially diastolic)?

- Lungs: are there basal crepitations? Remember that these are not specific for pulmonary oedema and cardiac failure.

Signs of pulmonary hypertension

This is suggested by the following.

- Raised JVP.

- Left parasternal heave (palpable right ventricle).

- Loud pulmonary component of the second heart sound.

Also note whether one leg is much more swollen than the other, which might indicate deep venous thrombosis.

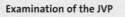

Examination of the JVP

- Do not finish your examination until you have found out where the JVP is. Make sure that you correctly position the patient, ensuring that he or she is at 45° with the head well supported by a pillow, thereby relaxing the neck muscles. Good lighting will help. Look for position, waveform characteristics (if in AF, then large waves must be *v* waves) and the effect of respiration.
- Remember that it is possible to miss a markedly elevated JVP: if you cannot see it and the neck appears 'full', then look again when the patient is sitting up at 90°.

Further discussion

Clinical diagnosis of heart failure can be difficult. Although any individual sign (eg elevated JVP) has a relatively low positive predictive value for the diagnosis, finding a constellation of signs makes left ventricular impairment much more likely. The diagnosis should always be confirmed by an objective assessment of cardiac function, generally in the form of an echocardiogram. Along with an ECG and CXR, this would be the first-line investigations to request in this case.

The following are important factors when considering the case of a patient with possible congestive cardiac failure.

- The presence of bilateral basal crackles on auscultation of the chest has a very poor positive predictive value for the presence of pulmonary oedema; a CXR is much more accurate.

- Remember that marked abnormality of renal and liver function tests commonly occurs in cases of congestive cardiac failure, and does not necessarily indicate primary disease in these organs.

- The severity of left ventricular dysfunction on echocardiography correlates poorly with the severity of the clinical syndrome of heart failure, but normal systolic left ventricular function on echocardiography should prompt a review of a diagnosis of heart failure.

⚠ When the cause of breathlessness is not obvious, consider chronic repeated pulmonary thromboembolism, which is a commonly missed diagnosis. Multiple small pulmonary emboli lead to progressive occlusion of the pulmonary arteriolar bed, classically presenting with breathlessness that becomes more severe in a stepwise manner. Pulmonary hypertension eventually leads to right ventricular failure and ankle swelling. Prominent pulmonary arteries may be the only finding on a CXR. Diagnosis is made by lung ventilation–perfusion scan or spiral CT scan of the chest.

1.2.3 Hypertension

Instruction

Please examine the cardiovascular system of this woman with hypertension.

General features

The main objectives of the examination are to assess for evidence of organ damage secondary to hypertension and to uncover a secondary cause of hypertension.

Comment on the patient's general appearance and particularly on any obvious appearances that might indicate a secondary cause of hypertension, eg obvious cushingoid appearance or features of acromegaly (unlikely to be in the cardiac station of PACES; more likely to appear in Station 5).

Cardiovascular examination

Pay particular attention to the following.

- BP: in a scenario such as this you should obviously offer to measure the patient's BP, but it is unlikely that the examiners will actually allow you to do so because of the time constraints of the station. However, if they do, make sure you do it properly. The patient is likely to have been lying on a couch for some time, but remember that they should be recumbent for at least 3 minutes before taking a reading and that the arm should be supported at the level of the heart when making the measurement. Make sure you use an appropriately sized cuff and offer to measure the BP in both arms (which will almost certainly be declined).

- JVP, apex beat, heaves, heart sounds and lungs: examine these

for any evidence of left ventricular hypertrophy or heart failure.

- Peripheral pulses: examine carefully, in particular for the radiofemoral delay of coarctation of the aorta. Also assess the presence and volume of all pulses as the patient may have peripheral vascular disease.

- Abdomen: feel for an abdominal aortic aneursym and listen over the renal arteries for bruits.

- Fundi: offer to examine for evidence of hypertensive retinopathy (again this will almost certainly by declined by the examiners in Station 3 as fundoscopy is frequently performed in Station 5).

When examining a patient with hypertension, consider the following.

- Essential hypertension: if the patient has elevated BP, evidence of left ventricular hypertrophy or hypertensive retinopathy and evidence of secondary causes is absent.
- Isolated clinic hypertension: look for anxiety, eg tachycardia. Is the BP lower when measured by the clinic nurse or the GP, or at place of work or at home? There must be no evidence of target organ damage.
- Renovascular disease: are there abdominal bruits, abdominal aortic aneurysm or other evidence of atherosclerosis?
- Coarctation: look for absent femoral pulses and radiofemoral delay, collaterals in the back muscles and a widespread systolic murmur heard best over the back.

Further discussion

You should be able to discuss the secondary causes of hypertension and in particular any obvious cause that you may have elicited from the examination. Particular emphasis

may be placed on the subsequent treatment of the patient's hypertension, including lifestyle changes, risk factor modification and medical management (see Section 2.17).

1.2.4 Mechanical valve

Instruction

This man has had cardiac surgery. Please examine his cardiovascular system.

General features

From the foot of the bed, can you hear the characteristic clicking sound of a ball-and-cage valve? Look for pallor or jaundice, which may be caused by haemolysis from a failing valve. Also check for bruising, which could suggest problems with anticoagulation use. Aside from the scar of cardiac surgery, look for scars on the upper chest suggestive of a pacemaker (atrioventricular block is more common following aortic valve surgery) and on the legs suggestive of vein harvest for coronary artery bypass grafting. Remember also to look for a mitral valvotomy under the left breast. Does the patient have any phenotypic features of conditions associated with aortic valve pathology, eg Marfan's syndrome?

Cardiovascular examination

The following are the key points to look for in the cardiovascular examination.

- Pulse: check rate and rhythm. Is the patient in sinus rhythm? Atrial fibrillation is very common after cardiac surgery. A collapsing pulse suggests significant aortic regurgitation and valve failure. A slow rising pulse suggests valvular stenosis.

TABLE 11 TYPES OF PROSTHETIC HEART VALVE

Mechanical	Biological
Ball and cage (Starr–Edwards)	Porcine (Carpentier–Edwards)
Single disc (Björk–Shiley or Medtronic Hall)	Pericardial
Bileaflet (St Jude or Carbomedics)	Homograft
	Autologous (pulmonary autograft)

- BP: a wide pulse pressure suggests aortic regurgitation and a narrow pulse pressure outflow tract obstruction (offer to check this at the end of your examination).

- Signs of congestive cardiac failure: an elevated JVP, displaced or prominent apex beat, parasternal heave, added heart sounds, basal crackles and ankle swelling may be a result of prosthetic valve failure.

- Mechanical aortic valve: if present the second heart sound will be prosthetic and loud. There will always be abnormal forward flow with a mechanical valve and therefore an ejection systolic murmur will be present, the intensity of which has no bearing on the function (or dysfunction) of the valve. Listen carefully for an early diastolic murmur suggestive of valve failure and remember that a shorter duration of the diastolic murmur indicates severe regurgitation.

- Mechanical mitral valve: if present the first heart sound will be prosthetic and a diastolic flow murmur may be heard. However, these are not typically as loud as the prosthetic sound and flow murmur associated with a mechanical aortic valve. A systolic mitral regurgitant murmur may be due to a prosthetic or paraprosthetic leak.

- Biological valves: these do not produce the harsh metallic sounds of mechanical valves.

Further discussion

Prosthetic aortic or mitral valves can be mechanical or biological (Table 11).

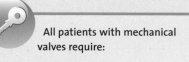

All patients with mechanical valves require:

- lifelong anticoagulation;
- prophylaxis against endocarditis.

All mechanical heart valves need anticoagulation to prevent valve thrombosis and the resulting complications. However, despite the best anticoagulation control, the incidence of systemic emboli is 1% per patient-year. The recommended INR is 2.0–3.0 for bileaflet valves and 2.5–3.5 for other disc and Starr–Edwards valves.

Endocarditis is a feared complication of all prosthetic valves. The greatest risk of infection is immediately following surgery: from 12 months onwards the annual incidence is 0.4%. The causative organisms are most likely to be coagulase-negative staphylococci and *Staphylococcus aureus* in the early period (see Section 2.8, Table 34). The mortality from prosthetic valve endocarditis is 60% and the condition is difficult to treat with medical therapy alone; hence urgent referral to a cardiothoracic surgical centre is required. To prevent endocarditis, dental care must be meticulous in patients with prosthetic heart valves

and antibiotic prophylaxis as detailed in the *British National Formulary* is mandatory.

Haemolysis from mechanical valves is more common than from bioprosthetic valves. It may be acute or chronic, and may be related to valve failure. Presentation is typically with anaemia and mild jaundice. Blood films show a microangiopathic haemolytic picture (see *Haematology*, Section 2.1.7). Infective endocarditis must be excluded. Management may vary from regular transfusions to repeat valve surgery.

Replacement of a prosthetic valve should only be considered in patients who are symptomatic with objective evidence of valve failure. It is a high-risk procedure and may not provide a better outcome than an expectant approach in both the elderly and those with significant comorbidity.

1.2.5 Pansystolic murmur

Instruction

This man has a murmur. Please examine his cardiovascular system.

General features

Comment on the patient's general appearance and in particular if he appears short of breath at rest, cyanosed or has a phenotype suggesting a particular valvular abnormality, eg Marfan's syndrome (this can be associated with mitral regurgitation as well as aortic regurgitation). Look carefully for surgical scars, remembering especially that the left thoracotomy scar of mitral valvotomy is easy to miss (especially in women, when it can be hidden under the fold of the breast).

Cardiovascular examination

Check for stigmata of endocarditis. Pay attention to dental hygiene. Check if the patient is in atrial fibrillation. Look for signs of heart failure, particularly elevation of JVP and displacement of the apex. Do not forget to examine for a parasternal heave suggesting pulmonary hypertension. Remember the following when trying to decide the cause of the pansystolic murmur.

- Mitral regurgitation: a thrusting displaced apex beat suggests volume overload of the left ventricle, which means that the murmur is probably mitral. The murmur will typically be loudest in expiration, most prominent at the apex and radiate to the axilla. A soft first heart sound and loud third sound would support the diagnosis.

- Ventricular septal defect (VSD): you should suspect this condition if the murmur is loudest in inspiration and best heard over the lower left sternal edge. In cases of VSD the apex is undisplaced, the first sound normal and no third heart sound is heard.

- Tricuspid regurgitation: typically the murmur is loudest over the lower left sternal edge during inspiration. Giant *v* waves will be present and a pulsatile liver edge. The apex is not displaced and a third sound not heard.

Differential diagnosis of a pansystolic murmur:

- mitral regurgitation;
- VSD;
- tricuspid regurgitation.

Further discussion

The commonest causes of mitral regurgitation are mitral valve prolapse and ischaemic heart disease. Other causes are rheumatic heart disease, previous mitral valvotomy and dilated cardiomyopathy.

Features of the examination that would suggest severe mitral regurgitation include a third heart sound, displaced apex beat, signs of heart failure and signs of pulmonary hypertension. An echocardiogram will confirm the diagnosis and (probably) aetiology, as well as the severity, by giving information about the haemodynamic consequences of the mitral leak. This is particularly the case for left ventricular dilatation, impaired left ventricular systolic function and pulmonary hypertension.

Patients with mild or moderate disease should be reviewed annually in a cardiac clinic. All patients should be given advice regarding antibiotic prophylaxis against endocarditis. Many patients with mitral regurgitation will require lifelong anticoagulation with warfarin.

Surgery is indicated in those with severe mitral regurgitation and symptoms. For asymptomatic cases, surgery is recommended if there is evidence of left ventricular dilatation, impaired left ventricular systolic function or pulmonary hypertension. The outcome is generally better if the mitral valve can be repaired rather than replaced, but suitability for repair will depend on the complexity of the valvular disease. Coronary angiography is required prior to surgery to look for coexistent coronary artery disease.

1.2.6 Mitral stenosis

Instruction

This woman has had increasing shortness of breath over the past 6 months. Please examine her cardiovascular system.

General features

Comment on the patient's general well-being and in particular if she is short of breath at rest or cyanosed. Look for surgical scars, particularly a mitral valvotomy under the left breast. Does the patient have a malar flush?

Cardiovascular examination

Check for stigmata of endocarditis. Pay attention to dental hygiene. In mitral stenosis (MS) the following may be seen.

- Pulse: atrial fibrillation (AF) is very common in MS.

- Signs of heart failure: elevated JVP and giant *v* waves due to secondary tricuspid incompetence (also hepatomegaly, ascites and ankle oedema).

- Apex beat: tapping (palpable first heart sound) that is not displaced.

- Parasternal heave: suggests pulmonary hypertension.

- Heart sounds: the first is loud, then there is a loud pulmonary second sound and an opening snap followed by a mid-diastolic rumbling murmur (with presystolic accentuation if the patient is in sinus rhythm) localised to the apex and heard loudest in expiration with the patient in the left lateral position. A Graham Steell early diastolic murmur due to secondary pulmonary regurgitation may be heard.

Further discussion

By far the commonest cause of MS is rheumatic heart disease. The murmur of MS may be difficult to hear, so be alert for clues prior to auscultation. If a patient in PACES is in AF and their face looks as though it has a malar flush, then MS is much more likely to be the diagnosis than it might be in routine clinical practice. Note that the murmur of MS is accentuated with exercise, but tachycardia may make it more difficult to hear. The presence of an opening snap suggests the mitral valve (MV) is still pliant. The closer the murmur is to the second heart sound, the more severe the stenosis.

Transthoracic echocardiography confirms the diagnosis and allows an assessment of severity (see Section 2.5.3).

Patients with mild or moderate disease should be reviewed annually in a cardiac clinic. All patients should be given advice regarding antibiotic prophylaxis against endocarditis. All patients with MS require lifelong anticoagulation with warfarin unless there are very pressing contraindications.

Surgery is indicated for severe MS with limiting symptoms, embolic events or an episode of pulmonary oedema. If this is planned, a transoesophageal echocardiogram should be performed to assess the degree of valve calcification, to check for the presence of mitral incompetence and to examine for thrombus in the left atrial appendage. Patients with minimal MV calcification (no more than mild mitral regurgitation and no left atrial appendage thrombus) should be considered for percutaneous mitral valvotomy. Otherwise, the patient requires MV replacement. In general, mechanical and not tissue MV prostheses are required (see Table 11). Coronary angiography is required prior to surgery to look for coexistent coronary artery disease.

1.2.7 Aortic stenosis

> ## Instruction
>
> This woman has chest tightness on effort. Please examine her cardiovascular system.

General features

Comment on the patient's general well-being and in particular if she is short of breath at rest or cyanosed. Look carefully for surgical scars.

Cardiovascular examination

Check for stigmata of endocarditis. Pay attention to dental hygiene. Check for signs of heart failure, noting particularly that in cases of aortic stenosis the following may be observed.

- Pulse: this will be regular, slow rising and small volume due to narrow pulse pressure. Reduced arterial compliance in older patients may negate these findings. Atrial fibrillation is less common than with mitral valve disease.

- BP: narrow pulse pressure.

- JVP: prominent *a* wave.

- Apex: this is usually undisplaced and heaving; it may have a double beat due to additional left atrial impulse. Displacement suggests left ventricular dilatation. A systolic thrill may be palpable over the aortic region and carotids.

- Heart sounds: the dominant feature is likely to be a harsh ejection systolic murmur in the aortic region, radiating to the neck and loudest in expiration. Typically the murmur quietens across the precordium and becomes loud again at the apex (Galliverdin's sign). First heart sound may be normal or soft. Second heart sound may be single (there is no aortic component from a calcified aortic valve that does not move) or with reversed splitting due to delayed aortic valve closure (if the aortic valve cusps are still mobile). Fourth heart sound may be present.

In late presentation, classic signs may lessen and left ventricular failure and secondary pulmonary hypertension dominate.

 In aortic stenosis the murmur is not a guide to severity – look for clinical signs that reflect the haemodynamic significance.

Further discussion

The differential diagnosis of aortic stenosis include the following.

- Innocent systolic murmur, eg aortic sclerosis.

- Pulmonary stenosis: dominant indications are a murmur loudest in inspiration, palpable right ventricular heave and signs of right heart failure. Usually congenital in origin, eg tetralogy of Fallot. Always consider in a cardiac patient who looks cyanosed.

- Hypertrophic cardiomyopathy (HCM): if you suspect this look for jerky impulse and a double apex beat. Patients with HCM are often young.

Features present in aortic stenosis that would not be expected in aortic sclerosis include:

- low pulse pressure;
- slow rising pulse;
- carotid thrill;
- radiation of murmur to neck;
- abnormal heart sounds;
- forceful/displaced apex (unless there is another possible explanation, eg hypertension).

Symptoms of aortic stenosis include angina, shortness of breath and syncope. Transthoracic echocardiography confirms the diagnosis and enables an assessment of severity (see Section 2.5.1). Note, however, that the aortic valve gradient will be underestimated in patients with heart failure, so a dynamic assessment with dobutamine stress may be required in this situation. Coronary angiography is required prior to surgery to look for coexistent coronary artery disease.

Patients with mild or moderate disease should be reviewed annually in a cardiac clinic. All patients should be given advice regarding antibiotic prophylaxis against endocarditis.

All patients with symptoms due to aortic stenosis require aortic valve replacement because the prognosis is poor for sufferers who remain untreated. In particular, the onset of heart failure is a very poor prognostic sign and such patients should be considered for urgent valve replacement. Mechanical valve prostheses (see Table 11) are generally preferred unless the patient is elderly, increased risks of bleeding on anticoagulation are present, or the patient is a young woman who wishes to become

pregnant in the future. In the latter situation patients will often elect to have a tissue valve: this eliminates the need for teratogenic warfarin during their childbearing years but accepts that valve replacement will need to be performed again at a later date.

1.2.8 Aortic regurgitation

Instruction

This woman is short of breath. Please examine her cardiovascular system.

General features

Comment on the patient's general well-being and in particular if she is short of breath at rest or cyanosed. Look for previous surgical scars. Look for a marfanoid habitus or features of arthropathy, especially ankylosing spondylitis.

Cardiovascular examination

Check for stigmata of endocarditis. Pay attention to dental hygiene. Check for signs of heart failure, noting particularly that in aortic regurgitation (AR) the following may be observed.

- Pulse: this would be regular, collapsing in nature and large volume. Atrial fibrillation is less common than with mitral valve disease.

- BP: wide pulse pressure. This may be associated with a number of eponymous signs (Table 12).

- Apex: thrusting and displaced (volume overload). A systolic thrill may be palpable over the aortic region and carotids.

- Heart sounds: the dominant finding is an early diastolic murmur best heard over the lower left sternal edge during expiration while the patient is sitting forward. There is almost always an accompanying ejection systolic murmur. An Austin Flint murmur, which needs to be distinguished from the murmur of mitral stenosis, is a rumbling mid-diastolic murmur caused by the aortic regurgitant jet hitting the mitral valve leaflets. The second heart sound is single (no aortic component), but P2 may be loud. The third heart sound may be heard.

TABLE 12 CLINICAL SIGNS OF THE WIDE PULSE PRESSURE SEEN IN AORTIC REGURGITATION

Sign	Clinical observation
De Musset's	Head nods with each pulsation
Quincke's	Capillary pulsation visible in nail beds
Duroziez's	Double 'to-fro' (systolic and diastolic) murmur heard over femoral arteries when auscultation with firm pressure from stethoscope
Corrigan's	Visible carotid neck pulsations
Müller's	Pulsating uvula
Hill's	Pistol shot sounds over femoral arteries when auscultation with light pressure from stethoscope
Traube's	Pistol shot sounds over femoral arteries

Further discussion

Causes and associations of AR

Chronic:

- Bicuspid aortic valve.
- Marfan's syndrome.
- Infective endocarditis.
- Arthritides – ankylosing spondylitis, rheumatoid and Reiter's syndrome.
- Hypertension.
- Syphilis.

Acute:

- Dissection of aorta.
- Infective endocarditis.
- Failure of prosthetic valve.
- Acute rheumatic fever.

Symptoms of AR include angina, shortness of breath and lethargy. Transthoracic echocardiography confirms the diagnosis (see Section 2.5.2), may reveal the aetiology and enables assessment of severity. If there is a suggestion of significant dilatation of the proximal aorta from CXR or echocardiography, a cardiac MRI scan should be considered. Coronary angiography is required prior to surgery to look for coexistent coronary artery disease.

Patients with mild or moderate disease should be reviewed annually in a cardiac clinic. All patients should be given advice regarding antibiotic prophylaxis against endocarditis.

Asymptomatic patients with severe AR should be considered for surgery if there is evidence of declining left ventricular systolic function or left ventricular dilatation. The onset of heart failure is a poor prognostic sign. Mechanical valve prostheses (see Table 11) are generally preferred unless the patient is elderly, increased risks of bleeding on anticoagulation are present, or the patient is a young woman who

wishes to become pregnant in the future. In the latter situation patients will often elect to have a tissue valve: this eliminates the need for teratogenic warfarin during their childbearing years but accepts that a valve replacement will need to be performed again at a later date.

In acute AR there is often no murmur due to very rapid equalisation of pressures between the aorta and the left ventricle in early diastole. The only murmur that sounds like AR is pulmonary regurgitation, which can be distinguished because it is louder in inspiration and usually associated with signs of right heart compromise.

1.2.9 Tricuspid regurgitation

Instruction

This man has a murmur. Please examine his cardiovascular system.

General features

Comment on the patient's general well-being and in particular if short of breath at rest or cyanosed. Look for previous scars on the chest and more widely over the skin for evidence of intravenous drug abuse.

Cardiovascular examination

Check for stigmata of endocarditis. Pay attention to dental hygiene. Check if the patient is in atrial fibrillation. Note that in tricuspid regurgitation (TR), the following may be observed.

- Signs of heart failure: JVP elevated with giant *v* waves.

- Apex: undisplaced and with parasternal heave.

- Heart sounds: a pansystolic murmur that is loudest in

inspiration and typically most prominent at the lower left sternal edge. A loud pulmonary component of the second heart sound would suggest pulmonary hypertension.

- Other signs: palpable pulsatile liver, sacral and peripheral oedema. Look for evidence of chronic lung disease as TR may be caused by cor pulmonale.

Further discussion

Causes of TR

- Right ventricular (RV) dilatation due to RV failure:
  (a) Mitral valve disease.
  (b) Pulmonary hypertension.
  (c) Intracardiac shunt.
  (d) RV infarction.
- Infective endocarditis (intravenous drug abuse).
- Carcinoid syndrome.
- Congenital, eg Ebstein's anomaly.
- Trauma.
- Myxomatous change.

The character of the JVP establishes the presence of TR, but the examiner will expect you to be able to discuss the differential diagnosis of a pansystolic murmur: mitral regurgitation, ventricular septal defect and TR (see Section 1.2.5).

An echocardiogram will confirm the diagnosis and severity of TR. It is possible to estimate the pulmonary artery pressure from the velocity of the tricuspid regurgitant jet. If pulmonary hypertension is suspected to be the cause of TR, then CXR, lung function tests and lung ventilation–perfusion scanning (or spiral CT) should be pursued.

Surgery is rarely indicated, even for severe TR. However, when the cause is endocarditis it should be considered if there is a large vegetation (>1 cm), persistent sepsis despite the patient taking antibiotics, or evidence of embolisation. In patients undergoing mitral valve surgery, tricuspid annuloplasty is sometimes performed in the presence of severe TR and dilatation of the annulus (>5.0 cm). All patients should be given advice concerning antibiotic prophylaxis against endocarditis.

1.2.10 Eisenmenger's syndrome

Instruction

This woman has become breathless on minimal exertion. A doctor noted that she had a murmur as a child. Please examine her heart.

General features

A large left-to-right shunt causes increased pulmonary blood flow, which in turn causes increased pulmonary vascular resistance and right ventricular (RV) hypertrophy. Eventually the pulmonary resistance exceeds the systemic resistance, and the blood flow is reversed causing a right-to-left shunt with resulting cyanosis.

Look for cyanosis and evidence of stroke in a young person. Is there a sputum pot? Look specifically for haemoptysis.

Cardiovascular examination

Look specifically for the following.

- Cyanosis.

- Clubbing: seen more dramatically in cyanotic congenital heart disease than in any other context.

- Pulse: atrial fibrillation or flutter are common.

- JVP: this will always be significantly raised. Are there flutter waves?

- RV heave.

- Listen for RV gallop rhythm and loud P2.

- Pulmonary or tricuspid regurgitation.

- Ankle oedema.

Once Eisenmenger's syndrome has developed, the murmur of the original shunt will have disappeared.

Further discussion

Eisenmenger's syndrome is a clinical diagnosis aided by ECG (particularly for RV hypertrophy), CXR (for cases of prominent pulmonary arteries and peripheral pruning), echocardiography and cardiac catheterisation. Echocardiography enables the shunt to be visualised and an assessment of RV pressure to be made.

Optimal treatment of patients with Eisenmenger's syndrome is provided by a congenital heart disease specialist service, and may involve the following.

- Continuous oxygen, which acts as a vasodilator.

- Aspirin for patients with polycythaemia to reduce the risk of stroke.

- Venesection for symptomatic polycythaemia.

- Atrial arrhythmias: these are common but may be lethal and can often be treated with catheter ablation (see Section 3.4).

- Ventricular arrhythmias: patients at high risk may require an implantable cardioverter defibrillator (see Section 3.4).

- Transplantation is an option in selected cases.

- Counselling: this can include advice regarding pregnancy and delivery risks for both mother and fetus. Contraceptive advice is also important. In a case where the patient is pregnant, the early opinion of a fetal medicine obstetrician and congenital heart disease specialist are vital.

- Antibiotic prophylaxis: patients with shunts need antibiotic prophylaxis prior to dental procedures or other instrumentation.

Early detection and closure of haemodynamically significant left-to-right shunts is important in order to prevent Eisenmenger's syndrome from developing. Other options include pulmonary artery banding to limit the flow to the lungs and prevent the development of pulmonary hypertension. When Eisenmenger's syndrome is established, the 10-year survival rate is 80% and the 25-year survival rate 40%. Poor prognostic features include syncope, low cardiac output, hypoxaemia and RV failure.

> Patients with Eisenmenger's syndrome should be told to avoid volume depletion, systemic vasodilators, altitude, heavy exertion and pregnancy. They should also be advised to take antibiotics before dental or other procedures.

> **Who was Eisenmenger?**
> In 1897 Dr Victor Eisenmenger reported the case of a 32-year-old man who had showed exercise intolerance, cyanosis, heart failure and haemoptysis prior to death. At post-mortem a large ventricular septal defect and an overriding aorta were found. Eisenmenger described the link between a large congenital cardiac shunt defect and the development of pulmonary hypertension for the first time.

1.2.11 Dextrocardia

Instruction

This patient has a congenital heart condition. Please examine his heart.

General features

This instruction raises many possibilities, making general inspection from the end of the bed particularly important in this case. Are there any obvious dysmorphic features that may indicate a well-known congenital condition? Is the patient cyanosed, which may indicate a cyanotic congenital heart lesion or Eisenmenger's syndrome (see Section 1.2.10)? Are there any obvious surgical scars? Look carefully all over the torso.

Cardiovascular examination

You will need to keep an open mind as you approach this case and may need to focus on particular aspects of the examination depending on what you discover. Key points to look for include the following.

- Pulse: check all peripheral pulses to ensure that they are present and equal. Previous surgery may cause absent pulses, and coarctation of the aorta or stenoses may cause delayed or weakened pulses. Is the pulse irregular and/or tachycardic? Atrial arrhythmias are very common in patients with congenital cardiac conditions, especially if they have been surgically corrected.

- JVP: this may be significantly elevated with right heart conditions or pulmonary hypertension. Tricuspid regurgitation (TR) may be evident (giant *v* wave).

- Precordium: examine for thrills and heaves.

- Apex beat: identify the location and nature of the apex beat. If you cannot feel it in the normal position, percuss the area of cardiac dullness and remember to feel the right side of the chest to identify dextrocardia.

- Heart sounds: careful auscultation will reveal any added sounds/murmurs (Table 13). If you suspect dextrocardia, auscultate over the right side of the chest as well as the left.

- Signs of congestive heart failure: is there any evidence of pulmonary oedema? Is there peripheral oedema or hepatic enlargement, or a pulsatile liver of TR? This is not an uncommon finding with complex congenital conditions.

Further discussion

This patient had the relatively rare condition of dextrocardia with no other associated cardiac abnormalities. Keeping an open mind would have led to a successful outcome in this instance when the apex beat was difficult to feel and the heart sounds very quiet. This was the only abnormality on examination and so the case would easily confuse if the abnormal apex beat had been missed. There are increasing numbers of patients with surgically corrected complex congenital conditions surviving to adulthood. With a methodical approach to the examination it

TABLE 13 KEY CLINICAL SIGNS WITH CONGENITAL HEART DISEASE

Congenital condition	Clinical signs
Dextrocardia	Quiet/absent sounds on left side of chest. Area of cardiac dullness shifted. Apex felt on the right side
Ventricular septal defect (VSD)	Palpable thrill at left sternal edge. Loud pansystolic murmur
Atrial septal defect (ASD)	Wide fixed splitting of second heart sound (does not vary with respiration) and soft ejection systolic murmur over pulmonary area
Pulmonary stenosis (PS)	Right ventricular (RV) heave and thrill in second right space. Split second heart sound (not fixed) and systolic click may be heard
Coarctation of the aorta	Systemic hypertension, reduced lower limb or left arm pulses and radiofemoral delay
Surgically corrected transposition of the great arteries	Mustard or Senning operations are indicated by RV heave, single second heart sound and pansystolic murmur of TR. Switch-operation patients may have ejection systolic murmurs of supravalvular PS or aortic stenosis
Congenitally corrected transposition	Raised JVP and pansystolic murmur of TR. Signs of systemic (right in this situation) ventricular dysfunction
Ebstein's anomaly	JVP often normal even with severe TR. First and second heart sounds widely split. Often third and fourth heart sounds present
Eisenmenger's syndrome	Cyanosed and clubbed. Will have clinical features of underlying shunt, ie ASD, VSD or patent ductus arteriosus, although these may not be apparent if the shunt has reversed

Note: some patients will have extensive surgical scars.
TR, tricuspid regurgitation.

should be possible to identify many of the clinical signs. It is not always necessary to obtain the exact diagnosis, as the complexity of some of these cardiac conditions can be exceptional.

1.3 Communication skills and ethics

1.3.1 Advising a patient against unnecessary investigations

Scenario

Role: you are a junior doctor in a cardiology outpatient clinic.

Miss Jenny Pinto, aged 28 years, has been referred to the clinic for investigation of palpitations. She had previously not been worried about these symptoms, but recent knowledge of the deaths of two relatives following sudden collapses has made her very concerned. At her first appointment it became clear from her history that the palpitations were consistent with ventricular ectopic beats. Examination was normal, as was a routine 12-lead ECG. Echocardiography showed her heart to be normal and a 24-hour ECG demonstrated ectopic beats when she was symptomatic. She is keen to have further investigations, but these would not be appropriate.

Your task: to reassure Miss Pinto that her condition is benign and explain that further investigations are not necessary.

Key issues to explore

What is the patient's main concern? Why does she want further investigation? Does her desire stem from the actual symptoms or the perceived risk from the condition in view of her family history?

Key points to establish

Reassure the patient that the diagnosis of ectopics is certain, as her symptoms have been clearly correlated with ectopics on the 24-hour ECG. Additional reassurance is often provided when patients understand that most people have ectopic beats at some stage every day, the majority of whom are unaware of them. Some people have a lot more ectopics than others, but this does not signify anything if the heart is normal. In this case we know from investigations that her heart is normal and further tests will add nothing to this.

It is important that the patient understands her symptoms are not being dismissed. An explanation that ectopic beats can be very debilitating in some people can reassure. Further, knowing the symptom is benign often leads to a significant improvement in the degree of intensity and awareness the patient feels.

Appropriate responses to likely questions

Patient: what can I do to make them go away?

Doctor: in many cases they will just settle down without needing to do anything. Some people find that they are worse after alcohol or after drinks containing caffeine. It might be worthwhile trying to reduce your intake of these to see whether the symptoms improve. Other people

find relaxation tricks such as taking a few deep breaths or lying down can be helpful.

Patient: are there any tablets that you can give me to help with them?

Doctor: there are drugs that can help suppress the symptoms, but these ectopic beats are, essentially, a normal heart rhythm. We would not generally advise patients to take any medication unless absolutely necessary, because you can end up with more symptoms from the side effects of the medication than the actual palpitations themselves. If you are desperate to take something for these then beta-blockers may help. I can explain how they work and what side effects they might cause.

Patient: am I likely to die suddenly like my relatives?

Doctor: it is difficult to answer this question without further knowledge of exactly what was responsible for the deaths of your two relatives. However, we have very carefully assessed your heart and can find no problems that would give us cause for concern at all. I can certainly reassure you that the palpitations will not cause you to die.

Patient: I am really worried about these symptoms. Would it be possible to have a second opinion?

Doctor: of course you can. Either your GP or I can organise this for you, but I would emphasise that all of the investigations have been reassuring and we know that these ectopic beats, whilst unpleasant, are not in any way life-threatening, but if you'd like to have a second opinion, then I can help arrange this.

1.3.2 Explanation of uncertainty of diagnosis

Key issues to explore

What is the wife's current level of understanding of events? What are her concerns and expectations regarding her husband's condition and treatment?

Key points to establish

Firstly, establish that you have the patient's consent to talk to his wife about his condition. Explain that the cause of the collapse is uncertain, but initial assessment has so far been reassuringly normal, as have the appropriate investigations.

Reassure her that this is a common presentation and that the vast majority of syncopal episodes have a benign cause. Explain that sometimes an exact diagnosis is not determined, and the importance of investigations is to rule out the more serious causes for which there are effective treatments rather than to pinpoint the specific cause.

Appropriate responses to likely questions

Wife: what caused my husband to collapse?

Doctor: at the moment it is not possible to give an exact cause, but the most common cause of collapse is a simple faint. We will make a plan to do further tests, mainly to rule out other causes.

Wife: does this mean that this will never happen again?

Doctor: unfortunately there is no guarantee that the symptoms will not reoccur, but the fact that he is well now, that there are no abnormalities when we examine him, and that the initial tests, the EGG (an electrical tracing of his heart), a CXR (a chest X-ray) and blood tests, are all normal, makes it less likely that there is a serious underlying cause.

Wife: you said he needed more tests: what are these?

Doctor: it's very unlikely that they will show anything worrying, but to be on the safe side we plan to organise for a 24-hour tape recording of his heart beat to check that it doesn't go too fast or too slow at any time, and an echocardiogram – that's a special scan – to look at the heart in more detail than you can see on the CXR. We plan to do these with your husband as an outpatient.

Wife: can't these tests be done before he goes home?

Doctor: I'm afraid that we can't do them right away. Your husband seems well now and when the consultant saw him earlier on we agreed that we didn't need to keep him in hospital and would do the tests as an outpatient.

Wife: can he drive?

Doctor: not at the moment. However, if he has no recurrence of his symptoms then he can return to driving in 4 weeks (see Section 2.19). However, if there are any further symptoms then he should await the results of his remaining investigations and clinic review before recommencing driving.

Wife: will a pacemaker help?

Doctor: at this stage there is no evidence that a pacemaker would be helpful. The results of his tests will help decide whether this needs to be considered in the future.

Wife: what happens if he collapses again at home?

Doctor: as I've explained, we don't think that this is likely or we wouldn't be suggesting that he goes home. If he does collapse, then – the same as if you or I were to collapse – you would need to call the doctor or an ambulance.

1.3.3 Discussion of the need to screen relatives for an inherited condition

been previously fit and well. Examination on admission revealed a normal pulse rate, but his BP was elevated persistently at 160/95 mmHg. There was a soft ejection systolic murmur over the left sternal edge. His ECG was normal apart from large-voltage complexes consistent with left ventricular hypertrophy. He was discharged and prescribed atenolol for his hypertension, and arrangements were also made for him to have a 24-hour ECG and an echocardiogram as an outpatient. The 24-hour ECG was normal but the echocardiogram demonstrated severe hypertrophic cardiomyopathy (HCM) with an outflow tract gradient of 50 mmHg, following which an urgent appointment for the cardiac clinic has been made. His GP has told him that the condition can affect the family, and he is concerned about this.

HCM is typically an autosomal dominant disorder with very variable manifestations: some people with the condition have no problems, but others die suddenly. Further investigation, eg electrophysiological studies, will be advised.

Your task: to explain the diagnosis of HCM and the potential genetic implications of the condition.

Key issues to explore

Has the patient had any further symptoms since discharge? What does he understand about his condition and what are his main concerns regarding his family?

Key points to establish

Establish that there are two main issues to be explored: firstly, the impact of HCM on the patient and the potential need for him to have further investigations; secondly, the hereditary nature of the condition. It is important to understand precisely why the patient is concerned about the impact of the diagnosis on his family. Is his main concern the impact of his health (or ill-health) on the family? Has he understood the genetic aspect of the condition? Or are both issues of concern to him? Both are very important, but an understanding of the patient's main concern will allow a more productive consultation.

Appropriate responses to likely questions

Patient: I feel great now. Does this mean I don't need any further tests?

Doctor: that is really good news and an excellent sign, but it is important that we do further tests of your heart as some patients with this condition can have very serious problems later on.

Patient: does this mean I am going to die?

Doctor: that's not what I said, but a small number of patients with this condition are at risk of dangerous heart rhythm problems and sudden blackouts. The further tests will help us assess whether you are at risk of this. If you are, then there are a number of ways that we can reduce this risk.

Patient: have I given this to my children?

Doctor: I assume that none of your children have had any heart problems so far? [Patient confirms that they have not.] But yes, this condition can be passed on to your children.

Patient: what are the chances that my children have it?

Doctor: because of the way it runs in the family the chances for each child are about 50/50. So at some stage it will be important for you to have your children seen by a specialist, when a simple test like an ultrasound scan of the heart may allow the diagnosis to be made. However, it's not always possible to say that a child definitely does not have the condition.

Patient: is there a blood test that will enable a diagnosis to be made?

Doctor: at the moment there is no single test that will give a definite diagnosis. There have been a lot of advances in the genetic testing of blood samples that may allow us to get this answer in the future, and we can refer you to a clinical geneticist who will be able to give you more information on the inherited aspect of the condition.

1.3.4 Communicating news of a patient's death to a spouse

Scenario

Role: you are a junior doctor on a coronary care unit.

Mr Smith, a 40-year-old man, is admitted from work with a large anterior myocardial infarct, which is treated with thrombolysis. Unfortunately he arrests and, despite prolonged attempts at resuscitation, he dies. His wife arrives 5 minutes after he dies.

Your task: to inform Mrs Smith that Mr Smith is dead.

Key issues to explore

What does the patient's wife know already? She will be more prepared for bad news if she knows he is gravely ill than if she doesn't know why he is in hospital. Explaining an unexpected death is one of the most difficult communication tasks that a medical professional has to perform: if it is done with compassion and sensitivity it can ease the inevitable distress that family and friends will go through.

Key points to establish

Find a quiet room, if possible a relatives' room, and ask the nurse looking after the patient to accompany you. Leave your pager with someone else so that you are free of interruptions. There is no hiding from the fact that you must inform Mrs Smith that her husband has had a heart attack and unfortunately has not survived. State that you and the team did what you could, and say how sorry the whole team is. Demonstrate empathy: if it feels appropriate hold her hand or touch a non-threatening area, such as the arm or the shoulder. Wait until asked to explain details, but keep it simple. Allow her to cry with dignity, such as by handing her some tissues. Do not be afraid of silence, but if this becomes uncomfortable it is often helpful to make an open statement, such as 'This must have come as a shock'.

In finishing the discussion, explain that should further questions arise you will be happy to answer them. Also say that you will have to notify the coroner, which is routine following any unexpected death, and that the nursing staff will provide her with information about practical matters such as death certification.

Appropriate responses to likely questions

Wife: what's happened?

Doctor: [After ascertaining that she knows that her husband was brought into hospital as an emergency, but not that he has died; and speaking quietly, slowly and deliberately to let the information sink in.] Your husband was brought to the hospital as an emergency. He was very unwell: he had suffered a big heart attack. We gave him the best treatment we could – an injection of a drug designed to open up the artery that had blocked off – but I'm afraid that things did not go well. The damage to his heart was too great, it couldn't beat properly and, despite us doing everything we could, he passed away.

Wife: you mean he's dead?

Doctor: yes. I'm very sorry, but I'm afraid he's dead.

Wife: why did this happen?

Doctor: I don't know why it happened, but he had a big heart attack. This must mean that the blood vessels going to his heart muscle were narrowed, and that one of them blocked off and gave him a heart attack.

Wife: but people can survive heart attacks, why didn't he?

Doctor: you're right, many people do survive heart attacks, but I'm afraid that many also don't. Sometimes the heart attack is so big that it damages too much of the heart muscle for the heart to work at all; and sometimes the heart attack affects the wiring mechanism that makes the heart beat in a regular manner, so that instead of pumping in a normal way the heart can't pump at all. I'm sorry to say that both of these things happened in your husband's case.

Wife: why couldn't you bring him back to life?

Doctor: we did absolutely everything we could to restart his heart, but he had suffered such a large heart attack that this wasn't possible. We tried everything we could to resuscitate him, but I'm afraid that it didn't work.

Wife: did he suffer?

Doctor: no – it was very quick and he was unconscious throughout, so he wasn't aware of what was going on and he would not have suffered.

Wife: will he have a post-mortem?

Doctor: it is unlikely that he will have to have a post-mortem. We will need to inform the coroner, which is something that we have to do after any unexpected death, and very occasionally they will insist on a post-mortem. However, I think this is very unlikely in this case, because we know why your husband died. If you would like further information about his health and how he died then we can request a hospital post-mortem, but it may be difficult for you to discuss this now. We can talk about this again later if you want to.

1.3.5 Explanation to a patient of the need for investigations

Scenario

Role: you are a junior doctor working on a cardiology ward.

Mr Hugh Jones, aged 23 years, has congenital heart disease. He was admitted from clinic for further investigations into the cause of his breathlessness. The view of the cardiac team is that it will not be possible to give best advice about prognosis and treatment without information from a cardiac catheterisation study, but he is refusing to consent.

Your task: to determine what concerns Mr Smith has and explain the purpose of further investigation.

Key issues to explore

First find out what the patient knows about his condition: he may be concerned that nothing can be done or be in denial about the seriousness of the problem. Then establish what he knows about cardiac catheterisation and his fears about the procedure: some patients are worried about pain and discomfort, whereas others worry about complications. Try and put any such fears in perspective. Explain any alternative investigative strategies that are available, but also why a cardiac catheterisation study is needed to give him best advice about his condition. If possible offer him information booklets and if there is a specialist nurse available, ask him or her to speak with the patient.

Key points to establish

Mr Smith does not have to undergo any investigation or treatment unless he agrees to it. He will still receive care even if he does not undergo the investigations recommended, but a proper investigation may improve the care that can be given to him and thus alleviate some of his symptoms.

Appropriate responses to likely questions

Mr Smith: I feel fine.

Doctor: I hear what you say, but you went to the doctor because your breathing isn't as good as it should be and it looks as though this is due to a problem with your heart.

Mr Smith: but the problem isn't very bad.

Doctor: I know that things aren't terrible at the moment, but we have found a problem with the heart that could be serious and which may get worse. It may be that treatment now can improve things so that they don't get any worse, or the rate of any deterioration can be slowed down so that you will feel well for longer.

Mr Smith: can you guarantee that the problem can be sorted?

Doctor: no, I'm afraid that I can't. Until we know exactly what the problem is, we won't be able to tell you.

Mr Smith: I still don't like the idea of a cardiac catheter. Is there an alternative?

Doctor: yes, we can and will do scans that will give us some information. However, cardiac catheterisation gives us the most important information, such as the amount of oxygen in the chambers of the heart, which we cannot get in any other way. We wouldn't recommend this if there were better alternatives.

Mr Smith: will it hurt?

Doctor: the procedure may be uncomfortable while the local anaesthetic is being given. This lasts a few minutes and after this it should not be uncomfortable. It's a bit like going to the dentist: the injection is unpleasant, but then things go numb.

Mr Smith: could I die during the procedure?

Doctor: that's very unlikely indeed. This is a routine procedure, although as you can imagine any procedure involving the heart carries a small risk, but it is very small. The risk of death is 1 in 4,000, which means that 3,999 survive out of 4,000 people undergoing the procedure.

1.3.6 Explanation to a patient who is reluctant to receive treatment

Scenario

Role: you are a junior doctor in a medical outpatient clinic.

Mrs Jessica Yelland, aged 30 years, has been found to be significantly hypertensive when she came to her GP's family planning clinic. Her BP has been measured on several occasions and found to be consistently in the region of 180/100 mmHg. It has been explained to her that she has high BP that requires investigation and treatment, but she feels well and only wants a prescription for the oral contraceptive pill, not any tests or medication.

Your task: to inform Mrs Yelland why investigations and treatment are required.

Key issues to explore

The key to a successful outpatient consultation will be to understand the reason why the patient does not want further investigation or treatment. Does she feel that investigation and treatment are unnecessary because she feels well? Is she afraid of what may be found? Is she concerned about the effects of treatment?

Key points to establish

It is very important to establish a rapport with this woman so that she will trust you and thus hopefully follow the recommended management plan. Explain to her that hypertension is a common and often asymptomatic condition that is frequently detected on routine screening, or incidentally as part of investigations for other medical problems. It is important that she understands what hypertension is and why it should be taken seriously, even in the absence of any complaints or limitations: the potential harmful effects of long-term high BP must be explained.

She will need reassurance and an explanation that investigations are necessary to exclude a secondary cause of high BP, which might mean that the hypertension can be cured and that she would not need long-term treatment. If no specific cause for hypertension is found, then simple changes to her lifestyle may be adequate to treat her BP. But in some situations this is not enough and she may require medication.

Your advice should be accompanied by provision of reading material and help with associated programmes for smoking cessation, weight loss and dietary advice. But remember that most patients diagnosed wih hypertension perceive themselves as being healthy and leading a normal lifestyle with no day-to-day limitations; hence starting treatment and addressing lifestyle issues can be difficult and in some cases unacceptable.

Appropriate responses to likely questions

Patient: I feel very well and only went to the doctor for a prescription, so I can't have much of a problem, can I?

Doctor: high blood pressure is a very common condition that can affect up to 20% of people. As in your case, high blood pressure is often discovered when someone has their blood pressure measured for an entirely unrelated problem. The fact that it was discovered for that reason does not mean that having high blood pressure is unimportant.

Patient: what will happen if I have nothing done?

Doctor: over a period of many years high blood pressure can result in serious damage to many important organs in the body. For example, if untreated it can lead to major heart problems and strokes, and very rarely it can result in problems with the eyes that can affect normal vision and in extreme cases may result in blindness. However, all these problems can be avoided by achieving good blood pressure control.

Patient: what causes high blood pressure?

Doctor: a good question, and I wish I could give you a good answer. For most patients we don't know, but in some cases it can be caused by problems with the kidneys or glands so we will recommend some tests – blood tests and urine tests – to see if this might be the case for you.

Patient: how can you tell if high blood pressure is causing damage to the body?

Doctor: by examining you and doing tests. For instance, we can look in your eyes to see if it is having an effect on the blood vessels at the back of the eye; we can do an ECG – an electrical tracing of the heart – or an echocardiogram – a special scan of the heart – and see if it is having an effect there; and we can do urine and blood tests to check kidney function.

Patient: what is the treatment likely to consist of?

Doctor: the first thing is for us to look at your lifestyle to see whether we can help you make it more healthy to bring your blood pressure down. Examples of things that can help are ensuring you take regular exercise, stopping smoking and looking at your diet. But it is likely that tablets will also be needed.

Patient: am I always going to have high blood pressure?

Doctor: not everyone who is started on medication for blood pressure continues with high blood pressure for the rest of their life. In some situations the changes to their lifestyle may mean that they do not need to continue taking medication long term. The treatment is something that your doctor will want to review on a regular basis.

Patient: will one tablet cure me?

Doctor: it might do, but a significant number of patients actually require a combination of tablets. We will start you off on one tablet and then review your blood pressure, and only add in additional tablets if required.

Patient: what if I get side effects from the pills?

Doctor: there are lots of different sorts of blood pressure pills, and we want to make sure that we get one that suits you. If you do get side effects from the first one that we try, I'd like you to tell me so that we can try and find one that suits you better.

Patient: can I still take the oral contraceptive pill?

Doctor: yes, as long as we can get your blood pressure under control.

1.4 Acute scenarios

1.4.1 Syncope

Scenario

A 75-year-old woman presents in the Accident and Emergency Department with a history of sudden collapse. This occurred unexpectedly while she was shopping and there have been no previous similar episodes. When the paramedic team arrived at the scene she was alert and orientated, and all observations were normal and have remained so.

Introduction

How common are unexplained collapses?

These are a very common clinical problem, and account for up to 3% of attendances at Accident and Emergency departments and 1% of hospital admissions. A difficult aspect of managing patients such as this is that there are many causes of syncope, both cardiac and non-cardiac (Table 14).

Who are the high-risk patients?

Untreated cardiac-related syncope has a 1-year mortality rate of 20–30%, making it of paramount importance to identify this group of patients as early as possible. A carefully taken history may exclude a large proportion of these and a meticulous examination may elicit the cause. A history from a witness should be obtained if at all possible – it might be invaluable.

History of the presenting problem

Did the woman really have a syncopal episode, or did she just trip up? If syncope is likely, direct questions should be targeted towards the causes listed in Table 14. One of the most important of these is seizures. It is essential therefore to differentiate between seizures and cardiac syncope. Seizures are associated with the following:

- blue face (not pale);

- convulsive movements (usually, but not always);

- tongue biting;

- incontinence;

- unconsciousness for less than 5 minutes;

- drowsiness and disorientation for a variable length of time on recovery.

A detailed description of the events leading up to the syncopal episode, and a description of the syncopal episode itself and of the recovery phase may provide information to establish the cause. Be very particular in your enquiries: 'Can you remember exactly what you were doing before you collapsed?' Do not accept 'I was out shopping'. Ask: 'Were you sitting down . . . standing up . . . had you just turned your head?' This history should be obtained from the patient, any witness and preferably both.

Specific questions about symptoms that would suggest a cardiac cause include the following.

- Did you feel sweaty or nauseous before the episodes?

- Did you get palpitations, chest pain or breathlessness beforehand?

And if someone has had more than one episode.

- How long have these episodes being going on for and how many have you had?

- Are the episodes becoming more frequent?

- Have you had fits of any sort before?

- Is there anything that brings on the symptoms?

Which conditions make the patient at high risk of recurrent syncope or death?

- Aortic dissection: was syncope associated with chest pain? Is there a history of hypertension? Has the patient had any previous vascular conditions?

- Pulmonary embolism: has the patient had a period of immobility, or had any operations recently? Has there been a previous history of thromboembolism?

- Aortic stenosis: has a murmur been noticed in previous

Type	Cause
Non-cardiac	Seizures*
	Postural hypotension*
	Situational (micturition, defecation, cough and swallow)*
	Cerebrovascular
	Psychogenic (anxiety, panic, somatisation and depression)
Cardiac	Bradyarrhythmias (including vasovagal)*
	Tachyarrhythmias*
	Left ventricular outflow obstruction (aortic stenosis and hypertrophic cardiomyopathy)
	Pulmonary obstruction (pulmonary embolism and pulmonary hypertension)
	Cardiac tamponade
	Aortic dissection
	Other rarities, eg atrial myxoma

TABLE 14 CAUSES OF SYNCOPE

* commonest causes.

examinations? Is there a history of dyspnoea? Is there a history of exertional presyncope?

Specific treatments are available for all these conditions, making it important to consider them when taking a history, even though they are unlikely.

Other relevant history

Identification of any underlying cardiac disease places the patient in a high-risk group for recurrent syncope. Establish whether there are other symptoms suggestive of cardiac abnormality.

- Is there a history of angina/myocardial infarction?

- Is there any cardiac family history?

- Is there a history of rheumatic fever?

- Are there any risk factors for ischaemic heart disease?

Also ask if she is taking any medication and, if so, what? Are there any that might predispose her to syncope, eg diuretics that could cause postural hypotension, or agents that might predispose her to arrhythmia (check all drugs in the *British National Formulary*)?

Examination

General features

Look for evidence of injury caused by the syncope, and concentrate specifically on cardiovascular and neurological assessment.

Cardiovascular system

Take careful note of the following:

- Peripheral perfusion.

- Pulse rate and rhythm.

- Peripheral pulses, including left radial and femorals.

- Pulse character: is it slow rising?

- BP: is there a postural drop and is it the same in both arms?

- JVP.

- Cardiac apex.

- Are there carotid bruits (or bruits elsewhere)?

- Heart sounds and murmurs.

- Lung bases.

- Liver edge.

- Peripheral oedema.

What is the significance of any abnormal cardiac signs? They increase the chances of a cardiac cause of syncope.

What other bedside examinations may help reach a diagnosis? Ask the patient to move her neck through its full range of movement: if this provokes feelings of presyncope or dizziness, then this suggests vertebrobasilar ischaemia as a likely cause for her syncope. Consider carotid sinus massage whilst recording an ECG rhythm strip to investigate carotid sinus sensitivity, but be extremely cautious in those patients who are at risk of atheromatous carotid disease.

Neurological system

The presence of any focal neurological signs would raise the possibility that syncope was caused by a cerebrovascular event, but does not prove that this is the case. A cardiac cause of syncope could have led to cerebrovascular ischaemia.

Investigation

 Remember that patients with syncope are likely to be in a high state of anxiety and it is essential that all other explanations are carefully considered before attributing the problem to psychogenic causes.

What would you do next for this woman?

She will need to be admitted for further investigations and management, the nature of which will be determined by your initial history and examination. If you feel that her syncope is most likely to be neurological in origin, then investigation should be pursued as described in *Neurology*, Section 1.1.3. However, in the absence of a firm diagnosis, a cardiac cause of the syncope can never be totally excluded without thorough investigation.

What are the immediate investigations required for a patient with probable cardiac syncope?

Of patients with cardiac syncope, 10% will have an identifiable abnormality on their 12-lead ECG that suggests a cause. Look for the following:

- sinus rate;

- PR interval;

- QRS axis;

- QRS width;

- QT interval (long QT syndromes);

- left ventricular hypertrophy;

- right ventricular hypertrophy;

- P-wave morphology;

- evidence of pre-excitation (Wolff–Parkinson–White syndrome);

- evidence of acute (or old) myocardial infarction;

- Brugada syndrome (partial right bundle-branch block and ST elevation V1–V3).

On the CXR, look for the following:

- cardiac size and shape;

- prominent pulmonary vasculature;

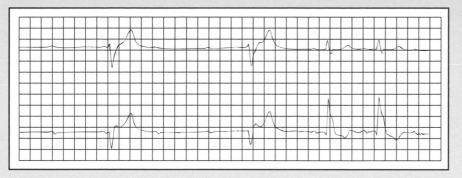

▲**Fig. 19** Complete heart block demonstrated on a Holter monitor.

- pulmonary oedema;

- aortic outline (is the mediastinum of normal width?).

Blood tests are rarely useful in the diagnosis of syncope, but cardiac enzymes, FBC, electrolytes, renal and liver function tests, and inflammatory markers will usually be requested as a 'screen'. Electrolyte disturbance (particularly hypokalaemia) might predispose to arrhythmia and syncope. Raised inflammatory markers may indicate a systemic problem.

Further investigations

What further investigations should you consider during hospital admission?

It is more than likely that the ECG, CXR and screening blood tests will not demonstrate any clear cause of this patient's syncope, in which case consider the following.

- Ambulatory monitoring: 24-hour Holter monitoring and patient-activated devices may be useful for excluding tachyarrhythmias and bradyarrhythmias (Fig. 19) (see Section 3.3).

- Echocardiography: this may indicate structural or functional cardiac abnormality. Transthoracic echocardiography (Fig. 20) is usually adequate, but in some instances transoesophageal echocardiography may be required, eg when aortic dissection is being considered.

- If pulmonary embolism is plausible, check the patient's blood gases and organise lung ventilation–perfusion scanning or CT angiography (see Section 3.8).

- If aortic dissection is possible, request a CT scan of the chest.

What should you do for those with recurrent unexplained syncope?

Consider referral for specialist investigations such as tilt-table testing and electrophysiological tests (see Section 3.2).

Management

If a cardiac cause of syncope is established, what management is indicated?

- Bradyarrhythmias: consider permanent pacemaker (see Section 3.5).

- Tachyarrhythmias: pharmacological therapy, ablation or implantable cardioverter defibrillator (ICD) (see Sections 2.2.2 and 3.4).

- Valvular disease: consider surgical intervention (see Section 2.5).

- Pulmonary embolism: will need anticoagulation (see Section 2.18 and *Haematology*, Section 3.6).

- Hypertrophic cardiomyopathy: give advice on lifestyle changes and pharmacological therapy, and

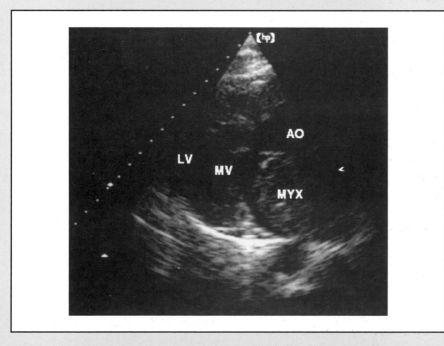

▲**Fig. 20** Transthoracic echocardiogram of an atrial myxoma. The myxoma (MYX) is seen to occupy most of the left atrium and is almost prolapsing through the mitral valve (MV) into the left ventricle (LV). The aorta (AO) is seen above the left atrium. This would be an exceedingly rare cause of syncope.

consider an ICD if there are any features suggestive of a high risk of sudden death (see Section 2.4.1). If there is significant left ventricular outflow tract obstruction, then consider referral for surgical myomectomy or alcohol septal ablation (see Section 2.4.1).

What should you do if no cause for syncope is established and the patient is asking to go home?

If after 24–48 hours there has been no recurrence of presyncope or syncope, the patient has 'mobilised' satisfactorily on the ward and serial 12-lead ECGs show no change, then the patient should be discharged home with the following:

- reassurance that nothing terrible has been found, but also a clear statement that no firm diagnosis has been made, meaning that patient and doctors must remain alert;

- a letter for the patient's GP;

- instructions to report recurrence of presyncope or syncope immediately;

- arrangements for 24-hour ambulatory monitoring (and perhaps echocardiography) if it has not been possible to obtain this during the patient's brief admission.

> Most patients will be aware of the serious nature of most cardiac causes of syncope. It is essential to be aware of the psychological needs of such patients. Reassurance and appropriate information at an early stage may prevent problems at a later stage in their management.

1.4.2 Stroke and a murmur

Scenario

A 58-year-old woman who is married with two sons and works as a part-time teacher presents with a left-sided hemiparesis of sudden onset. She had previously been fit and well. However, a murmur had been noted, but not investigated, when she was 45 years old and undergoing a minor gynaecological procedure. There is no past medical history or family history of note. She is on no medication.

Introduction

A stroke can be a devastating condition with high morbidity and mortality. It is not possible at presentation to predict accurately the degree of recovery that this woman will make. However, it is important to identify whether she is at high risk of further events, and in particular whether she is at risk of cardiac embolic stroke. Most strokes are related to cerebrovascular atheromatous disease and not to cardiac disease, but most cardiac causes of embolic stroke are treatable, indicating that further events in this group are potentially preventable. History or examination will detect most cases where there is a cardiac cause for stroke.

> Consider the causes of cardiac embolic stroke when taking a history and examining a patient who has had a stroke:
>
> - 'non-valvular' atrial fibrillation (AF);
> - acute myocardial infarction (MI) with mural thrombus;
> - mechanical prosthetic valves;
> - rheumatic heart disease;

- dilated cardiomyopathy;
- infective endocarditis;
- paradoxical embolism;
- left atrial myxoma;
- calcific aortic stenosis;
- aortic arch atheroma.

History of the presenting problem

The first priority will be to confirm the diagnosis of stroke, then to focus on possible causes. With regard to identification of cardiac causes of stroke, establish whether there have been any previous thromboembolic events. Is the patient known to have any cardiac condition? Does she have any cardiac symptoms? Specifically, is there a history of palpitations suggestive of AF?

Other relevant history

In most cases it will be obvious if there is any pre-existing cardiac condition, but ask the patient the following.

- Are you known to have an irregular pulse?

- Have you had angina or a heart attack?

- Have you had rheumatic fever?

- Have you had any heart operations?

- Has a murmur ever been heard?

- Did you have a 'hole in the heart' as a child?

Examination

General features

In the absence of previous cardiac conditions and with an entirely normal clinical examination, the likelihood of stroke being cardiac in origin is small. It is therefore vital that examination of the cardiovascular system is thorough. A patient with a recent stroke may have difficulty in cooperating with

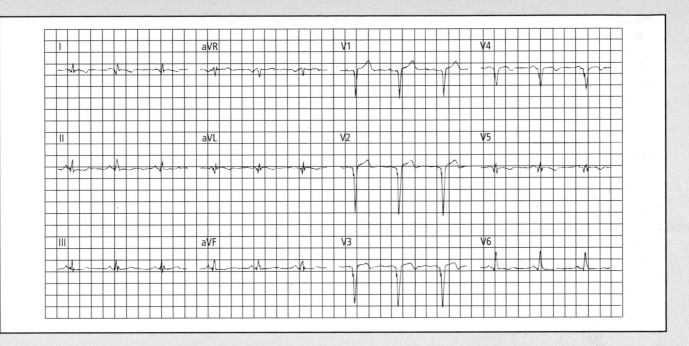

▲ **Fig. 21** ECG demonstrating anterior Q waves and poor R-wave progression across the chest leads. This is most probably secondary to a previous large anterior MI. Left ventricular mural thrombus is possible in this scenario.

you during the examination, eg rolling the patient on to the side to listen for mitral stenosis may be difficult if he or she has a hemiparesis. However, it is important not to compromise the quality of your examination – seek help in moving the patient if necessary.

It is unlikely that there will be many signs from a general examination that will help in establishing whether the cause was cardiac.

- The patient with a previous MI or dilated cardiomyopathy might be dyspnoeic as a result of cardiac failure, but there are many other causes of breathlessness, including aspiration pneumonia, in someone who has just suffered a stroke.

- The patient with infective endocarditis or atrial myxoma may have fever and peripheral stigmata, but these are uncommon conditions (see Section 1.4.7).

- Look carefully for any signs of previous cardiac surgery,

particularly if the patient is unable to give a history. Do not forget to examine the back and the breast crease where there may be scars from previous mitral surgery (valvuloplasty).

Cardiovascular system

Take careful note of the following.

- Pulses: check the rhythm and character. In particular, is there AF? Is it possible that this woman has had an aortic dissection?

- BP: this is often elevated in someone who has just had a stroke.

- Heart sounds: this woman is said to have a murmur – listen carefully for both mitral stenosis and aortic incompetence, which are easy murmurs to miss. You are most unlikely ever to hear the 'tumour plop' of an atrial myxoma, but it is absolutely certain that you will not if you never listen!

Consider non-thromboembolic cardiovascular causes for her stroke, eg aortic dissection involving the

carotid arteries or vasculitis of the cerebral vessels (very rare).

Investigation

In most cases, simple non-invasive investigations will provide the information needed to establish a cardiac cause of a stroke.

ECG and CXR

Every patient who has a stroke should have a 12-lead ECG and a CXR. The ECG may provide valuable clues to the aetiology of thrombus (Fig. 21).

Echocardiography

This should be requested if there is a clinical, ECG or chest radiographic indication of cardiac abnormality (Fig. 22). If the heart is structurally normal on transthoracic echocardiography and no other cause of stroke is found, a transoesophageal echocardiogram should be requested to look for aortic arch atheroma, patent foramen ovale (PFO) (Fig. 23) or left atrial appendage thrombus (Fig. 24). CT or MRI of the chest

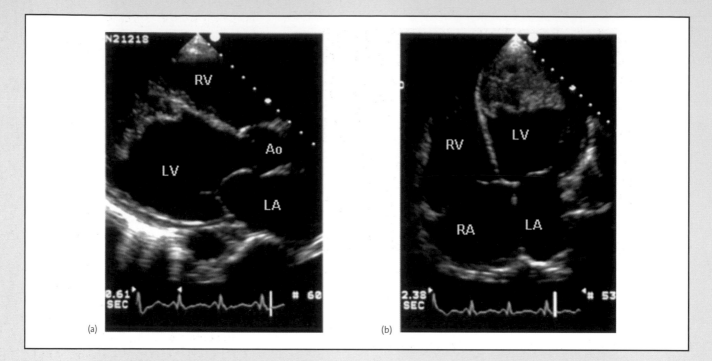

▲ **Fig. 22** Transthoracic echocardiogram of an apical thrombus after MI. LA, left atrium; LV, left ventricle; RA, right atrium; RV, right ventricle; Ao, aorta.

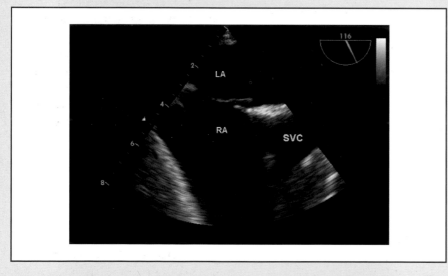

▲ **Fig. 23** Transoesophageal echocardiogram of a PFO. LA, left atrium; RA, right atrium; SVC, superior vena cava.

may rarely be required to define a structural abnormality.

Blood tests

- FBC (if polycythaemia or thrombocytosis is possible).

- Electrolytes.

- Renal and liver function tests.

- Inflammatory markers: if these are raised and there is no other mundane explanation, consider endocarditis, myxoma and vasculitis, and perform appropriate specialist blood tests.

- Blood cultures (if any suspicion of endocarditis).

Brain CT scan
This is required to exclude haemorrhage, aneurysm or

tumour. Evidence of multiple cortical infarcts in different vascular territories and a structurally normal heart on transthoracic echocardiography should raise the possibility of PFO if carotid artery disease is not found.

Management
The patient will require care appropriate to the disability produced by their stroke (see *Medicine for the Elderly*, Section 2.8; *Acute Medicine*, Section 1.2.30; and *Neurology*, Sections 1.4.2 and 2.8.1). Particular attention to anticoagulation, restoration of sinus rhythm (in some cases) and surgical correction of cardiac lesions (in rare cases) will be required in patients with a cardiac cause for stroke.

Anticoagulation
Consider if the stroke is confirmed as ischaemic on brain CT scan and a cardiac cause has been identified. The balance of benefit versus risk in the acute setting is difficult: leaving

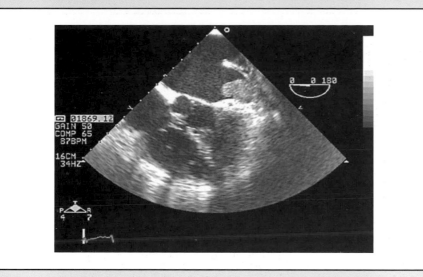

▲ **Fig. 24** Transoesophageal echocardiogram of thrombus in left atrial appendage.

the patient without anticoagulation keeps her at risk of further thromboembolism, but anticoagulation puts her at increased risk of haemorrhagic transformation of a cerebral infarct. There are no good data to determine when anticoagulation should be started. Assuming that the patient is recovering from a stroke, most physicians would begin with heparin (intravenous or low-molecular-weight) at some time between 7 and 14 days, with a view to long-term warfarin therapy if the thromboembolic risk persists.

- Strokes may be haemorrhagic, even in those at risk of thromboembolism.
- Some features are more likely with cerebral haemorrhage than with infarction, such as nausea/vomiting, cerebral irritation and depressed conscious level.
- Ischaemic and haemorrhagic strokes cannot be distinguished with certainty on clinical grounds and a brain CT scan should always be performed before commencing anticoagulation.

Antiarrhythmics

After anticoagulation, restoration of sinus rhythm should be the primary target in those with AF. Pharmacological cardioversion is preferable to DC cardioversion in this context so as to avoid general anaesthetic after a recent stroke (see Section 2.2.2).

Closure of PFO

Percutaneous closure is recommended if no other cause of stroke is found, there are recurrent episodes despite anticoagulation and a large PFO is demonstrated by echocardiography.

Surgical correction of cause

Repair of an aortic dissection, replacement of an infected valve or removal of an atrial myxoma may be necessary immediately. There is high risk of further cerebral insult when the patient goes on cardiac bypass, but this has to be balanced against the potential risk of not treating the underlying condition. In those with valvular pathology, it is usual to allow time for the patient to make as complete a recovery as possible from the stroke before considering surgery.

1.4.3 Acute chest pain

Scenario

A 55-year-old Glaswegian merchant seaman presents with chest tightness after unloading his ship of heavy goods.

Introduction

If the patient is still in pain, the first concern is to rule out life-threatening emergencies such as myocardial infarction (MI) or aortic dissection where treatment can be life-saving. Quickly assess the patient's haemodynamic status, including checking for bradycardia and tachycardia, and measuring the BP. Obtain an initial brief history and conduct a quick examination whilst the ECG is being recorded.

History of presenting problem

This patient's pain was associated with heavy exertion, but it is important to determine answers to the following questions if they do not emerge spontaneously.

- When did it start?

- What were you doing when it started?

- What was it like? Characteristically ischaemic pain is described as tight, squeezing or crushing. It may be helpful to offer suggestions, but it is important to realise that patients may find it difficult to describe pain, especially if it is severe.

- How bad was the pain? Severity should be recorded on a scale of 1 to 10.

- How long did it last? Pain that last for only a few seconds or constantly for days is unlikely to be cardiac.

- Did it start suddenly? If so, consider aortic dissection, although this is also typical of non-cardiac pain related to anxiety. Or did it build up rapidly over minutes? This is more typical of cardiac ischaemia.

- Did the pain go anywhere else? In particular, did it radiate in a manner typical of ischaemic cardiac pain?

- Was it sharp and stabbing in nature? If yes, consider causes of pleuritic chest pain.

- Has the patient experienced unusual breathlessness or chest tightness on exertion previously?

- Beware of pain which comes on at rest or during sleep: both unstable angina and acute coronary syndromes may occur at rest.

Also ask about associated symptoms, such as breathlessness, sweating, nausea, faintness and whether the pain was frightening, all of which are features of cardiac ischaemia.

> A patient with stable angina who then presents with increasing frequency and severity of angina ('crescendo angina') is likely to have an unstable plaque and should be admitted, even if pain-free when seen.

Differential diagnoses

Aortic dissection A sudden onset of severe pain radiating to the back, which may be described as 'tearing', should ring alarm bells and the patient should be evaluated for dissection. This is more likely in patients with known hypertension.

Digestive pain (reflux oesophagitis or peptic ulceration) Ask whether the pain was associated with the bringing up of wind or an acid taste in the mouth. Also enquire about

any previous history of indigestion, use of treatments for indigestion (eg antacids) or previous investigations for indigestion (barium meal or endoscopy test). Remember that severe epigastric pain can be caused by myocardial ischaemia as well as the abdominal conditions usually considered (peptic ulceration, biliary pain, pancreatitis and intestinal ischaemia).

Musculoskeletal This tends to be very localised and affected by the position of the sufferer, unlike ischaemic pain, which is not. It may occur after strenuous exertion, which often leads to anxiety that this has 'brought on a heart attack'.

Pericarditis This is unlikely in this case, but ask whether the patient has had any 'flu-like' symptoms. The pain tends to be sharper than ischaemic cardiac pain and is usually eased by sitting forward.

Anxiety This can manifest itself as pain, but severe pain may cause patients to become anxious, so beware of dismissing the patient's symptoms. Patients may develop tingling in the fingers due to hyperventilation in response to chest pain.

Other relevant history

Does the patient have known coronary artery disease? Ask about history of angina, MI and cardiac catheterisation/revascularisation procedures (percutaneous coronary intervention or coronary artery bypass surgery). If not, are they at high risk of coronary disease? Note previous vascular events: does the patient have a history of stroke or peripheral vascular disease? Consider risk factors for coronary disease, including family history, smoking, diabetes mellitus, hypercholesterolaemia and hypertension.

Examination

General features

All patients with chest pain need prompt rapid assessment. How does the patient look: well, ill, very ill or about to die? Patients with MI usually look very ill (or worse).

After checking vital signs, examine particularly for epigastric tenderness and guarding: patients with perforations or pancreatitis may present in this way and be misdiagnosed. Where the patient does not have a life-threatening condition, palpation for tenderness that reproduces the pain is useful.

Cardiovascular system

This is frequently normal in patients with acute central chest pain. However, a full examination is essential, looking in particular for features that would be diagnostically useful.

- Pulses: unequal radial pulses and unequal BP in the arms may indicate aortic dissection.

- Heart sounds: an early diastolic murmur of aortic regurgitation may indicate dissection; a pericardial rub would suggest pericarditis.

Investigation

Appropriate investigations are the key to proving a diagnosis of an acute coronary syndrome.

ECG

An entirely normal ECG at presentation does not exclude serious underlying coronary disease. Look in particular for:

- ST-segment elevation/left bundle-branch block (MI) (Fig. 25);

- ST-segment depression [non-ST elevation MI (NSTEMI) or unstable angina] (Fig. 26);

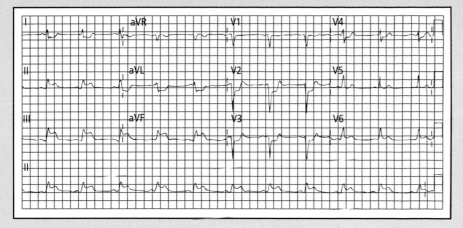

▲**Fig. 25** Acute inferior MI. The ECG shows ST-segment deviation in the inferior leads (II, III and aVF). ST-segment depression in leads V2 and V3 may indicate posterior extension.

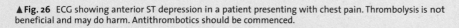

▲**Fig. 26** ECG showing anterior ST depression in a patient presenting with chest pain. Thrombolysis is not beneficial and may do harm. Antithrombotics should be commenced.

- T-wave inversion (NSTEMI or unstable angina);

- concave ST-segment elevation in multiple leads that do not conform to a single coronary artery territory (pericarditis).

Biochemical markers
Troponins are markers of myocyte necrosis and should be measured at 12 hours in order to diagnose MI (see Section 3.7).

Other blood tests
FBC, creatinine and electrolytes, glucose, cholesterol and, in patients with epigastric pain, amylase should be measured.

Chest radiograph
Is the mediastinum widened (aortic dissection) or is there pulmonary oedema?

Management

Ischaemic cardiac pain
Patients will usually already have received aspirin 300 mg. Give oxygen and analgesia if the patient is still in pain. Further management will depend on the diagnosis:

- unstable angina/NSTEMI (see Section 2.1.2);

- ST-elevation MI (see Section 2.1.3).

Persisting pain without ECG abnormalities and no other clear diagnosis
Reassure the patient, give analgesia, and admit for overnight observation with repeat ECG and troponin at 12 hours.

 Do not discharge patients who present with undiagnosed chest pain without a further ECG and troponin test at 12 hours – unstable ischaemic heart disease can be difficult to diagnose clinically and is easily missed.

Pain resolved but diagnosis uncertain
Patients who attend hospital with chest pain that is not clearly musculoskeletal should stay for further assessment, with a troponin test and ECG at 12 hours after the pain. A negative troponin test will not rule out important coronary disease, so an investigation to look for ischaemia (eg exercise test) should be arranged as an outpatient. The patient should be advised to seek medical help immediately if the pain recurs after discharge.

Difficult cases of chest pain may be due to coronary vasospasm (Fig. 27). Features of spasm include:

- normal coronary angiogram or 'minor irregularities';
- paroxysms of crushing central chest pain at rest;
- affects postmenopausal women the most;
- relieved by glyceryl trinitrate;
- does not limit exercise;
- may be associated with syncope;
- usually benign unless associated with ECG changes or ventricular arrhythmias.

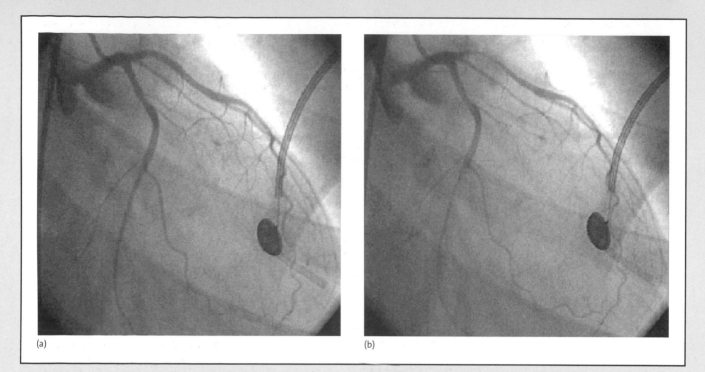

(a)   (b)

▲ **Fig. 27** Left coronary angiogram demonstrating coronary vasospasm. This 34-year-old woman presented with chest pain and anterior ST-segment elevation on the ECG. Shortly afterwards, she had a ventricular fibrillation arrest. After resuscitation, the ECG returned to normal. (**a**) Initial angiography showed a normal left coronary artery. (**b**) Intracoronary ergometrine induced localised spasm of the proximal left anterior descending coronary artery and reproduced the chest pain with ECG changes.

 Oesophageal pain is difficult to distinguish from cardiac pain. Cardiac pain may be relieved by belching. It is inadvisable to discharge a high-risk patient with a clinical diagnosis of oesophageal pain.

1.4.4 Hypotension following acute myocardial infarction

Scenario

Mr Jones is a 60-year-old man who was admitted with an acute inferior myocardial infarction (MI), which was treated with aspirin, clopidogrel and thrombolysis. Ninety minutes after thrombolysis he was still in pain and there was no change in the elevation of ST segments in the inferior leads. He underwent percutaneous coronary intervention (PCI) to the right coronary artery via the right femoral artery. He was reviewed the following morning once the coronary care team were happy with his progress. His creatine kinase (CK) was 4,010 IU/mL and troponin I >50 IU/mL (both grossly elevated) and an angiotensin-converting enzyme (ACE) inhibitor was prescribed. However, the coronary care nurses ask you to review him before giving the first dose of the ACE inhibitor because his systolic BP has fallen to 70 mmHg.

Introduction

Hypotension after MI requires rapid assessment and intervention. The combination of clinical examination, ECG and CXR will usually determine the diagnosis.

History of the presenting problem

Pay particular attention to the following.

- How quickly did the hypotension arise? Sudden onset of hypotension usually indicates a catastrophic event, whereas pump failure is more gradual.

- Does the patient have chest pain? This may indicate reinfarction or cardiac rupture.

- Drugs: streptokinase is a cause of hypotension, which usually occurs in the first 20 minutes of administration. Other than this, drugs are rarely the cause of severe hypotension unless the patient is fluid depleted, but look for a temporal relationship.

- Breathlessness: this may indicate pulmonary oedema or, more rarely in this situation, pulmonary embolism.

- Volume depletion: has the patient received diuretics? Examine the fluid charts.

Examination

General features
Assess the general condition. If the patient appears on the verge of arresting, call the resuscitation team immediately: do not wait until the heart has definitely stopped. Check the Glasgow Coma Scale to confirm the baseline. Assess pain level (if any).

Cardiovascular system
The following are important.

- Peripheral circulation: does the patient have cold feet and hands? How far up the arms and legs is perfusion impaired? Severe peripheral shutdown indicates a poor prognosis.

- BP: recheck the measurement, and record in the left arm as well as the right. Could the patient have an aortic dissection presenting with an inferior MI?

- JVP: if it is grossly elevated, consider right ventricular infarction, ventricular septal defect (VSD), tamponade or pulmonary embolism (PE).

- Heart sounds: a gallop rhythm suggests left ventricular failure. A new pansystolic murmur suggests VSD or mitral regurgitation from chordal or papillary muscle rupture.

- The groin: could the patient be bleeding into the leg or abdomen from the femoral puncture?

- Urine output: an essential aid for assessment of end-organ perfusion.

Investigations
Routine investigations will help establish the diagnosis.

- ECG: arrhythmia or reinfarction?

- CXR: look for pulmonary oedema, and also for widening of the mediastinum.

- Arterial blood gases: these will confirm oxygenation and ventilation. Hypoxia in the presence of a normal CXR suggests PE.

- Other blood tests: creatinine and electrolytes will document renal function; FBC will be used to assess for blood loss (could the patient be having a gastrointestinal bleed following thrombolysis?) or sepsis (unlikely in this context).

- Echocardiography: this is essential to assess left and right ventricular function, mitral regurgitation, VSD and tamponade.

When contemplating the results of these investigations, consider the diagnoses listed in Table 15.

Management
Rapid assessment and diagnosis are vital: delay can be disastrous. Early consultant advice is important. Continuous monitoring of rhythm and BP and of hourly urine output is essential. Serum creatinine and electrolytes should be checked at least daily.

- Stop drugs which cause hypotension, except beta-blockers in patients with heart failure who have been taking them long term, as there is a risk of mortality on rapid cessation.

- Monitor pulse oximetry and give high-flow oxygen.

- Assess and treat the underlying condition if possible: patients with VSD or mitral regurgitation require urgent cardiothoracic surgical referral.

- Attempt to chemically cardiovert new-onset atrial fibrillation by correcting potassium and magnesium levels, and administering intravenous amiodarone. These patients should receive therapeutic heparin.

- Most patients are not fluid depleted after MI, but in a hypotensive patient with clear lung fields who is not hypoxic it is reasonable to give a fluid bolus of 250 mL 0.9% saline intravenously and then reassess. This can be repeated if necessary. However, if there is no response it is important to seek further advice and consider inserting a PA catheter to guide fluid management.

- The combination of pulmonary oedema and hypotension indicates a poor prognosis. If there is evidence of pulmonary oedema, you must not administer fluid as this could be fatal. Give furosemide 80 mg as an intravenous bolus. Central venous access should be obtained, inotropes started and consultant advice sought. Intra-aortic balloon pumping may be helpful, particularly if revascularisation may be feasible in the future. Notify the intensive care unit, as ventilation may be required.

Further comments
Hypotension after MI is a serious problem with a high mortality. Remember that the patient must be kept as comfortable as possible: explain what needs to be done and why, and give analgesia in small doses (eg diamorphine 2.5 mg iv) as often as needed. The patient's relatives should be contacted.

TABLE 15 DIFFERENTIAL DIAGNOSIS OF SUDDEN HYPOTENSION FOLLOWING MI

Differential diagnosis	Features
Right ventricular infarction	Inferior MI High JVP with hypotension Clear CXR
Acute mitral regurgitation	Pansystolic murmur, although this may be absent if there is rapid equalisation of pressure between left atrium and left ventricle Severe pulmonary oedema Echocardiography will be diagnostic (Fig. 28) Pulmonary artery (PA) catheter may confirm this diagnosis by revealing a giant *v* wave
Acquired VSD	Very high JVP Pansystolic murmur Pulmonary oedema, but less severe than acute mitral regurgitation Echocardiography will detect location
Intermittent ischaemia from severe ischaemic heart disease	Severe coronary disease (especially critical left main-stem disease) Recurrent chest pain associated with widespread ischaemic changes on ECG High risk of death; refer patient for urgent revascularisation
Pump failure	Raised JVP Pulmonary oedema Echocardiogram shows poor left ventricular function, but no evidence of VSD or mitral regurgitation PA catheter may be helpful if there is doubt about left ventricular filling. In general, fill with cautious boluses of fluid until PA wedge pressure is 15 mmHg; if the patient is hypotensive and anuric despite PA wedge >15 mmHg, start inotropes
Retroperitoneal bleeding	This may be spontaneous in response to thrombolytic and antiplatelet agents, but may also occur from a leaking femoral artery puncture site after angiography and PCI Tachycardia Low BP and JVP Good BP response to fluids Evidence of dropping haemoglobin on serial tests Consultant advice should be sought regarding urgent CT scan of the abdomen, and stopping glycoprotein IIb/IIIa antagonists
Gastrointestinal bleeding	Recognised complication of thrombolytic and antiplatelet agents Tachycardia Low BP and JVP Good BP response to fluids Evidence of dropping haemoglobin on serial tests Watch for melaena

MI, myocardial infarction; PCI, percutaneous coronary intervention; VSD, ventricular septal defect.

1.4.5 Breathlessness and collapse

Scenario

A 55-year-old woman is brought to hospital by ambulance. Her husband called 999 this morning when he found her acutely breathless at home. She had a brief syncopal episode on being moved into the ambulance, but is now conscious, although extremely dyspnoeic. Her BP is only 80 mmHg systolic. You are bleeped urgently by the Emergency Department to assess and instigate initial management.

Introduction

What is the differential diagnosis in this patient? Common causes (Table 16) should be considered as you assess and resuscitate the patient. Preliminary assessment will direct specific investigations and treatment. Pulmonary embolism (PE) should be high on the list of diagnoses for a patient such as this, particularly if there is no prior history of cardiorespiratory disease. The episode of syncope is of particular concern and confirms the life-threatening nature of this presentation.

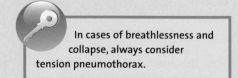

In cases of breathlessness and collapse, always consider tension pneumothorax.

History of the presenting problem

If you can obtain a history from the patient and/or her husband, ask

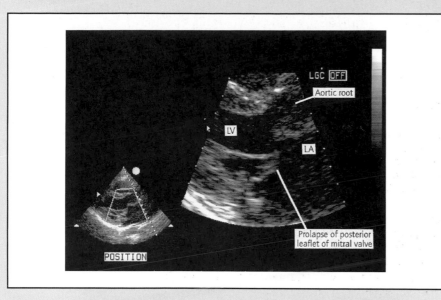

▲ **Fig. 28** Transoesophageal echocardiogram showing prolapse of the posterior mitral valve leaflet (indicated) into the left atrium (LA) after papillary muscle rupture. LV, left ventricle.

TABLE 16 DIFFERENTIAL DIAGNOSIS OF ACUTE DYSPNOEA AND HAEMODYNAMIC COLLAPSE

General cause	Comment	Specific cause
Cardiac	Common	MI/complications (acute mitral regurgitation, VSD, acute left ventricular failure)
		Arrhythmia (VT)
	Less common	Aortic dissection
		Cardiac tamponade
		Acute aortic regurgitation
Cardiorespiratory	Common	Massive PE (occluding >50% of pulmonary vasculature)
Respiratory	Common	Acute life-threatening asthma
	Less common	Tension pneumothorax[1]
Other	Common	Sepsis
	Less common	Intra-abdominal catastrophe
		Severe haemorrhage ('air hunger')
		Anaphylaxis

1. Remember that although tension pneumothorax is uncommon, this diagnosis should be considered before all others because immediate treatment is life-saving.
MI, myocardial infarction; VSD, ventricular septal defect; VT, ventricular tachycardia.

---

particularly about the following, doing so at the same time as you examine and organise initial investigations such as ECG, arterial blood gases and CXR.

- Did the breathlessness have a sudden or gradual onset? Sudden onset suggests pneumothorax, massive PE, acute valve dysfunction, dissection or arrhythmia.

- Is there central chest or interscapular pain? This suggests MI or aortic dissection, respectively.

- Presence of pleuritic chest pain or haemoptysis: either suggests smaller PEs preceding a larger one.

- Are there any symptoms suggestive of pulmonary oedema, such as orthopnoea, paroxysmal nocturnal dyspnoea or pink frothy sputum?

- Does the patient have a history of asthma and has it been getting worse?

- Has the patient suffered from abdominal pain, vomiting, haematemesis or melaena: could there have been an intra-abdominal catastrophe?

- Symptoms suggestive of sepsis: the most common infective cause of hypotension and breathlessness would be septicaemia and acute respiratory distress syndrome, but with 'flu-like illness also consider pericardial effusion with sudden decompensation.

- Exposure to a known allergen.

- Drugs: illicit or prescribed.

> When dealing with patients who are very ill, history-taking, examination, investigations and treatment should all begin together. Finishing a very complete history at the same time as the patient expires is to be avoided!

Other relevant history

This is not the time for a lengthy medical history, but ask about the following.

- PE or deep venous thrombosis and the relevant risk factors (see Section 2.18).

- Cardiac: MI, angina, previously undiagnosed anginal pain, valve disease, rheumatic fever, 'heart murmur' (and if so any recent dental work or surgery – could she have acute valve dysfunction caused by infective endocarditis?) and hypertension (risk factor for ischaemic heart disease and aortic dissection).

- Respiratory: asthma, chronic airflow obstruction and pneumothorax.

- Abdominal: peptic ulcers, pancreatitis and gallstones.

- Anaphylaxis: allergy to anything?

- Drugs: a useful rapid check of past medical history in this context.

If no history is available, check bags and pockets for inhalers, glyceryl trinitrate, etc.

Examination

General features

🔑 If the patient looks *in extremis*, call for help from the intensive care unit or the cardiac resuscitation team immediately. Do not wait until she has a cardiac arrest if she looks as though she is deteriorating.

Immediately assess the following.

- Vital signs: pulse (rate and rhythm), BP, respiratory rate and temperature.

- Is there cyanosis? Check pulse oximetry (but do not remove the high-flow oxygen to 'check value on air' in someone who is desperately ill).

- Is there swelling of the lips and tongue (anaphylaxis)?

- Conscious level: establish baseline Glasgow Coma Score.

Cardiovascular system

🔑 Is there a tension pneumothorax? Look for asymmetry of the chest, shift of trachea from midline, shift of mediastinum from midline (percuss area of cardiac dullness) and silent chest on one side (with a few breath

sounds in the opposite axilla). These signs are not subtle, but they require a clear head to recognise in the context of a patient who is desperately ill.

- Does the pulse become impalpable on inspiration? This indicates severe paradox, so consider life-threatening asthma or tamponade.

- Where is the JVP? A high JVP suggests a cardiac or respiratory cause for collapse, whereas a low one suggests bleeding, intra-abdominal catastrophe or sepsis.

- Specifically look for evidence of massive PE: high JVP, right ventricular heave and tricuspid regurgitation.

- Heart sounds: is there a pansystolic murmur? If so, consider acute mitral regurgitation or VSD (see Section 1.4.4)?

Respiratory system

Are there reasonable breath sounds in both lungs? If there are many crackles and/or bronchial breathing, consider pulmonary oedema, pneumonia or adult respiratory distress syndrome.

Abdominal

Peritonism indicates an intra-abdominal catastrophe. Feel deliberately for an abdominal aortic aneurysm.

Investigation

The following investigations are required immediately in all patients who present with severe hypotension and breathlessness.

Blood tests

Check fingerprick blood glucose immediately in anyone who is severely ill. Check arterial gases.

Take samples for FBC, electrolytes, renal and liver function tests, cardiac enzymes and blood cultures.

ECG

Look for the following (and repeat after 1 hour, or sooner if clinically indicated).

- Arrhythmia (see Section 2.2).

- Localised ST-segment elevation of acute MI (see Section 2.1.3).

- ECG changes compatible with acute PE, the most common being sinus tachycardia and T-wave inversion in leads V1–V4. The 'typical' right-axis deviation and 'S1Q3T3' are actually quite unusual (see Section 2.18).

- Generalised low voltages of pericardial effusion (see Section 2.6).

Chest radiograph

Look for pneumothorax, pulmonary oligaemia (resulting from PE), pulmonary oedema, consolidation, effusions, heart size, mediastinal shift and the widened mediastinum of aortic dissection.

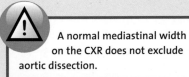 ⚠ A normal mediastinal width on the CXR does not exclude aortic dissection.

Echocardiography

This is the examination of choice for effusion, valve regurgitation and VSD, and for assessing ventricular function. Remember that right ventricular dysfunction in the context of acute severe dyspnoea and hypoxia is highly suspicious of massive PE.

Other investigations

As determined by clinical assessment and the findings of preliminary tests, eg pulmonary CT angiography for suspected massive PE, or CT of the abdomen if an abdominal cause is likely.

Management

Key priorities when you reach the patient include the following.

- Resuscitate (*A*irway, *B*reathing and *C*irculation) and secure venous access while taking a history.

- Give high-flow oxygen.

- Exclude tension pneumothorax: insert a large-bore cannula into the silent side of the chest (second intercostal space, mid-clavicular line or mid-axillary line, above the level of the nipple) if this is the clinical diagnosis (see *Acute Medicine*, Sections 1.2.14 and 3.5; and *Respiratory Medicine*, Sections 3.2 and 3.4)

- Exclude other diagnoses that can be established quickly, eg arrhythmia or acute MI with definitive ECG changes.

General supportive measures will be required by all patients, in particular rapid restoration of intravascular volume in those who are volume depleted (low JVP and postural hypotension when lying and sitting, as standing will clearly not be possible).

Specific management depends on the diagnosis.

- PE: the two major treatment options for massive PE with haemodynamic collapse are thrombolysis and surgical embolectomy (see Section 2.18).

- Arrhythmia (see Section 2.2).

- Complications of MI (see Section 2.1).

- Tamponade: urgent pericardiocentesis (see Section 2.6.2).

- Asthma (see *Acute Medicine*, Section 1.2.9 and *Respiratory Medicine*, Section 2.2.2).

- Intra-abdominal catastrophe: call for surgical help immediately. Resuscitate the patient while considering surgery – do not say you will resuscitate the patient and then call the surgeons.

- Anaphylaxis (see *Acute Medicine*, Section 1.2.33 and *Rheumatology and Clinical Immunology*, Section 1.4.2).

Also, if you do not know the diagnosis, give broad-spectrum antibiotics to cover sepsis (see *Infectious Diseases*, Section 1.3.2).

Arrange for the patient to be transferred to an appropriate high-dependency area for continuing management (high-dependency unit, critical care unit or intensive treatment unit).

Further comments

Communication

After making your clinical assessment, performing immediate investigations and initiating management, you will need to speak to the patient's husband to explain the situation.

1.4.6 Pleuritic chest pain

Scenario

A 50-year-old woman gives a 1-day history of left-sided pleuritic chest pain and progressive breathlessness on minimal exertion. Routine observations reveal her temperature is 37.9°C, pulse 80 bpm, BP 130/80 mmHg and respiratory rate 18/minute. You are asked to see her in the Medical Assessment Unit.

Introduction

The differential diagnosis of the patient presenting with pleuritic pain is shown in Table 17. The two most important acute diagnoses to consider in this case are obviously pulmonary embolism (PE) and pneumonia, although pneumothorax

TABLE 17 DIFFERENTIAL DIAGNOSIS OF PLEURITIC CHEST PAIN

Frequency	Cause
Common	PE Pneumothorax Pneumonia Musculoskeletal: rib fracture, costochondritis, Bornholm myalgia (Coxsackie B virus, self-limiting), non-specific
Less common	Autoimmune/rheumatic disease Pericarditis Neoplasia: primary or secondary Herpes zoster ('shingles', difficult to diagnose before the rash)

PE, pulmonary embolism.

also needs to be considered. A CXR will easily exclude a pneumothorax and infection if the infective process is advanced to have formed pulmonary changes. However, the diagnosis of PE, be it an early infection or an atypical infection, that does not result in typical radiographic changes may be difficult.

Beware of the following in a patient with pleuritic chest pain.

- A low-grade fever (<38°C) does not necessarily indicate infection; it can be associated with inflammation of any cause, including pulmonary infarction.
- Pneumonia may present in a variety of ways and sputum production is not generally an early feature.
- Rib fracture tends to be associated with a clearly memorable episode of trauma and is therefore not usually a diagnostic difficulty, but remember the possibility of pathological fracture.

History of presenting problem
Bear in mind the diagnoses listed in Table 17 when taking the history. Which is most likely?

Description of the pain

- Character: it is important to ensure that the pain is definitely pleuritic, ie sharp, localised and exacerbated by deep inspiration and coughing.

- Onset: was it sudden and associated with coughing or straining (this would indicate pneumothorax or PE), or gradual? Did it follow a 'flu-like illness (suggesting pneumonia or Bornholm myalgia) or an incident of chest trauma (suggesting a pneumothorax or rib fracture)?

- Position: it is important to identify the location of pain and any radiation.

Associated clinical features

- Dyspnoea: when did this occur in relation to the pain? A sudden onset of pain and breathlessness together supports PE (although different timing does not exclude it). How severe is the breathlessness (occurs at rest/patient cannot walk/patient cannot hurry)?

- Cough: a non-specific symptom, but production of purulent sputum indicates likely infection and haemoptysis is a feature of PE, pneumonia and (exceedingly unlikely in this case) malignancy.

- Fever: sweats, rigors and temperature >38.5°C would suggest pneumonia. It could also be a feature of autoimmune disease (although unlikely in this case).

- Unilateral leg pain, swelling or tenderness: all of these are suggestive of venous thrombosis and strongly support the diagnosis of PE in this clinical context.

Other relevant history
Have there been similar previous episodes? This is always a good question to ask – the patient may tell you the diagnosis! Enquire specifically about previous history of pneumothorax, PE or deep venous thrombosis and autoimmune/rheumatic disease.

Pursue other risk factors for PE, such as recent immobility, surgery, travel, dehydration, smoking and a family history of PE, and deep venous thrombosis or hypercoagulable states. In a woman, ask about pregnancy or use of the oral contraceptive/hormone-replacement therapy.

Also consider risk factors for pneumothorax (chronic respiratory disease, recent flights or diving) and for pneumonia (exposure to others with the condition and travel, which is especially relevant for atypical pneumonias such as *Legionella*).

Examination

General features
The first priority is always to establish how unwell the patient is.

- Is she breathless at rest?

- Does she look cyanosed? Check pulse oximetry.

- Can she speak easily?

- Check peripheral perfusion and confirm pulse, BP, respiratory rate and temperature.

In this case the routine observations do not indicate that the patient is severely compromised, although she clearly has significant symptoms: examination can therefore be completed before a decision regarding investigation. In patients who appear very unwell with cardiorespiratory compromise, history-taking, examination, investigations and treatment would all begin concurrently (see Section 1.4.5).

Note any of the following.

- Habitus: tall thin 'marfanoid' young men have an increased risk of spontaneous pneumothorax.

- Labial herpes: this is often seen in pneumonia.

- Signs of autoimmune or rheumatic disease, eg joint deformity in rheumatoid arthritis or butterfly rash in systemic lupus erythematosus.

Cardiovascular system
Note particularly the following.

- Pulse: rate and rhythm. Tachycardia would be expected in a patient such as this and is non-specific. Atrial fibrillation can occur secondary to PE or pneumonia, but is once again non-specific.

- Signs of right ventricular dysfunction, such as elevated JVP, left parasternal heave, loud P2 and pansystolic murmur of tricuspid regurgitation. Any or all of these would support the diagnosis of a large PE, but a patient presenting with a small peripheral PE causing lung infarction and pleurisy (as perhaps in this case) would not be expected to have any of these findings.

- Heart sounds: is there a pericardial rub?

- Calf swelling and tenderness: measure both sides. A difference of >2 cm may indicate venous thrombosis and would strongly support the diagnosis of PE in this clinical context. However, an absence of swelling does not rule out a PE.

Respiratory and other systems

Thoracic wall tenderness or rib crepitus Exquisite local tenderness clearly suggests a musculoskeletal cause, but there can be local tenderness with pleurisy. Rib crepitus proves that a rib has been broken.

Expansion, percussion and auscultation of the chest Is there a pleural rub? This can be very localised. Ask the patient to point to the place that hurts most and listen here and just around it. In pneumothorax expansion may be reduced, the percussion note may be hyperresonant and breath sounds may be diminished on the affected side. However, with a small pneumothorax examination may be normal. If there is consolidation

secondary to an infection, percussion will be dull and localised course crackles and/or bronchial breathing may be heard.

If you suspect a PE, examine the abdomen for masses and organomegaly, along with the breasts in a woman or the testes in a man.

> To hear a pleural rub, ask the patient to point to the place that hurts most and listen here and just around it – you may miss it if you do not take care to do this.

Investigation

The most important investigations in making the diagnosis will be imaging of the chest. Look at the CXR carefully for the features listed in Table 18.

ECG

Look for arrhythmia, right ventricular strain and pericarditis (see Section 3.1). Remember that the ECG is most likely to be normal in someone with PE, and also that pain and fear are the most common causes of sinus tachycardia in a

patient presenting to hospital (sinus tachycardia will be the most likely finding in this case).

Blood tests

FBC, electrolytes, renal and liver function tests and a clotting screen would be routine in all cases with this presentation. Blood cultures, atypical respiratory serology screen, inflammatory markers and tests for autoimmune rheumatic disease may all be indicated in some patients. Note that measurement of D-dimers is not an appropriate investigation in this situation: the clinical probability of PE is high and clinical decision-making will (or should) not be affected by the result since imaging to exclude PE will be required.

> - Do not measure D-dimers if the clinical probability of PE is high: definitive imaging is required whatever the result might be.
> - Do measure D-dimers if the clinical probability of PE is low. Patients can be reassured that they are extremely unlikely to have had a blood clot in their lungs if the result is normal, and further imaging is not required.

TABLE 18 SIGNS TO LOOK FOR ON THE CXR IN THE PATIENT WITH PLEURITIC CHEST PAIN

Radiological sign	Comment
Pneumothorax	Look very carefully at the lung apex and bases. Is there an area within the chest that does not have any lung markings? Can you see a line indicating the edge of the lung? Are you absolutely sure?
Lobar oligaemia	A rare sign, but suggesting large PE
Pleural effusion	This may be small and visible only as blunting of the costophrenic angle. This would be consistent with the diagnosis of PE or pneumonia
Wedge-shaped peripheral infarcts	Typical of PE (but rare)
Consolidation	Typical of pneumonia
Ribs and bony structures	Look carefully at anterior and posterior aspects of ribs for fracture lines and more obvious displacement

PE, pulmonary embolism.

Arterial blood gases

If the patient is unwell or pulse oximetry indicates oxygen saturation <95%, check arterial blood gases. Some would recommend that this be performed for all patients presenting with pleuritic chest pain. Typical findings in cases of PE where the patient presents with pleurisy are normal Po_2 (but there may be hypoxia) and reduced Pco_2, both as a result of hyperventilation.

Sputum

If present, sputum should be sent for microscopy, culture and sensitivity, and also for cytology and acid-fast bacilli (indicating tuberculosis) if the clinical picture is appropriate.

Other imaging

If a confident diagnosis cannot be made to explain the pleuritic pain and breathlessness, then ventilation–perfusion lung scanning (see Section 3.9) or pulmonary CT angiography (see Section 3.8) is required.

Management

> If the probable diagnosis is PE, then give anticoagulation (low-molecular-weight heparin) immediately while you are waiting for confirmatory investigations.

This depends on the specific diagnosis.

- PE (see Section 2.18; see also *Acute Medicine*, Section 1.2.10 and *Haematology*, Section 3.6).

- Pneumothorax (see *Acute Medicine*, Sections 1.2.14 and 3.5; and *Respiratory Medicine*, Sections 3.2 and 3.4).

- Pneumonia (see *Acute Medicine*, Section 1.2.11; *Infectious Diseases*, Section 1.3.4 and *Respiratory Medicine*, Section 1.4.1).

- Musculoskeletal pain: analgesia and reassurance. Particularly in the case of rib fracture, adequate analgesia is essential to allow the patient to inspire fully and avoid hypostatic pneumonia. Local intercostal nerve blocks can be very effective.

- Pericarditis (see Section 2.6).

> If you diagnose a PE for which there is no obvious cause (eg postoperative), perform rectal (and, in a woman, pelvic) examination and consider pelvic ultrasonography to exclude masses causing deep venous thrombosis by compression.

1.4.7 Fever, weight loss and a murmur

Scenario

A 26-year-old man with a previous history of intravenous drug abuse presents with a 6-week history of recurrent sweats and weight loss. He comes to the Emergency Department because he is feeling increasingly unwell. On examination he is tachycardic and has a swollen, hot and tender left knee joint and a faint pansystolic murmur at the left sternal edge. You are called to assess him.

Introduction

Possible causes of this presentation are shown in Table 19. However, in the presence of a murmur, whether new or not, the diagnosis of infective endocarditis (IE) must be the favoured differential diagnosis. This remains the case even though the patient is, according to the scenario, no longer using intravenous drugs

and may be septic from a primary infection of his knee joint. A careful history and examination are essential to help rule out other non-infective and non-cardiac causes for his symptoms, although these would clearly be very unlikely in this case.

History of the presenting problem

The history (and examination) will be dominated by consideration of the most likely diagnosis (IE), but clues may emerge that take you in another direction. Bear the diagnoses listed in Table 19 in mind as you take the history and examine the patient.

Gauge the severity of the patient's debilitation. In acute IE, the fever is high with rigors and prostration. Ask 'Have you had attacks of really bad shivering and shaking? Have you sweated so much that you had to change your clothes or the sheets on the bed?' The current history is more suggestive of a subacute presentation, which is associated with a low-grade fever, malaise and weight loss.

It is clearly critical to explore whether the patient has been injecting drugs at any point over the past 2–3 months, emphasising the point that even a single episode may be enough to result in a very dangerous infection. Also enquire about dental procedures or medical investigations (particularly if invasive), which are other well-recognised risk factors for endocarditis.

Ask the patient about symptoms of heart failure: has he been breathless when walking, at rest or lying flat in bed at night? Have his ankles become swollen? These signs may be insidious. If present they raise the possibility of haemodynamic compromise from aortic or mitral regurgitation. Sudden episodes

TABLE 19 **DIFFERENTIAL DIAGNOSIS OF FEVER AND WEIGHT LOSS OF 6 WEEKS' DURATION**

Category	Common example	In presence of a murmur
Infective	Infective endocarditis Tuberculosis Liver abscess Primary joint infection/osteomyelitis Soft-tissue infection Rheumatic fever (very unlikely in UK)	Infective endocarditis is the most likely
Autoimmune disorders and/or vasculitis	SLE Rheumatoid arthritis Polymyalgia rheumatica Potentially any other vasculitic condition	SLE (also some other rheumatic disorders) can affect the heart valves and cause substantial diagnostic difficulty
Malignancy	Lymphoma Hypernephroma	Atrial myxoma possible, but extremely rare. Marantic endocarditis is possible

SLE, systemic lupus erythematosus.

of pulmonary oedema may be suggestive of significant valve degeneration.

Ask about chest pain and haemoptysis: myocardial infarction is rare in endocarditis, but can arise from coronary artery embolism. Pleuritic chest pain and/or haemoptysis would suggest pulmonary abscess or infarction, commonly from tricuspid valve endocarditis. In this patient, where tricuspid endocarditis is a real possibility, there might be mycotic pulmonary emboli from the right side of the heart. Remember that pulmonary tuberculosis (TB) and (much less likely in this case) other lung pathologies such as malignancies can also present with haemoptysis.

Other relevant history

Endocarditis has a very wide range of extracardiac manifestations (see Section 2.8), and hence many other aspects of the history could be relevant. For instance, the swollen knee joint could be secondary to infective seeding from bacteraemia or the result of a mycotic embolus from the heart (in the latter, the infection would have to affect a left-sided cardiac valve). Ask about systemic manifestations of the other conditions listed in Table 19, especially autoimmune disorders, TB and (in this case because of the knee problem) joint/bone infections.

The following can be seen with both IE as well as autoimmune disorders:

- skin rashes;
- changes in the nails;
- blood in the urine;
- back or abdominal pain;
- changes in vision;
- sudden periods of arm or leg weakness;
- episodes of difficulty speaking.

Although uncommon, vasculitic rashes can occur with IE, but they are not specific and may occur with several of the differential diagnoses.

Also rare, but much more suggestive, are transient changes in the hands and feet: painful lesions in the finger or toe pulps (Osler's nodes) or painless ones in the palms or soles (Janeway's spots or lesions).

The glomerulonephritis that may accompany IE or autoimmune conditions often results in microscopic haematuria, which goes unnoticed by the patient, although macroscopic haematuria (a symptom that can also be caused by renal infarction or hypernephroma) is also possible.

Back pain may simply result from myalgia, but severe loin pain suggests renal infarction, abscess or tumour, although the latter is not normally painful. Similarly, pain in the left hypochondrium radiating to the left shoulder may result from splenic infarction or abscess.

Regarding other infective causes, ask the patient the following questions.

- Have you had a cough? Does this produce any phlegm or blood?
- Have you travelled abroad recently?
- Have you ever had TB? Have you been in contact with anyone who has TB?
- Have you had any injuries to your knee?
- Did your cough or knee injury start before or after your sweats and temperature?
- Have you had any swollen glands? Have you had any problems with the blood or the lymph glands in the past?
- Have you had arthritis?
- Have you had any odd illnesses in the past?

Concerning past history, also ask the following.

- Has anyone ever told you that you have a 'mumur' or 'hole' in your heart?

- Have you had rheumatic fever?

- Have you had any antibiotics recently? Are you absolutely sure about that? (A common reason for negative blood cultures in endocarditis is partial treatment with antibiotics, which render the blood cultures sterile but do not cure the condition.)

Examination

General features

Just as the history may be relatively non-specific, the examination findings may also be so. As always, get an overall impression. Patients with IE are likely to look unwell, although elderly patients presenting atypically may simply be confused.

General points must include the following.

- Temperature: a fever of <39°C is typical of endocarditis, although higher is occasionally seen.

- Pallor and anaemia: these can suggest chronic disease.

- Look at the hands, feet, skin, conjunctiva and mucous membranes for splinters/vasculitic manifestations of endocarditis.

🔑 Examination of the patient with chronic fever, malaise and weight loss

- How does the patient look?
- A thorough examination of all systems is essential.
- Look carefully for skin rashes and nail changes.
- Look carefully for signs of embolic phenomena.
- Is there lymphadenopathy?
- Is there evidence of significant valvular regurgitation?
- Can you feel the patient's spleen?

Cardiovascular

Take particular note of the following.

- Peripheral perfusion.

- Pulse: check rate (often tachycardic as in this case), rhythm and character ('collapsing' pulse in significant aortic regurgitation).

- JVP: this may be elevated if there is tricuspid valve regurgitation (often seen in right heart infective endocarditis) and/or heart failure.

- Apex: will be hyperdynamic in sepsis and if displaced is suggestive of long-standing heart disease.

- Heart sounds: are there any murmurs or added sounds? The pansystolic murmur could be tricuspid or mitral regurgitation, but take care to listen carefully for aortic and/or pulmonary incompetence. Be aware that a difficult murmur/funny sound could (extremely rarely) be a 'tumour plop'.

Other systems

Check specifically for the following.

- Lymphadenopathy: this is not a feature of endocarditis and would point towards another infective cause or a lymphoproliferative condition.

- Chest: are there any signs at all? Consider TB but remember, as stated previously, that right heart IE may give rise to pulmonary mycotic emboli.

- Abdomen: can you feel the spleen? The splenic tip or a mildly enlarged spleen can be felt in endocarditis, but a moderately or grossly enlarged spleen would favour lymphoma as the diagnosis. Is the liver palpable or

tender (consider liver abscess), and can you feel a renal mass (hypernephroma)?

- Neurological: are there any focal signs? These are likely to have been caused by emboli from an infected valve in this clinical situation.

- Fundi: is there any evidence of endocarditic lesions (see Section 2.8)?

Investigations

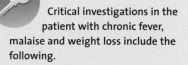 **🔑 Critical investigations in the patient with chronic fever, malaise and weight loss include the following.**

- Blood cultures: at least three taken 1 hour apart from separate well-cleaned sites.
- FBC, erythrocyte sedimentation rate (ESR) and C-reactive protein (CRP): is there evidence of systemic inflammation?
- Urine: look for haematuria and proteinuria, which suggest glomerulonephritis (autoimmune, vasculitic or endocarditic).
- Chest radiograph: look for TB, lung abscess or lymphadenopathy.
- Echocardiography: check for evidence of endocarditis.

The following are the key investigations in the patient with chronic fever, malaise and weight loss.

Blood cultures

These are the single most important investigation and should be carried out as soon as possible. Three or more blood samples should be taken from separate sites at different times, ideally over 24 hours. Seriously ill patients thought to have endocarditis should have samples taken over 1–2 hours and then be given antibiotics.

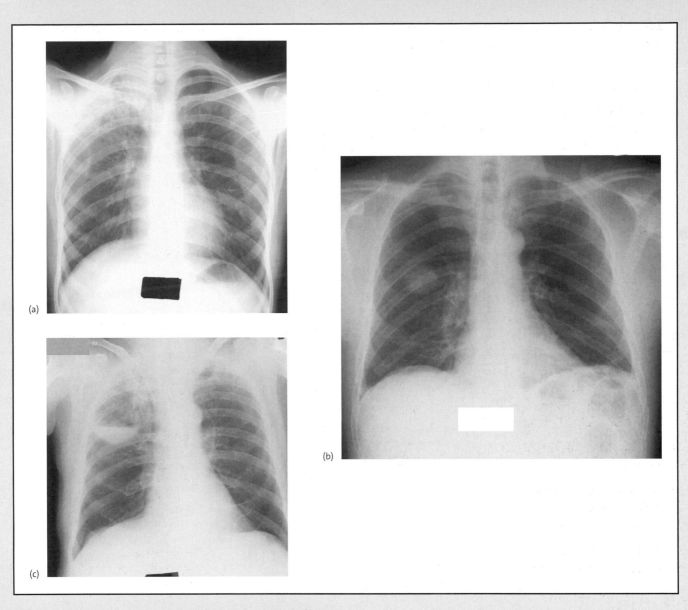

▲ **Fig. 29** Chest radiographs demonstrating (**a**) TB, (**b**) lung tumour and (**c**) abscess.

Other blood tests

FBC, inflammatory markers (ESR and CRP), electrolytes, and renal, liver and bone function in all cases. A range of further studies, in particular serological tests for other infective conditions or autoimmune disease, may be indicated if there are appropriate clues from the history or examination.

Urine

Use dipsticks to detect haematuria and proteinuria in all cases, microscopy to look for casts (indicating renal inflammation), and culture and sensitivity if dipsticks show abnormality.

ECG

Look particularly for evidence of conduction disturbance (consider aortic root abscess in this context) and atrial fibrillation.

Chest radiograph

Look for pulmonary oedema, heart contour, pulmonary abscess, pneumonia, mediastinal lymphadenopathy or (unlikely here) lung tumour (Fig. 29).

Echocardiography

This is crucial for the detection of vegetations (or cardiac tumours) and the assessment of valvular regurgitation and paravalvular abscesses. Transoesophageal echocardiography may be needed (Fig. 30) if good views cannot be obtained on transthoracic echocardiography. This is

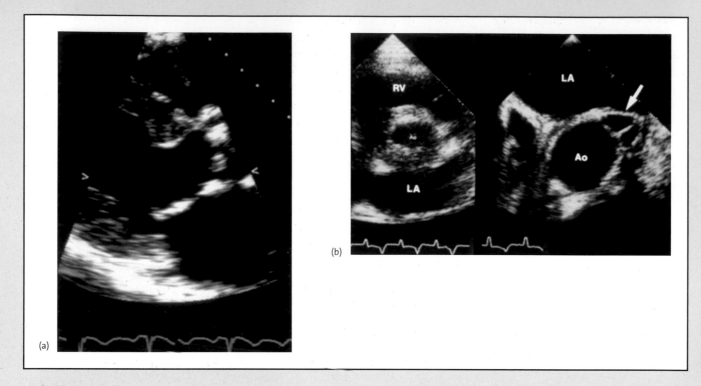

▲ **Fig. 30** (a) Aortic vegetation and (b) para-aortic abscess (arrow). Ao, aorta; LA, left atrium; RV, right ventricle. (Courtesy of Dr J. Chambers.)

particularly relevant if the patient has prosthetic heart valves or the clinical suspicion for endocarditis is high even if transthoracic echocardiography is completely normal.

Management

This depends on the specific diagnosis.

- IE: see Section 2.8.1.

- Left atrial myxoma: see Section 2.9.

- See *Infectious Diseases, Haematology, Oncology,* and *Rheumatology and Clinical Immunology* modules for further information on the many diseases that can present with fever and which are differential diagnoses of IE.

1.4.8 Chest pain following a 'flu-like illness

Scenario

A 25-year-old woman presents to the Emergency Department complaining of a 4-day history of chest pain. She has been unwell with 'flu for the last week. You are asked to review the patient.

Introduction

The history immediately suggests an acute viral pericarditis. This is usually a mild and self-limiting condition, so the greatest danger arises from failure to recognise more serious pathology that presents in a similar manner (Table 20). You must initially decide whether the pain is caused by pericarditis, excluding other causes of chest pain along the way. If you decide it is, then you

TABLE 20 DIFFERENTIAL DIAGNOSIS OF PERICARDITIC CHEST PAIN

Comment	Diagnosis
Common	Acute pericarditis Musculoskeletal Oesophagitis
Must consider	Pneumonia Pulmonary embolism Autoimmune rheumatic disease
Do not completely forget	Myocardial ischaemia Aortic dissection

need to be aware of the more serious underlying causes of pericarditis and must not immediately assume viral aetiology.

As there is overlap between the symptoms of pericardial and pleural inflammation, you will need to consider pulmonary pathologies, particularly pneumonia and pulmonary embolism (PE). Remember that serositis is also a feature of some autoimmune rheumatic diseases, such as systemic lupus erythematosus and rheumatoid arthritis.

Both myocardial infarction and aortic dissection would be extremely unlikely in this patient, but because of their potentially fatal consequences they should always be considered, even if only briefly and to dismiss them, in any patient presenting with chest pain.

History of the presenting problem

Get as much information about the pain as possible. Ask the patient 'Show me where you feel it? What is it like? Does it go anywhere else?' If a clear description of the pain is not forthcoming, offer suggestions such as 'like a knife' or 'raw', both of which suggest pericarditic pain, or 'like a heavy weight' or 'squeezing', which do not. The pain of pericarditis is usually located retrosternally, and like angina it may radiate to the neck or shoulders.

Ask specifically about the following.

- Did the pain start suddenly?

- Do you have pain all the time?

- If not, when do you get it?

- Does it hurt when you breathe in?

- When you sit forward, does the pain change?

- Is the pain affected by lying down?

Pericarditic pain is usually continuous, but does not typically have a sudden onset, unlike PE. It is exacerbated by inspiration, movement and lying supine, and is typically eased by sitting forward. Aside from movement itself, there is no relationship with exertion, unlike angina.

Other symptoms

This woman has had 'flu-like symptoms recently, but ask any patient presenting with chest pain the following questions.

- Have you been feeling 'under the weather' or feverish recently?

- Do you feel breathless?

- Have you coughed up any phlegm? If so, what colour was it and did it contain any blood?

- Have you had any joint pains?

- Do you ever get an acid taste at the back of your mouth?

Although painful breathing may cause dyspnoea in pericarditis, prominent respiratory symptoms are clearly more in keeping with pulmonary pathology. Haemoptysis would suggest PE. The presence of arthralgia may simply reflect the associated viraemia, but could also be due to autoimmune rheumatic disease. Acid reflux suggests oesophagitis, as would a history of indigestion.

When taking a history from a young patient at low risk of ischaemic heart disease who presents with chest pain, look for the following patterns.

- Pericarditis: indicated by a continuous sharp or raw retrosternal discomfort, which is worse on lying down and relieved by sitting forwards. This is often accompanied by a history of a 'flu-like illness.

- Musculoskeletal pain: history of unaccustomed activity with chest wall tenderness.
- Oesophagitis: suggested by dyspeptic symptoms, particularly belching and reflux, and is worse at night.
- Pneumonia: fever (sometimes rigors), breathlessness, malaise and (sometimes) pleuritic pain; also a painful cough that is dry initially, but later productive of sputum.
- PE: sudden onset of pleuritic pain with breathlessness and haemoptysis.
- Myocardial infarction or aortic dissection: however unlikely you consider these to be in a young patient, think of them if the symptoms are 'ischaemic' or 'tearing' in nature.

Other relevant history

You will obviously ask whether there have been any similar episodes in the past and, if so, what diagnosis (if any) was made. This woman is very likely to have a viral pericarditis, but ask about other conditions that could be associated with acute pericarditis:

- rheumatoid arthritis and other autoimmune rheumatic disease;

- renal failure;

- hypothyroidism;

- rheumatic fever;

- tuberculosis (TB) and contact with TB;

- malignancy, eg breast;

- chest radiotherapy.

Examination

General features

As always, form an overall impression first. A patient with uncomplicated pericarditis is unlikely to look very unwell: he or she may be in pain, which may be severe, and is likely to be sitting forward rather than lying supine.

If the patient with suspected pericarditis is unwell, then you should assess immediately for evidence of tamponade, PE or pneumonia, which may be life-threatening.

In all cases check temperature (pyrexia indicates an inflammatory cause of pain), examine the sputum pot (haemoptysis suggests PE) and ask 'Does it hurt when I press on the chest where the pain is?' This would clearly suggest a local musculoskeletal cause, but remember that there can be tenderness in pleurisy.

Cardiovascular system

Perform a full cardiovascular assessment, taking particular note of the following.

- Peripheral perfusion: is this impaired? It should not be in uncomplicated pericarditis.

- Pulse: check rate, rhythm and character.

- BP: a significant (>10 mmHg) fall on inspiration (pulsus paradoxus) indicates cardiac tamponade.

- JVP: should be normal in uncomplicated pericarditis. Gross elevation could be due to cardiac tamponade or PE.

- Heart sounds: a pericardial rub would clinch the diagnosis.

Respiratory and other systems

- Look for chest signs suggestive of pneumonia or PE.

- Is the patient euthyroid?

- Are there any signs of malignancy, eg breast?

- Is there evidence of autoimmune rheumatic disorder, eg joint inflammation or deformity, or a rash?

When examining a young patient at low risk of ischaemic heart disease who presents with chest pain, look specifically for the following.

- Pericarditis: is there a pericardial rub? Look for an underlying aetiology.
- Is there evidence of cardiac tamponade? Look for poor peripheral perfusion, elevated venous pressure and tachycardia with a small-volume pulse exhibiting pulsus paradoxus (BP falls significantly on inspiration). This is an emergency and requires pericardiocentesis.
- Musculoskeletal pain: pain that is well localised and reproduced by local pressure on the chest wall.
- Pneumonia: fever with signs of focal lung consolidation. Listen for a pleural rub.
- PE: is there haemoptysis in the sputum pot? Listen for a pleural rub. Are there signs of pulmonary hypertension? (See Sections 2.12.1.)

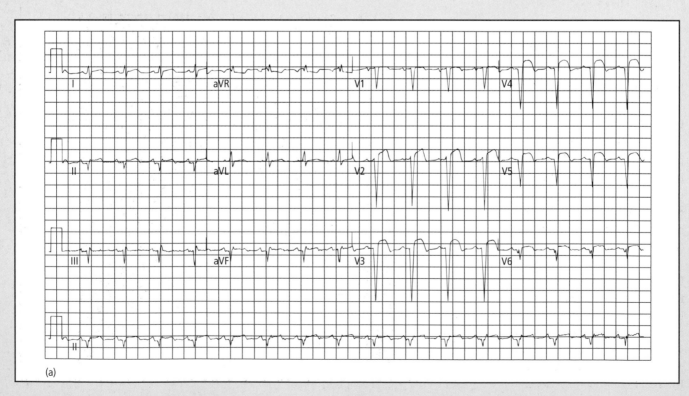

▲**Fig. 31** ECGs of (a) anterior myocardial infarction.

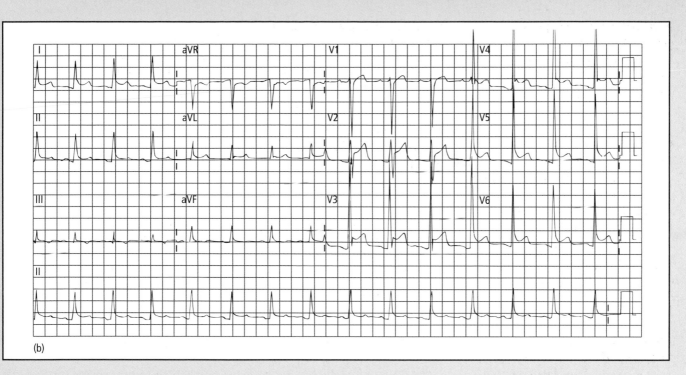

(b)

▲ **Fig. 31** ECGs of (**b**) acute pericarditis, where widespread ST-segment elevation, concave upwards, is seen.

- Aortic dissection: a rank outsider. However, does the woman look as though she may have Marfan's syndrome? Can you feel the left radial pulse? Is the BP the same in both arms? (See Section 2.11.1.)

Investigations

ECG

Along with chest pain and pericardial rub, the changes in the ECG encountered in acute pericarditis form a triad of characteristic findings that can establish the diagnosis (Fig. 31).

Blood tests

FBC, electrolytes, renal and liver function, thyroid function, inflammatory markers (erythrocyte sedimentation rate and C-reactive protein) and cardiac enzymes. If clinically indicated, check blood cultures and serology for evidence of autoimmune rheumatic disorders (see *Rheumatology and Clinical Immunology*, Section 3.2). Checking 'viral titres' is not generally useful.

Chest radiograph

Look for cardiomegaly, suggesting an effusion, and for any areas of consolidation or pleural effusion (Fig. 32).

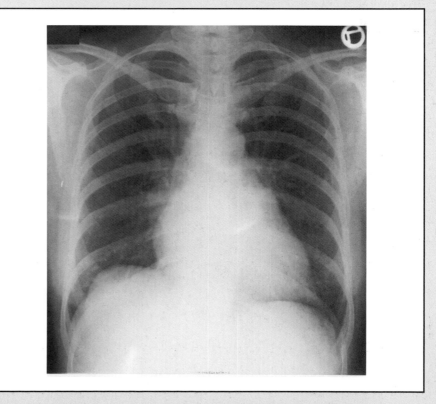

▲ **Fig. 32** Cardiomegaly. Note the increased cardiothoracic ratio in this posteroanterior film.

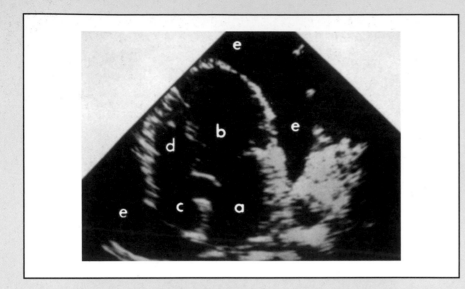

▲ **Fig. 33** Large pericardial effusion: the heart is surrounded by an echo-free space (e) formed by the effusion. a, left atrium; b, left ventricle; c, right atrium; d, right ventricle. (Courtesy of Dr J. Chambers.)

Echocardiography

An echocardiogram that reveals a small amount of pericardial fluid can be very helpful in making the diagnosis of pericarditis, but the absence of pericardial fluid does not exclude this diagnosis. This investigation is mandatory, and urgent if the cardiac shadow is enlarged and you suspect cardiac tamponade (Fig. 33).

Other tests

Ventilation–perfusion scanning should be performed if clinically indicated.

Management

Management depends on the specific diagnosis. Uncomplicated viral pericarditis is a self-limiting illness. If patients are reasonably well, they should be reassured that they have not had a heart attack and can be discharged home with simple analgesia, NSAIDs often being particularly effective. Follow-up in a few weeks' time should be organised to ensure that the symptoms have settled. Admission is warranted if the pain is severe, if there is evidence of a large pericardial effusion or tamponade (a medical emergency) or if treatment of an underlying aetiology is indicated.

2.1 Coronary artery disease

Coronary artery disease (CAD) is the cause of two of every 10 deaths in the UK, accounting for 114,000 deaths in the UK in 2005. In the UK 260,000 people have a myocardial infarction every year.

2.1.1 Stable angina

Aetiology/pathophysiology/pathology

Atheromatous plaques in the coronary arteries reduce blood flow. The myocardial oxygen supply cannot meet the demand, resulting in myocardial ischaemia and chest pain (angina pectoris).

Epidemiology

The prevalence of angina in the UK is estimated as 3% of the population, ie 2,000,000 individuals.

Clinical presentation

Common

- Predictable exertional central chest tightness.

- Worse in cold weather and after meals.

- May radiate to jaw or the left arm.

- Pain resolves with rest.

Uncommon

- Exertional dyspnoea (angina equivalent). This is more common in females.

Physical signs

Examinations are often normal, but watch for signs of aortic stenosis and anaemia, and check the peripheral pulses and BP.

Investigations

Figure 34 shows an investigation algorithm.

- Resting ECG: this is often normal and does not exclude coronary disease.

- Exercise ECG: this may show exercise-induced ischaemic changes, confirming the diagnosis and giving objective evidence of exercise capacity and prognosis (see Section 3.1.1).

- Stress imaging includes myocardial nuclear perfusion, stress echocardiography and magnetic resonance stress imaging. This may be used in patients unable to exercise or who have bundle branch block (see Section 3.11).

- Cardiac catheterisation (see Section 3.12).

- Blood tests: FBC and fasting lipids.

Patients who have chest pain without diagnostic ECG changes during exercise testing may have important coronary disease. It is important to stratify patients by their presentation and risk

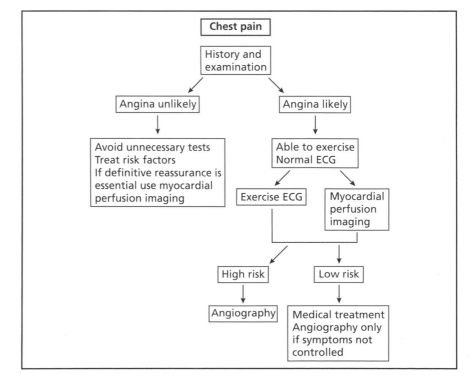

▲ **Fig. 34** Algorithm for patients presenting with suspected stable angina.

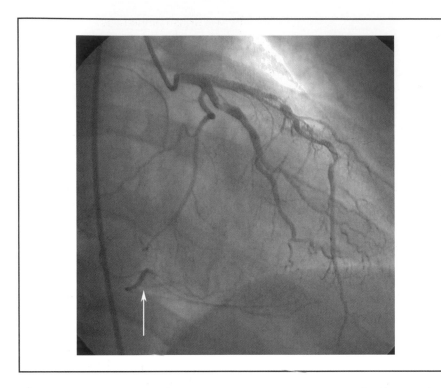

▲ **Fig. 35** Left coronary arteriogram demonstrating major stenosis in two major vessels with retrograde filling of a blocked right coronary artery (arrow) via collaterals. This patient has three-vessel coronary disease.

factors into low- and high-risk groups. Patients at high risk of CAD with exertional chest pain but without diagnostic ischaemic changes should proceed to diagnostic cardiac catheterisation (Fig. 35). Those at low risk of ischaemic heart disease should undergo stress imaging to search for ischaemia. If these investigations demonstrate ischaemia, then cardiac catheterisation should be considered.

Treatment

Lifestyle advice
Encourage regular exercise. Prophylactic sublingual glyceryl trinitrate (GTN) administered before exertion may be helpful. Stress the importance of stopping smoking.

Medical therapy
First-line therapy is with aspirin, GTN spray, beta-blockers and a statin. Angiotensin-converting enzyme inhibitors should be prescribed to patients with normal left ventricular function and ischaemic heart disease.

Revascularisation
There are two methods of revascularisation: coronary artery bypass grafting (CABG) and percutaneous coronary intervention (PCI) involving angioplasty and stenting. Currently, the evidence is that CABG confers prognostic advantage in certain groups, with diabetics showing a particular improvement in:

- left main-stem stenosis (>50%);
- proximal left anterior descending stenosis (>70%);
- three-vessel disease, especially with impaired left ventricular function.

PCI is carried out more commonly than CABG, and is currently indicated for symptomatic stenoses of >70%. At present an improvement in life expectancy has not been demonstrated, but trials are ongoing. Patients who are unfit for CABG may be considered for PCI. See Fig. 36 for an investigation algorithm.

Prognosis
Generally, stable CAD confers a good prognosis. Cardiac catheterisation of patients identified to be at high risk by non-invasive stress testing will identify those with prognostically important disease.

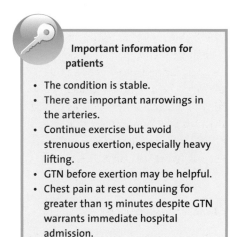

Important information for patients

- The condition is stable.
- There are important narrowings in the arteries.
- Continue exercise but avoid strenuous exertion, especially heavy lifting.
- GTN before exertion may be helpful.
- Chest pain at rest continuing for greater than 15 minutes despite GTN warrants immediate hospital admission.

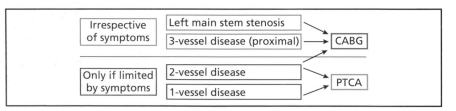

▲ **Fig. 36** Algorithm for interventional treatment of coronary artery disease. PTCA, percutaneous coronary angioplasty.

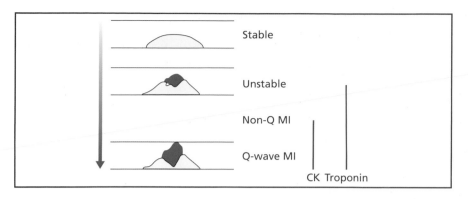

▲ Fig. 37 Schematic diagram illustrating the sequence of events within a coronary artery during an acute coronary syndrome. Fissuring or erosion of an atherosclerotic plaque (yellow) leads to thrombosis (red), a rapid reduction in coronary blood flow and myocardial infarction. Sustained occlusion of the coronary artery leads to Q-wave (transmural) infarction. Highly sensitive troponin assays can detect microembolic heart muscle damage, enabling identification of those at higher risk of further infarction. CK, creatine kinase.

2.1.2 Unstable angina and non-ST-elevation myocardial infarction

Aetiology/pathophysiology/ pathology

An atheromatous plaque within a coronary artery reduces the blood flow to such an extent that there is ischaemia at rest (unstable angina). The plaque may fissure or erode exposing the dense lipid core. The lipid is very thrombogenic, causing platelets to clump on it. If the thrombus is not sufficient to occlude the artery, it reduces blood flow downstream and pieces of the thrombus may break off and pass downstream to lodge in small end vessels, causing non-ST-elevation myocardial infarction (Fig. 37).

Clinical presentation

- Rapid onset of central chest pain at rest, unrelieved by glyceryl trinitrate (GTN).

- Pain may escalate, and occur with increasing frequency and severity (crescendo angina).

- Pain may radiate to jaw and arm.

- Severe breathlessness may reflect pulmonary oedema due to transient impairment of left ventricular function.

Physical signs

Often there are no abnormalities on examination, but other causes of chest pain may be excluded.

Investigation

- ECG: often normal, but look for ST-segment changes and T-wave inversion. T-wave inversion alone has no prognostic significance.

- Cardiac biomarkers (see Section 3.7).

- Cardiac catheterisation (Fig. 38) (see Section 3.12).

Differential diagnosis

After excluding ST-segment elevation myocardial infarction, other diagnoses should be considered. These are the same as the differential diagnoses for ST-segment elevation myocardial infarction.

Treatment

The aim of treatment is to limit myocardial damage by 'pacifying' the vulnerable plaque with medication. Patients who fall into high-risk groups undergo cardiac catheterisation.

Emergency

- Aspirin, sublingual GTN followed by an infusion, beta-blocker, low-molecular-weight heparin

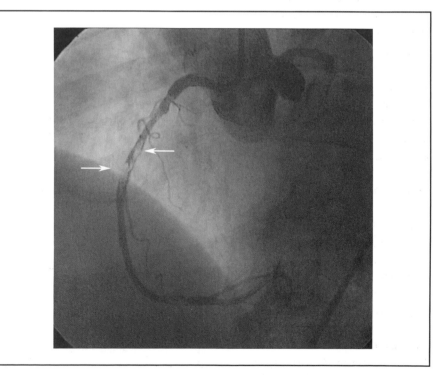

▲ Fig. 38 Right coronary angiogram in a patient with non-ST-elevation myocardial infarction. There is extensive thrombus present, seen as filling defects within the lumen (arrows).

and a statin. Chronic obstructive pulmonary disease and peripheral vascular disease are not contraindications to beta-blockers, and these groups benefit greatly from cardioselective beta-blockers.

- Clopidogrel (with an initial loading dose).

- Glycoprotein IIb/IIIa antagonists are recommended for patients with unstable symptoms and a positive troponin assay.

In-hospital management

Continue antianginals and antithrombotics. Patients who do not have elevated troponin are diagnosed with unstable angina and do not require urgent cardiac catheterisation unless they fall into a high-risk group (see below). Cardiac catheterisation with a view to revascularisation is indicated in high-risk groups:

- positive troponin assay;

- ongoing ischaemic pain;

- ST-segment changes with pain;

- recurrent unstable angina;

- ventricular arrhythmias.

Long-term treatment

Patients admitted with unstable angina are treated medically, and if the pain settles they are assessed in the same way as patients with stable angina. Medications should be continued, and if the troponin is positive clopidogrel is continued for 1 year.

Complications

Common

- Recurrent angina.

- Myocardial infarction.

Uncommon

- Pulmonary oedema.

- Ventricular arrhythmias.

Prognosis

The risk of death or non-fatal myocardial infarction is 7% at 6 months with appropriate revascularisation of high-risk cases.

2.1.3 ST-elevation myocardial infarction

Aetiology/pathophysiology/pathology

Rupture of an atheromatous plaque exposes the rich lipid core to the circulating platelets and fibrin, which forms thrombus, occluding the artery. Occlusion will lead to full-thickness muscle necrosis. Transient occlusion leads to limited heart muscle death.

Epidemiology

- Approximately 300,000 myocardial infarctions occur every year in the UK.

- One-quarter of patients do not reach hospital.

- Death rates are declining.

Clinical presentation

Common

- Rapid onset, severe and crushing central chest pain radiating to the jaw/left arm that is unrelieved by glyceryl trinitrate (GTN) or oxygen.

- Acute breathlessness (pulmonary oedema).

- Cardiac arrest (ventricular fibrillation).

Uncommon

- Epigastric, arm or back pain.

- Collapse.

- Vomiting and sweating without pain.

- Painless infarct (diabetics and the elderly).

Physical signs

Common

Examination may be normal. Patients are pale, sweaty and often appear to be in pain. The patient may be hypotensive or hypertensive. Listen for pulmonary oedema.

Uncommon

Epigastric tenderness.

Investigations

- ECG: ST-segment elevation and new onset left bundle-branch block are indications for reperfusion treatment (Fig. 39).

- Biochemical markers (see Section 3.7).

- Cholesterol (level may drop after 24 hours for up to 3 months).

- Echocardiogram: indicated in cardiogenic shock.

Differential diagnosis

- Unstable angina/non-ST-elevation myocardial infarction.

- Thoracic aortic dissection.

- Musculoskeletal pain.

- Pain of gastric/oesophageal origin.

Treatment

Emergency

It is vital to start reperfusion treatment as soon as possible, either with thrombolysis or primary percutaneous coronary intervention (PPCI).

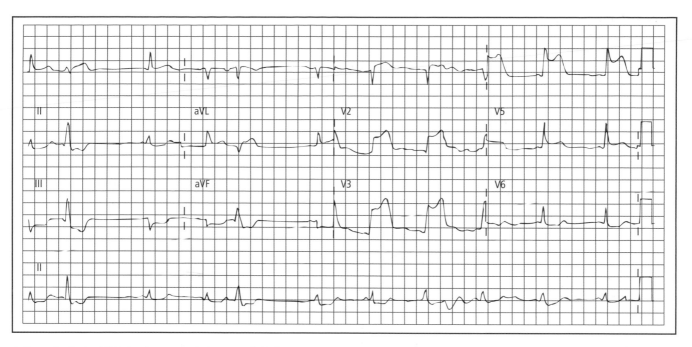

▲ **Fig. 39** Twelve-lead ECG showing acute anterior myocardial infarction.

Indications for thrombolysis

• ST-segment elevation >1 mm in the standard leads, >2 mm in the chest leads or new bundle branch block.
• Typical chest pain within 12 hours of onset.
• Bundle branch block: if there are no old ECGs and there is a good history for a myocardial infarction, then the patient should be thrombolysed.

Indications for PPCI

• ST-segment elevation >1 mm in the standard leads, >2 mm in the chest leads or new bundle branch block.
• Typical chest pain within 24 hours of onset.
• In the presence of cardiogenic shock, PPCI is more effective than thrombolysis.

• Take history whilst obtaining intravenous access.

• Simultaneous recording of ECG and observations by nursing staff.

• Oxygen, opiate analgesia and antiemetic.

• Aspirin 300 mg if no contraindications.

• Clopidogrel 600 mg.

• Once ST-segment elevation myocardial infarction (STEMI) is confirmed on ECG, quickly examine the patient and ensure there are no contraindications to thrombolysis/angiography and antiplatelet therapy.

• Transfer to coronary care unit after reperfusion initiated.

• Intravenous insulin for diabetics, or where blood glucose >11 mmol/L.

See Fig. 40.

Contraindications to thrombolysis

Consultant advice should be sought before deciding not to reperfuse a patient with STEMI, and PPCI should be considered. Prolonged resuscitation is not a contraindication unless there is obvious trauma. Oral consent to thrombolysis should be obtained from the patient, and the risk of haemorrhagic stroke should be explained. The following are considered contraindications to thrombolysis:

• active internal bleeding;
• active peptic ulcer;
• uncontrolled bleeding tendency;
• stroke in the last 6–12 months or any previous haemorrhagic stroke (obtain neurosurgical advice in the case of clipped subarachnoid haemorrhage aneurysm);
• aortic dissection;
• uncontrolled BP >180/110 mmHg (treat with intravenous GTN, then thrombolyse);
• major trauma or surgery within the past year.

Ninety minutes after thrombolysis the ECG should be recorded. If the ST segments do not show greater than 50% resolution, then rescue percutaneous coronary intervention may be appropriate. Obtain consultant advice.

Patients who present within 2 hours of pain have similar outcomes with both treatments. Thereafter, morbidity and mortality are lower with PPCI compared with thrombolysis. Patients in cardiogenic shock are best treated by PPCI and may have an intra-aortic balloon pump inserted.

Short term
Standard treatment should include the following.

- Beta-blocker: taken orally within 24 hours and continued indefinitely.

- An angiotensin-converting enzyme (ACE) inhibitor is of particular benefit in patients with left ventricular (LV) impairment, but improves the prognosis of all patients.

- Statin: for all patients unless contraindicated.

- Sliding insulin scale for patients with blood sugar >11 mmol/L or known diabetics.

- Warfarin: indicated for patients with atrial fibrillation, severe LV dysfunction due to risk of LV thrombus, or who exhibit presence of LV thrombus (Fig. 41).

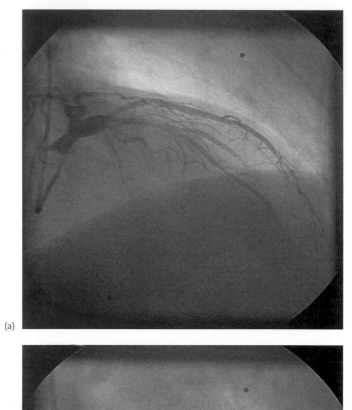

(a)

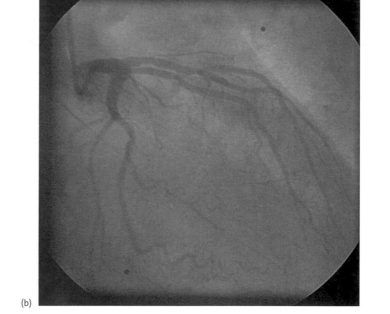

(b)

▲ **Fig. 40** Left coronary arteriogram showing a severe stenosis in the left anterior descending artery. **(a)** This patient had a prolonged ventricular fibrillation arrest due to an anterior myocardial infarct that was initially thrombolysed. **(b)** The stenosis has been stented.

- Clopidogrel: given for up to 30 days after thrombolysis, or for up to 12 months after PPCI.

- Cardiac catheterisation and revascularisation is recommended for all patients within 24 hours of STEMI. Definite indications include recurrent pain, reinfarction or small biomarker rises suggesting little damage from the infarct.

Long term
Continued secondary prevention is important. Glucose tolerance testing should be considered as a high proportion of patients have diabetes mellitus (30% of these

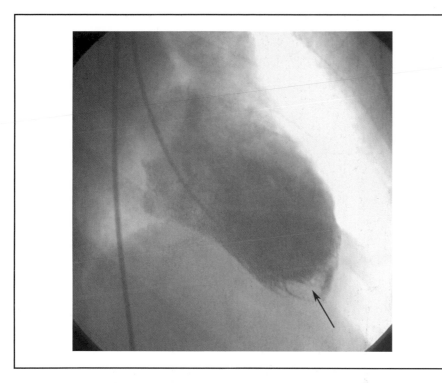

▲ **Fig. 41** Left ventriculogram showing apical mural thrombus (arrow) after anterior myocardial infarction.

patients are missed when fasting glucose alone is tested).

Complications

Common

- Haemorrhage induced by thrombolysis: transfuse as required.

- Haemorrhage from arterial puncture site: apply direct pressure, transfuse as required.

- Ventricular fibrillation/tachycardia: cardiovert promptly.

- Atrial fibrillation.

- Complete heart block.

- Pulmonary oedema.

- Cardiogenic shock: seek expert advice.

- Post-infarct unstable angina.

- Reinfarction.

- Post-infarct pericarditis: usually benign and responds to NSAIDs; echocardiogram is needed to exclude contained rupture.

- Stroke: urgent CT of head required.

- Deep vein thrombosis/pulmonary embolus.

Uncommon

- LV rupture (Fig. 42).

- Ventricular septal defect.

- Severe mitral regurgitation from papillary muscle rupture or ischaemia.

- Dressler's syndrome: fever, pleuropericarditis, anaemia, raised erythrocyte sedimentation rate, usually 1–4 weeks after infarct.

Prognosis

This is determined by LV function, comorbidity and whether the patient has been revascularised. Stress testing identifies patients with ischaemic myocardium who require cardiac catheterisation and revascularisation. Patients with poor LV function undergo repeat echocardiography at 6 weeks to see if remodelling has occurred. Of patients suffering a STEMI:

- 25% treated conservatively develop unstable angina;

- 10% treated conservatively have a further infarct;

- 25% with a first myocardial infarction do not reach hospital alive;

- 10% die before discharge;

- 10% die in the year after discharge.

Prevention

Primary
Prevention involves regular exercise, a healthy diet and stopping smoking.

Secondary

- Aspirin, beta-blocker, ACE inhibitor, statin and clopidogrel.

- Patients with poor LV function (ejection fraction <35%) undergo repeat echocardiography at 6 weeks to see if remodelling has occurred. If LV function remains poor, an implantable cardioverter defibrillator may be indicated (see Section 3.4.2).

- Patients with poor LV function may be treated with spironolactone or eplerenone if creatinine <180 μmmol/L.

Advice to patients

On admission:

- Inform the patient that he or she is having a heart attack and that effective treatment is available.
- Advise that the risk of treatment is less than the risk of the heart attack.
- Caution that the main risk is of bleeding, and that thrombolysis carries the risk of stroke.

On discharge:

- A good recovery is expected.
- Cardiac rehabilitation: patients are seen prior to discharge by the

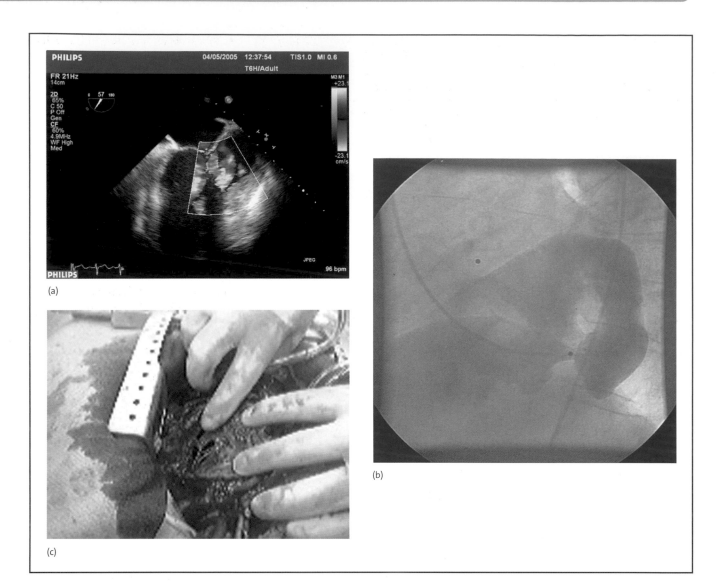

▲ **Fig. 42** Rupture of the inferior–posterior wall of the left ventricle (LV) after an acute myocardial infarction. (**a**) Transoesophageal echocardiogram showing flow through the defect in the LV wall. (**b**) Left ventriculogram: a pigtail catheter has been passed through the defect, outlining the LV, the defect and the pericardium. (**c**) LV at operation showing the hole on the inferior–posterior surface of the ventricle.

specialist nurses, an exercise programme is arranged and support to help them stop smoking is offered. Car drivers must cease driving for 4 weeks, and heavy goods drivers must inform the DVLA (Driver and Vehicle Licensing Agency) in the UK and must satisfy requirements prior to relicensing (see Section 2.19).

- The usual advice regarding fitness for sexual activity is that the patient should be able to climb one flight of stairs prior to intercourse.
- Smoking cessation is vital: it reduces risk of reinfarction by 50%.
- Always carry GTN, even if free of angina.

FURTHER READING

Hobbs FDR. Cardiovascular disease: different strategies for primary and secondary prevention. *Heart* 2004; 90: 1217–23.

– – – – – – – – – – – – – – – – –

Fox KAA. Management of acute coronary syndromes: an update. *Heart* 2004; 90: 698–706.

– – – – – – – – – – – – – – – – –

De Jaegere PP, Serruys PW and Simoons ML. Should all patients with an acute myocardial infarction be referred for direct PTCA? *Heart* 2004; 90: 1352–7.

– – – – – – – – – – – – – – – – –

Kristensen SD, Andersen HR, Thuesen L, *et al. Heart* 2004; 90: 1358–63.

2.2 Cardiac arrhythmia

2.2.1 Bradycardia

Aetiology

Virtually any condition that has a pathophysiological effect on the heart might affect normal electrophysiological properties and thus cause bradycardias. The more common conditions are listed in Table 21.

TABLE 21 POSSIBLE CAUSES OF BRADYCARDIA

Sinoatrial disease	Atrioventricular block
Ischaemic heart disease	Ischaemic heart disease
Idiopathic fibrosis	Aortic stenosis
Infective	Cardiomyopathy
Pericardial disease	Infection
Post radiotherapy	Sarcoidosis
Post cardiac surgery	Congenital
Trauma	Connective tissue disease
Antiarrhythmic drugs	Antiarrhythmic drugs
Amyloidosis	Post radiotherapy
	Post cardiac surgery
	Trauma
	Hypothermia

Pathology/pathophysiology

Sinoatrial dysfunction

- Abnormality of neurohormonal input to sinoatrial (SA) node, eg sympathetic/parasympathetic.

- Abnormality of SA node leading to slow or failed conduction to atrial tissue.

Atrioventricular block

- Abnormality in conduction through atrioventricular (AV) node.

- Failure to conduct rapidly throughout the ventricles.

Classification of bradycardias

Bradycardias can be divided clinically into SA dysfunction and AV block (Table 22).

Clinical presentation

Common

- Dizziness (presyncope).

- Syncope.

Uncommon

- Dyspnoea.

- Exertional fatigue.

- Heart failure.

Rare

Palpitations are unusual.

Physical signs

These include the following:

- slow regular/irregular pulse;

- cannon waves in complete heart block;

- beat-to-beat variation in intensity of first heart sound in complete heart block;

- hypotension;

- pulmonary oedema.

Consider using carotid sinus massage to provoke the bradycardia. Do not perform this in patients who have had a stroke or are known to have atherosclerotic carotid disease.

Investigations

In most cases the diagnosis will be made with one of the following:

- 12-lead ECG (see Section 3.1);

- Holter monitor (see Section 3.3);

- patient-activated device;

- tilt-table testing.

Treatment

Emergency/short term

In a patient with haemodynamic compromise consider the following:

- intravenous atropine;

- temporary pacing, either transvenous or transcutaneous (short-term measure).

Address any potential reversible causes of bradycardia:

- hypothyroidism;

- drugs (Fig. 43);

- hypothermia;

- electrolyte imbalance.

Long term

Consider whether permanent pacemaker implantation is appropriate (see Section 3.5).

TABLE 22 CLINICAL CLASSIFICATION OF BRADYCARDIAS

Sinoatrial dysfunction	Atrioventricular block
Sinus bradycardia	First degree
Vasovagal syndrome	Second degree: Mobitz I (Wenckebach's)
Carotid sinus hypersensitivity	Second degree: Mobitz II
Junctional rhythm	Third degree: complete

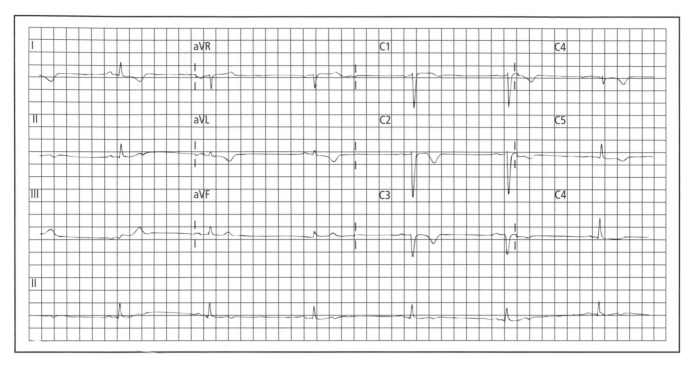

▲ **Fig. 43** Twelve-lead ECG of patient with ischaemic heart disease who presented with presyncope and was taking beta-blockers. Heart rate is <40/minute.

FURTHER READING

Zipes DP. Specific arrhythmias: diagnosis and treatment. In: Braumwald E, ed. *Heart Disease: A Textbook of Cardiovascular Medicine*, 6th edn. Philadelphia: WB Saunders; 2001: 815–90.

2.2.2 Tachycardia

For practical purposes it is easiest to divide tachyarrhythmias into:

- atrial tachycardia;

- atrial fibrillation/atrial flutter;

- atrioventricular nodal re-entry tachycardia (AVNRT) and atrioventricular re-entry tachycardia (AVRT);

- ventricular tachycardia (VT).

Aetiology/epidemiology

Atrial tachycardia

Atrial tachycardia is caused by an ectopic source of atrial tissue firing in a rhythmical manner faster than the sinus node. It is a rare cause of tachycardia. On an ECG it may look similar to sinus tachycardia but with abnormal P-wave morphology.

Atrial fibrillation/flutter

Atrial fibrillation affects 0.4% of the whole population, rising to 2–4% in people over 60 years old and >11% in those over 75 years old. Its causes are numerous:

- hypertension;

- ischemic heart disease;

- congestive heart failure;

- valvular heart disease;

- thyroid dysfunction;

- pulmonary abnormalities, eg pulmonary embolism;

- pericardial disease.

AVNRT/AVRT

These are the result of the presence of an additional conducting pathway, allowing a re-entry mechanism. In most cases, the electrical impulse is conducted antegradely (atrium to ventricle) via the atrioventricular (AV) node and retrogradely through the accessory pathway (concealed accessory pathway). If conduction is in an antegrade direction through the pathway (eg Wolff–Parkinson–White syndrome), pre-excitation is seen on the surface ECG.

Ventricular tachycardias

Almost any pathological process affecting the ventricles may predispose to VT:

- myocardial infarction (acute/chronic);

- dilated cardiomyopathy;

- hypertrophic cardiomyopathy;

- valvular heart disease (especially aortic stenosis and mitral prolapse);

- hypertension;

- congenital heart disease;

- long QT syndrome;

- cardiac tumours.

TABLE 23 CLINICAL FEATURES DISTINGUISHING ATRIAL FIBRILLATION FROM ATRIAL FLUTTER

	Atrial fibrillation	Atrial flutter
Pulse	Irregularly irregular	May be regular
JVP	Absence of *a* waves	Rapid flutter waves
First heart sound	Variation in intensity	Constant intensity

Pathophysiology/pathology

Tachyarrhythmias occur as a result of:

- abnormal automaticity, eg VT after myocardial infarction;

- triggered activity, eg VT with long QT syndrome;

- re-entry, eg atrial fibrillation, AVRT/AVNRT, VT, ventricular fibrillation.

Clinical presentation

Common

- Palpitations.

- Presyncope/syncope.

- Breathlessness.

- Chest pain.

Uncommon

Patients may complain only of lethargy.

Rare

Thromboembolism is unusual, except in atrial fibrillation.

Physical signs

Examination of sinus rhythm may be unremarkable. However, during tachycardia some physical signs may help to establish a diagnosis.

Atrial fibrillation/flutter

For the physical signs of atrial fibrillation/atrial flutter, see Table 23.

AVNRT/AVRT

Physical signs are not especially helpful in making the diagnosis:

- regular pulse;

- JVP may be raised, but waveform is normal;

- constant intensity of first heart sound.

Ventricular tachycardias

Patients may or may not be significantly compromised. Physical signs include:

- hypotension;

- cannon waves.

Investigations

Investigations aim to exclude a structural thoracic/cardiac or metabolic cause. Aside from an ECG, CXR, echocardiogram, thyroid function tests, renal function and electrolytes are appropriate in most cases.

Twelve-lead ECG

Documenting the arrhythmia with a 12-lead ECG will, in most cases, establish the diagnosis (see Section 3.1). In some cases where there is evidence of pre-excitation, the diagnosis can be relatively confidently made in sinus rhythm. Distinguishing some arrhythmias can be difficult.

- Atrial flutter versus atrial fibrillation: look for characteristic flutter waves (Figs 44 and 45).

- AVNRT versus AVRT: distinguishing these is rarely of clinical importance because, in most cases, management is similar (Fig. 46).

- VT versus AVNRT/AVRT with aberrant conduction (see Section 3.1).

Ambulatory monitoring

Documentation of an infrequent rhythm may be possible using 24-hour Holter monitoring or patient-activated devices (see Section 3.3).

Electrophysiological studies

See Section 3.2.

Treatment

There are many different classifications of antiarrhythmic agents. The Vaughan Williams classification is the most commonly used and is based on the cellular action of the drug (Table 24).

TABLE 24 VAUGHAN WILLIAMS CLASSIFICATION OF ANTIARRHYTHMIC DRUGS

Class	Action	Example
IA	Prolong action potential	Quinidine, procainamide, disopyramide
IB	Shorten action potential	Lidocaine, mexiletine
IC	Slow conduction	Propafenone
II	Block β-adrenergic receptors	Propranolol, atenolol, metoprolol
III	K^+ channel blockers, prolong repolarisation	Sotalol, amiodarone
IV	Block slow calcium channels	Verapamil, diltiazem, nifedipine

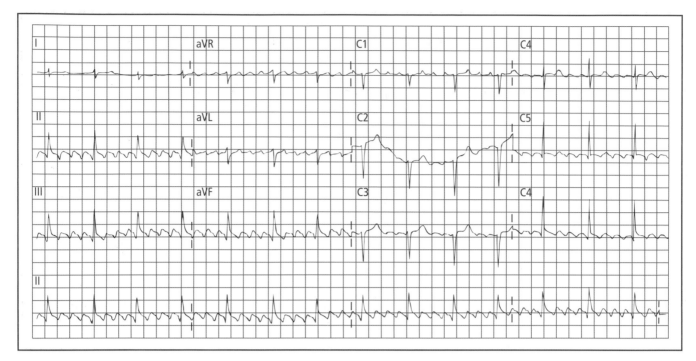

▲**Fig. 44** ECG of atrial flutter: note the characteristic saw-tooth appearance of the baseline.

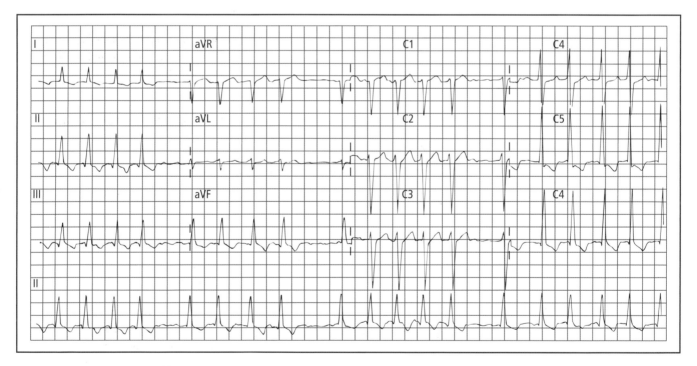

▲**Fig. 45** ECG of atrial fibrillation. Notice the 'chaotic' baseline in comparison with Fig. 44 and the complete irregularity of QRS complexes.

Emergency

Atrial tachycardia Most patients will not be compromised. DC cardioversion or intravenous amiodarone will restore sinus rhythm in the majority.

Atrial fibrillation/flutter If the patient is compromised, consider DC cardioversion or intravenous amiodarone.

AVNRT/AVRT Most will respond to intravenous adenosine.

Verapamil may be used if you are confident that the rhythm is not VT.

Ventricular tachycardias For resuscitation, see *Acute Medicine*, Section 1.2.1.

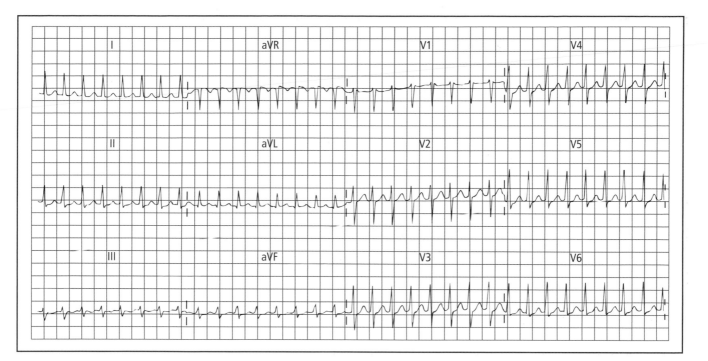

▲ **Fig. 46** ECG of AVNRT. Note the very rapid rate, regular rhythm and absence of discernible P waves.

Short term

Atrial tachycardia Consider the following:

- class I agent (if structurally normal heart and no coronary disease);
- beta-blocker;
- class III agent;
- calcium antagonist.

Atrial fibrillation/flutter The main aim of treatment is the restoration of sinus rhythm. This may be achieved pharmacologically or electrically with DC cardioversion. In all cases, the risk of thromboembolism and the requirement to anticoagulate should be considered. Consider the following:

- anticoagulation;
- DC cardioversion;
- class III agent;
- digoxin (rate control only);
- class I agent (if no coronary artery disease).

AVNRT/AVRT Consider the following:

- class IA and IC agents;
- class II (beta-blockers);
- class III (sotalol);
- class IV (verapamil).

Ventricular tachycardias Consider the following:

- class III agents;
- class I agents;
- class II agents;
- temporary pacing may prevent VT in patients with bradycardia-induced VT or long QT syndrome.

Long term

Most short-term drugs may be used long term, but more definitive therapies should be considered. Particular caution should be applied to commiting any patient to long-term use of amiodarone. Its side-effect profile is worse with chronic use.

Atrial tachycardia The focal origin of these arrhythmias makes them particularly suited to catheter ablation.

Atrial fibrillation/flutter Consider the following:

- anticoagulation;
- ablation for atrial flutter (see Section 3.4.1);
- ablation for paroxysmal atrial fibrillation (see Section 3.4.1);
- ablation of AV node and permanent pacemaker for atrial fibrillation not controlled with drugs (see Section 3.4.1).

AVNRT/AVRT Consider ablation (see Section 3.4.1).

Ventricular tachycardias Consider referral for ablation/implantable cardioverter defibrillator (see Section 3.4.2).

Complications

Atrial fibrillation/flutter
Thromboembolism is the most significant and devastating condition.

AVNRT/AVRT
Complications are uncommon, but with Wolff–Parkinson–White syndrome, rapid conduction of atrial fibrillation down an accessory pathway may precipitate ventricular fibrillation.

Ventricular tachycardias
Haemodynamic collapse and death is a potential risk in many cases of VT.

Prevention
Primary and secondary prevention of stroke/transient ischaemic attack (see *Neurology*, Sections 2.8.1 and 2.8.2).

FURTHER READING

Crystal E and Connolly SJ. Role of oral anticoagulation in management of atrial fibrillation. *Heart* 2004; 90: 813–17.

TABLE 25 CAUSES OF HEART FAILURE (APPROXIMATE RELATIVE FREQUENCY)	
Cause	**Relative frequency (%)**
Ischaemic heart disease	50
Valve disease	10
Hypertension	5
Dilated cardiomyopathy/unknown (see text)	35

2.3 Cardiac failure

Aetiology/pathophysiology/pathology
The common causes of heart failure are listed in Table 25.

Left ventricular (LV) systolic dysfunction is commonly associated with ventricular dilatation. Other causes include viral myocarditis, toxins (eg alcohol, cocaine and chemotherapeutic agents), metabolic abnormailites (eg thyroid disease and acromegaly) and inflammatory conditions (eg sarcoidosis and connective tissue disorders). In patients with idiopathic dilated cardiomyopathy, around 25% are thought to have a familial origin.

After a single episode of cardiac damage, eg a myocardial infarction (MI), LV dysfunction is often progressive even in the absence of further cardiac insults. This appears to result from the neurohumoral response to reduced cardiac output, which is initially compensatory but becomes detrimental in the long term (Fig. 47).

Epidemiology
The prevalence of heart failure is approximately 4 per 1,000 (28 per 1,000 in those aged over 65 years). Heart failure is the primary diagnosis in about 4% of general medical admissions to hospital. Increasing prevalence is the result of:

- an ageing population;
- better survival after MI;
- better survival with heart failure.

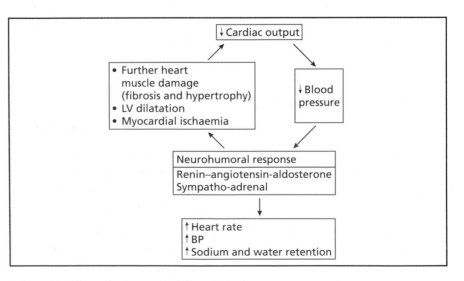

▲ **Fig. 47** The vicious cycle of progressive left ventricular damage.

Clinical presentation

Patients suffering from heart failure commonly present with the following:

- exertional breathlessness;
- fatigue;
- paroxysmal nocturnal dyspnoea;
- cough productive of clear frothy sputum;
- ankle swelling;
- orthopnoea.

> Severity of breathlessness in heart failure is graded according to the New York Heart Association (NYHA) classification.
>
> - NYHA class I: impaired LV function but asymptomatic on ordinary activity.
> - NYHA class II: symptoms resulting in slight limitation of ordinary activity.
> - NYHA class III: symptoms on minimal exertion, eg walking around the house.
> - NYHA class IV: symptoms present at rest.

Physical signs

The physical signs may include the following.

- Pulse: tachycardia or atrial fibrillation (AF).
- JVP: elevated. If it is up to angle of the jaw, then suspect tricuspid regurgitation (TR). Check for any systolic *v* waves that coincide with contralateral carotid; also check for pulsatile liver.
- Left parasternal heave (usually right ventricular hypertrophy, occasionally the result of greatly enlarged left atrium).
- Heart sounds: third heart sound (probably the most sensitive and specific physical sign for LV dysfunction, but has poor reproducibility). Pansystolic murmur of functional mitral regurgitation (other murmurs may be present and relate to aetiology).
- Basal lung crackles.
- Bilateral ankle oedema with or without ascites.

Investigations

ECG

A completely normal ECG is rare in heart failure. Look for:

- rhythm (eg AF);
- LV hypertrophy;
- previous MI;
- left bundle-branch block;
- left axis deviation.

Chest radiograph

In addition to excluding lung pathology, look for:

- heart size;
- pulmonary oedema;
- pleural effusions.

Blood tests

- Urea and electrolytes: associated hyponatraemia, hypokalaemia (diuretic treatment) and renal dysfunction.
- Liver function tests: often mildly deranged in chronic heart failure.
- Thyroid function tests (aetiology).
- Haemoglobin: mild anaemia common and associated with adverse outcomes. If present check haematinics.
- Brain natriuretic peptide (see Section 3.7): a normal value virtually excludes heart failure.

Echocardiography

Gold standard for diagnosis of heart failure; use for assessment of LV systolic function, filling pressures and valvular function (see Section 3.10).

Differential diagnosis

Consider the following:

- cor pulmonale;
- nephrotic syndrome;
- renal failure;
- liver failure.

Treatment

Emergency

In someone suffering from acute pulmonary oedema, carry out the following.

- Sit the patient up.
- Give oxygen (monitor blood gases).
- Give intravenous diamorphine (venodilator).
- Offload with intravenous infusion of nitrate titrated to maximum tolerated dose (but keep BP >90 mmHg systolic).
- Give intravenous furosemide in small aliquots (eg 40–80 mg).
- Check FBC, urea and electrolytes, and cardiac enzymes.
- Monitor clinical response including urine output (catheterise).
- Consider ventilatory support (continuous positive airway pressure or intubation) and/or inotropic support where appropriate.
- Invasive monitoring may be required if the patient gives a poor response (arterial line and central venous line, or pulmonary artery catheter).

Short term

Hospital treatment of decompensated chronic heart failure includes the following.

- Monitor fluid balance, daily weight (aim to lose 0.5–1 kg daily), and daily urea and electrolytes.

- No-added-salt diet.

- Intravenous loop diuretic, eg furosemide once or twice daily (dose will depend on prior exposure).

- Angiotensin-converting enzyme (ACE) inhibitor; angiotensin II receptor blocker can be used if ACE inhibitor not tolerated.

- Consider anticoagulation (AF and LV thrombus).

- Avoid calcium antagonists and NSAIDs.

If there is a good response, change to oral diuretics when approaching euvolaemia. Aim to continue hospital treatment until oedema is clearly improved and the patient is stable on oral therapy for 48 hours. In patients with impaired renal function it may be necessary to accept some residual oedema rather than precipitate acute-on-chronic renal failure. Do not use JVP as the sole guide for treatment because this is often persistently elevated as a result of TR.

If weight loss is not satisfactory on twice-daily furosemide, add a thiazide diuretic (bendroflumethiazide 2.5 mg or metolazone 2.5–5 mg daily) but watch renal function closely. If diuresis remains unsatisfactory, establish continuous intravenous furosemide infusion (eg 5–10 mg/hour). Fluid restriction should be held in reserve for resistant cases. Rarely, inotropes (dopamine or dobutamine) are required for a few days to assist diuresis.

Following discharge an early review is important to prevent re-decompensation. Check renal function and up-titrate medication.

Long term

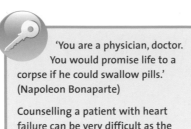

'You are a physician, doctor. You would promise life to a corpse if he could swallow pills.' (Napoleon Bonaparte)

Counselling a patient with heart failure can be very difficult as the prognosis is often poor. Yet education is key to enhancing patient compliance. It is important to judge each case individually and not give the patient unrealistic expectations.

Figure 48 shows long-term treatment options for those with heart failure. The following improve symptoms and life expectancy.

- ACE inhibitor for all patients, unless contraindicated (titrate to maximum tolerated dose).

- Beta-blocker, eg bisoprolol, carvedilol or nebivolol, in patients with stable NYHA II–IV

symptoms. Only start when clinically stable and euvolaemic: start low, go slow. Titrate to maximum tolerated dose. Hypotension may be avoided by reducing other drugs including diuretics where possible. If fluid retention occurs increase the loop diuretic. Try to continue the beta-blocker if at all possible, because side effects are usually transient.

- Candesartan (angiotensin receptor blocker) can be added in patients who remain symptomatic despite ACE inhibitors and beta-blockers.

- Spironolactone in patients with NYHA III–IV, creatinine <200 μmol/L and K^+ <5.5 mmol/L. Check electrolytes weekly for 2 weeks and stop spironolactone if K^+ <6.0 mmol/L.

- Digoxin does not prolong life, but improves symptoms and reduces hospital admissions in more severe cases of heart failure.

- Cardiac resynchronisation therapy (dual-chamber pacemaker with additional LV lead) may be considered in symptomatic

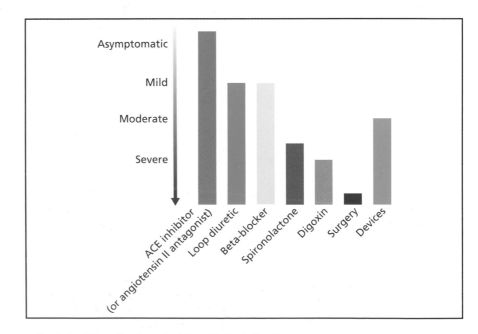

▲ **Fig. 48** Escalation of treatment for left ventricular dysfunction.

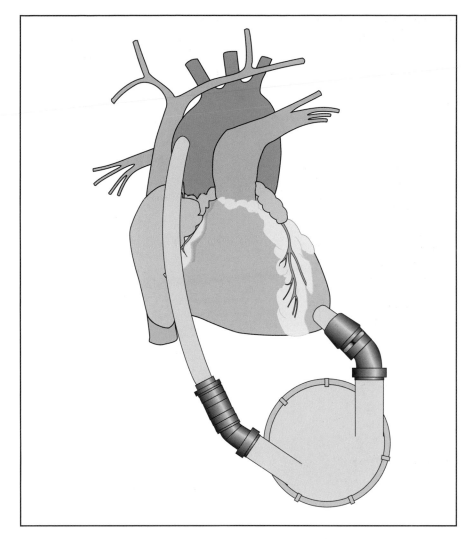

▲**Fig. 49** Left ventricular assist device.

patients with poor LV function and left bundle-branch block (see Section 3.4.3).

- Implantable cardioverter defibrillator (see Section 3.4.2) in selected patients.

Surgical intervention may be beneficial in carefully evaluated patients with valvular disease and those with ischaemic aetiology and ongoing angina. Cardiac transplantation (of which there are around 200 annually in the UK) is indicated for the following.

- Acute heart failure not responding to ventilation and inotropic support. A ventricular assist device (artificial heart) may

be used as a 'bridge to transplantation' if a suitable donor is not immediately available (Fig. 49). The function of the heart may improve (and transplantation avoided) when it is 'rested' by one of these devices. However, use of a ventricular assist device is frequently complicated by thromboembolism and infection.

- Chronic progressive heart failure in young patients with very poor prognosis and no comorbidity.

> '... it is infinitely better to transplant a heart than to bury it so it can be devoured by worms.' (Christiaan N. Barnard)

Complications

- AF.
- Ventricular tachycardia.
- Sudden death.
- Progressive heart failure.
- Renal impariment.

Prognosis

- Mortality related to ejection fraction and NYHA class.
- Chronic stable heart failure: overall annual mortality rate is 10%.
- Following hospitalisation, annual mortality rate is 30–50%.
- Mortality rate of NYHA IV is up to 60% in 1 year.

Prevention

Primary

- Prevention of MI (see Section 2.1).
- Prompt reperfusion therapy for acute MI.
- Avoid excess alcohol.

Secondary
ACE inhibitors, beta-blockers and spironolactone all reduce progression of heart failure and mortality.

> **Important information for patients**
>
> - Advise a no-added-salt diet.
> - Moderate alcohol intake.
> - Avoid heavy lifting (potentially arrhythmogenic).
> - May feel worse for a few days after starting beta-blocker, or if the dose is increased.
> - Must weigh themselves daily and report to their GP or increase dose of diuretic if they gain weight (>1–2 kg in 3 days or >2.5 kg in 2 weeks).
> - Education and monitoring ideally performed in conjunction with a specialist heart failure nurse.

FURTHER READING

Cowie MR and Zaphiriou A. Management of chronic heart failure. *BMJ* 2002; 325: 422–5.

Millane T, Jackson G, Gibbs CR, *et al.* ABC of heart failure: acute and chronic management strategies. *BMJ* 2000; 320: 559–62.

2.4 Diseases of heart muscle

2.4.1 Hypertrophic cardiomyopathy

Aetiology/pathophysiology/pathology

- Autosomal dominant.

- Mutations found in at least 10 genes (all encode contractile proteins, eg myosin β heavy chain and troponin T).

- Unexplained hypertrophy of the left (and occasionally the right) ventricle, which is usually focal, eg asymmetrical septal hypertrophy and apical hypertrophy.

- Mechanism of hypertrophy unknown: possibly secondary to impaired function of contractile proteins (ie a compensatory phenomenon).

- Degree of hypertrophy variable even between individuals with the same mutation.

- Left ventricular outflow tract obstruction may occur secondary to septal hypertrophy (Fig. 50).

- Mitral regurgitation may also be a feature, usually as a result of the Venturi effect in the presence of septal hypertrophy (Fig. 50).

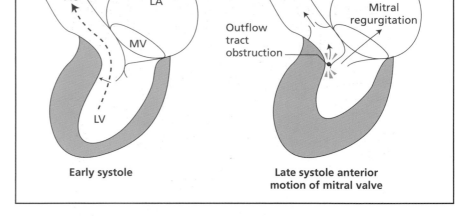

▲Fig. 50   Effect of asymmetrical septal hypertrophy in HCM. In late systole the septum contracts down on the outflow tract, obstructing flow and generating a gradient. This generates a negative pressure (Venturi effect) just proximal to the obstruction, sucking the mitral valve anteriorly (systolic anterior motion) and producing mitral regurgitation. AO, aorta; LA, left atrium; LV, left ventricle; MV, mitral valve.

Epidemiology

The prevalence of hypertrophic cardiomyopathy (HCM) is 1 in 500 and it is the most common single-gene cardiac disorder.

Clinical presentation

Common

- Exertional chest pain.

- Palpitations.

- Asymptomatic murmur.

- Abnormal ECG on screening.

Uncommon

- Syncope.

Rare

- Sudden death.

Physical signs

There may be no abnormal findings.

Common

- Jerky pulse.

- Prominent apical impulse.

- Systolic murmur at left lower sternal edge/apex.

Uncommon

- Fourth heart sound: often easier to feel (as a double apical impulse) than hear.

Investigations

The ECG and echocardiogram must be interpreted together because they provide complementary information.

ECG

The ECG is sensitive but not very specific. It varies from T-wave inversion to overt left ventricular hypertrophy (LVH).

Echocardiography

Echocardiography is specific but less sensitive than the ECG. Classically, there is asymmetrical septal hypertrophy with systolic anterior motion of the mitral valve leaflet, left ventricular outflow tract obstruction and secondary mitral regurgitation. Alternative patterns include apical, free wall or concentric LVH.

Ambulatory monitoring

This is used to identify the cause of palpitations or detect asymptomatic arrhythmia.

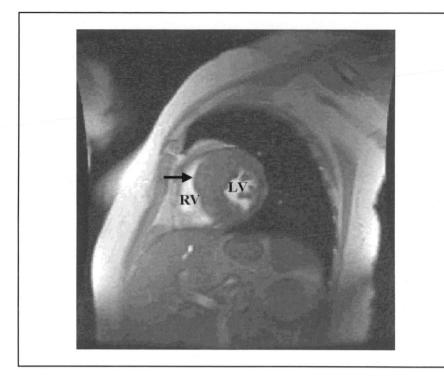

▲ **Fig. 51** MRI of the heart in short-axis view, showing asymmetrical hypertrophy of the interventricular septum in HCM (arrow). LV, left ventricular cavity; RV, right ventricular cavity.

Exercise ECG

This is used to provoke arrhythmia and assess the BP response (important for prognosis or for vocational driving licence).

Magnetic resonance imaging

MRI may confirm the diagnosis if echocardiographic images are not clear (Fig. 51).

 It is possible to have HCM without any hypertrophy. The diagnosis may be made on the family history plus an abnormal ECG.

Differential diagnosis

- Hypertensive cardiac hypertrophy: a concentric pattern of hypertrophy with documented hypertension.

- Athlete's heart: differentiation may be difficult because some highly trained athletes (especially weight-lifters, rowers and cyclists) have an identical pattern of physiological hypertrophy. However, this will regress if training is discontinued. A septal thickness >1.6 cm is likely to be pathological.

Treatment

No treatment is indicated in asymptomatic patients who do not have significant arrhythmia.

Antibiotic prophylaxis is generally recommended for dental and surgical procedures likely to produce a bacteraemia. Breathlessness and chest pain can be treated with beta-blockers or calcium antagonists, but often these only partially relieve symptoms. Severe breathlessness associated with a left ventricular outflow tract gradient may be treated in a number of non-medical ways.

- Surgical myectomy: partial excision of the hypertrophied

septum relieves gradient, but mortality rate is 1–2% at best.

- Percutaneous transluminal septal myocardial ablation is a promising new technique. A selected area of the obstructing septum is destroyed by alcohol injected into a carefully chosen septal artery (Fig. 52).

Complications

Common

- Atrial fibrillation: always anticoagulate because there is a high risk of thromboembolism. Atrial fibrillation is often poorly tolerated, so consider cardioversion along with antiarrhythmic drugs to maintain sinus rhythm. Note that digoxin is contraindicated if there is a significant left ventricular outflow tract gradient (>5 mmHg), so use a beta-blocker or calcium antagonist for rate control.

Uncommon

- Ventricular tachycardia (VT): sustained VT is associated with high risk of sudden death and requires an implantable cardioverter defibrillator (see Section 3.4.2).

- Progression to dilated cardiomyopathy: documented in up to 15% of early series, but certainly less common than this in modern practice.

- Sudden death.

Rare

- Endocarditis.

Prognosis

Risk of premature death is associated with the following:

- cardiac arrest or sustained VT;

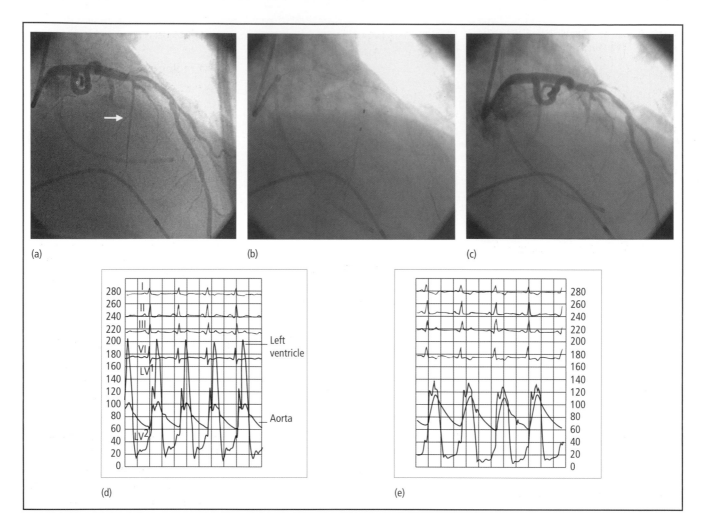

(a)   (b)   (c)

(d)   (e)

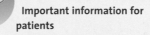 **Fig. 52** Septal ablation in hypertrophic obstructive cardiomyopathy. (**a**) A wire is passed through a coronary guide catheter into the target septal artery (arrow). A balloon catheter is passed, the wire is removed and the balloon inflated to occlude the artery. (**b**) Dye is injected into the lumen of the balloon catheter and into the distal septal artery to confirm correct positioning. (**c**) Absolute alcohol is then injected to destroy selectively the septal artery, leaving a stump. Simultaneous pressure recordings reveal a left ventricular outflow tract gradient (peak ventricular minus peak aortic pressure) of approximately 100 mmHg before the procedure (**d**), falling to 15 mmHg afterwards (**e**).

- syncope (especially when recurrent or associated with exertion);

- strong family history of sudden early death;

- diagnosis of HCM in childhood;

- VT on 24-hour ECG monitoring;

- BP drop on exercise;

- presence of certain high-risk mutations;

- extreme LVH (>3 cm).

Disease associations

Friedreich's ataxia and Wolff–Parkinson–White syndrome.

Important information for patients

- It is an inherited condition.
- There is a 50% chance of transmission to their children.
- It is benign in most cases, so reassure that it is low risk if appropriate.
- Continue as far as possible with a normal life, but avoid competitive physical sports.
- Seek medical advice in the event of palpitations, dizziness or blackouts.
- Carefully discuss before you begin screening: no treatment is indicated in the absence of symptoms and knowledge of the diagnosis will adversely affect life insurance, mortgages, etc.

Occupational aspects

Patients should not be professionals in sports requiring vigorous physical exertion. They may still hold vocational driving licences if they meet the DVLA (Driver and Vehicle Licensing Agency) criteria (see Section 2.19).

FURTHER READING

Frenneaux MP. Assessing the risk of sudden cardiac death in a patient with hypertrophic cardiomyopathy. *Heart* 2004; 90: 570–5.

- – – – – – – – – – – – – – – – – –

Maron BJ, Nishimura RA, Tajik AJ, *et al*. Efficacy of implantable cardioverter-defibrillators for the prevention of sudden death in patients with hypertrophic cardiomyopathy. *N. Engl. J. Med.* 2000; 342: 365–73.

Spirito P, Seidman CE, McKenna WJ, *et al*. The management of hypertrophic cardiomyopathy. *N. Engl. J. Med.* 1997; 336: 775–85.

2.4.2 Dilated cardiomyopathy

Aetiology/pathophysiology/pathology

This is a chronic progressive disorder of unknown aetiology, characterised by dilatation and systolic dysfunction of the left (and sometimes the right) ventricle. Some cases are probably the result of unrecognised alcohol abuse, 'burnt-out' hypertension or acute myocarditis. Familial dilated cardiomyopathy caused by mutations in cytoskeletal proteins has been described and is present in 35% of individuals with idiopathic cardiomyopathy. Dilated cardiomyopathy also complicates muscular dystrophy.

Clinical presentation

This condition presents with congestive cardiac failure or arrhythmia (atrial or ventricular).

Investigations

- ECG: often shows poor R-wave progression or left bundle-branch block.

- Echocardiography: dilated left ventricle with globally impaired contraction. Focal areas of hypokinesia suggest ischaemic damage or prior myocarditis.

- Cardiac catheterisation: ensures that there is no occult coronary disease and confirms diagnosis.

Treatment/prognosis

See Section 2.4.2.

FURTHER READING

Graham RM and Owens WA. Pathogenesis of inherited forms of dilated cardiomyopathy. *N. Engl. J. Med.* 1999; 341: 1759.

2.4.3 Restrictive cardiomyopathy

Aetiology/pathophysiology/pathology

This is a chronic progressive condition characterised by excessively rigid ventricular walls that impair ventricular filling (diastolic dysfunction). Contractile (systolic) function is preserved. Causes are divided into:

- myocardial, eg amyloid, sarcoid and storage diseases (often idiopathic);

- endomyocardial, eg endomyocardial fibrosis and hypereosinophilic syndrome.

Epidemiology

This condition is rare in Western countries. Endomyocardial fibrosis is common in the tropics, particularly in Africa.

Clinical presentation

Symptoms

- Breathlessness.

- Fatigue.

- Ankle swelling.

Signs

- Elevated JVP, which rises on inspiration (Kussmaul's sign).

- Third and/or fourth heart sound.

- Peripheral oedema.

- Ascites.

Investigations

Chest radiograph

The heart size may be normal or increased. Pericardial calcification suggests constrictive pericarditis rather than restrictive cardiomyopathy (see Sections 2.4.3 and 2.6.3).

Echocardiography

Ventricular cavities are usually not dilated, but atrial cavities are often greatly enlarged. Rapid ventricular filling may be seen at the onset of diastole, which stops abruptly in early diastole.

Cardiac catheterisation

May be diagnostic in restrictive cardiomyopathy. Rapid ventricular filling in early diastole produces a 'square root sign' appearance of the left ventricular diastolic pressure trace, which is also seen in pericardial constriction. However, other catheter data help differentiate the two conditions (Table 26).

Myocardial biopsy

Biopsy is sometimes useful to identify the cause of a restrictive cardiomyopathy.

Differential diagnosis

Restrictive cardiomyopathy must be distinguished from pericardial constriction, which is readily treated by surgery. Table 26 gives distinguishing features, but in up to 25% of patients it is not possible to differentiate the two conditions and in these circumstances exploratory surgery may be justified.

Treatment

The response of patients to medical treatment of heart failure is often poor. Successful combined heart and liver transplantation has been described in amyloid cardiomyopathy.

TABLE 26 FEATURES OF RESTRICTIVE CARDIOMYOPATHY AND PERICARDIAL CONSTRICTION

	Restrictive cardiomyopathy	Pericardial constriction
Third heart sound	Present	Absent
Pericardial calcification	Absent	In 50%
CT of the chest	Normal pericardium	Thickened pericardium
PA systolic pressure	Usually >50 mmHg	<50 mmHg
Diastolic pressure	LV > RV	LV = RV

LV, left ventricular; PA, pulmonary artery; RV, right ventricular.

Prognosis

The disease is generally relentlessly progressive with a high mortality.

FURTHER READING

Doughan AR and Williams BR. Cardiac sarcoidosis. *Heart* 2006; 92: 282–8.

Wynne J and Braunwald E. The cardiomyopathies and myocarditides. In Braunwald E, ed. *Heart Disease*. Philadelphia: WB Saunders, 2001: 1751–806.

2.4.4 Arrhythmogenic right ventricular cardiomyopathy

Aetiology/pathophysiology/pathology

Arrythmogenic right ventricular cardiomyopathy is a disease of primarily the right ventricular myocardium. It is characterised by myocyte death and replacement with fibro-fatty tissue. In some cases the left ventricle is also involved. Its aetiology is not known but 30–50% are thought to be familial (autosomal dominant) and recent studies have highlighted abnormalities in genes that code for cell adhesion molecules.

Clinical presentation

The condition usually presents with ventricular arrhythmias or sudden death and affects young adults. The ventricular arrhythmias arise from the right ventricle (commonly left bundle-branch block). In latter stages there may be progressive right ventricular dilatation leading to right heart failure and in some case biventricular failure.

Investigations

- ECG: may show ST abnormalities in the right precordial leads, although in some cases they may be normal.

- Echocardiography: often normal but may show dilatation of the right ventricle in some cases.

- MRI: best method of demonstrating fatty infiltration of the right ventricle.

- Electrophysiological studies: may induce ventricular arrhythmias (see Section 3.2).

Diagnosis is often difficult if the ECG and imaging are not conclusive. The main differential diagnosis is benign right outflow tract tachycardia, which can respond to beta-blockers.

Treatment

In the case of aborted cardiac death, the treatment is an implantable cardioverter defibrillator. Heart failure is treated in the usual way (see Section 2.3).

2.4.5 Left ventricular non-compaction

Aetiology/pathophysiology/pathology

This a recently described form of cardiomyopathy that is a result of persistence of the embryonic pattern of myocardial architecture. It is rare and has not been fully characterised. However, there are some associations with other inherited cardiomyopathies.

Clinical presentation

The most commmon presentation is in adulthood with signs and symptoms of congestive cardiac failure.

Investigations

Echocardiography can demonstrate a very trabeculated left ventricle.

Treatment/prognosis

See Section 2.3.

FURTHER READING

Hughes S and McKenna J. New insights into the pathology of inherited cardiomyopathy. *Heart* 2005; 91: 257–64.

2.5 Valvular heart disease

2.5.1 Aortic stenosis

Aetiology/pathophysiology/pathology

- Senile (calcific/degenerative): this is the most common form of aortic stenosis, especially in those aged over 65 years. Diabetes, hypercholesterolaemia and chronic renal failure are predisposing factors. Coexistent coronary artery disease is common.

- Congenital bicuspid valve: symptoms usually appear at the age of 40–50 years. There is a male predominance.

- Rheumatic heart disease: this is an unusual cause of aortic stenosis.

Stenosis results from a combination of fibrosis and calcification, with additional commissural fusion and reduced cusp separation. The increased left ventricular (LV) pressure load results in compensatory left ventricular hypertrophy (LVH) and diastolic dysfunction. Subendocardial ischaemia and fibrosis is common. Untreated, LV dilatation and failure will occur. There is an increased risk of ventricular arrhythmia. Atrial arrhythmias are usually poorly tolerated.

Clinical presentation

Common
Common symptoms are exertional angina, dyspnoea and syncope, and occasionally palpitations. There are symptoms of LV failure if presentation is late.

Uncommon

- Embolic phenomena from calcific emboli.

- Gastrointestinal bleeding (idiopathic/angiodysplasia).

- Infective endocarditis.

Physical signs
See Section 1.2.7.

Investigations

ECG
Look for LVH (85% of cases) and, rarely, conduction disturbance.

Chest radiograph
May be normal. Poststenotic aortic dilatation may be seen. Suspect aortic (or mitral) regurgitation or LV dilatation if cardiomegaly is present.

Echocardiography
Echocardiography determines whether the valve is tricuspid, bicuspid or rheumatic in appearance. The degree of valve thickening, leaflet mobility and calcification (Fig. 53) can be determined. Continuous-wave Doppler enables estimation of the pressure drop across the aortic valve and the aortic valve area (Table 27). LVH and LV dilatation with reduced systolic function will be seen with severe disease.

Coronary angiography
Coronary angiography will be required in most cases to assess the coronary arteries before surgery. The peak–peak withdrawal gradient across the aortic valve can also be determined.

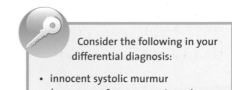

Consider the following in your differential diagnosis:

- innocent systolic murmur (pregnancy, fever, anaemia and thyrotoxicosis);
- aortic sclerosis;
- mitral regurgitation;
- hypertrophic obstructive cardiomyopathy;
- atrial or ventricular septal defect;
- pulmonary stenosis.

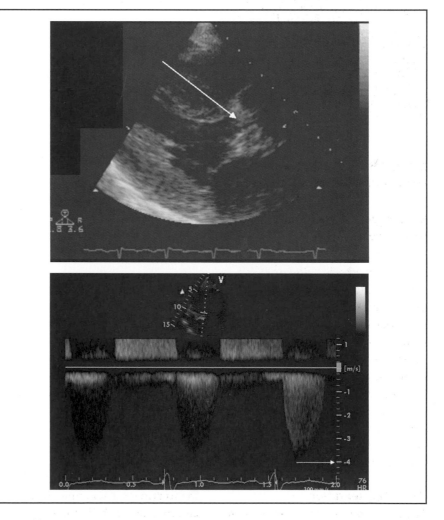

▲ **Fig. 53** (a) Calcific aortic stenosis. In this parasternal long-axis view, the aortic valve cusps (arrow) appear markedly thickened and calcified. Note the hypertrophy of the septum and posterior wall. (b) The peak velocity across the valve is 4 m/s. The calculated peak valve gradient is 64 mmHg.

TABLE 27 GRADING OF AORTIC STENOSIS BY AORTIC VALVE GRADIENT AND AREA

Aortic stenosis	Peak aortic valve gradient (mmHg)	Aortic valve area (cm^2)
Mild	<50	>1.5
Moderate	50–70	1.1–1.5
Severe	>70	<0.8–1.0

Treatment

> Severe aortic stenosis is associated with a peak gradient of >70 mmHg. However, with LV impairment the aortic valve gradient may underestimate the degree of stenosis. In this situation, valve area is a more reliable measurement and a dynamic assessment of the valve gradient with dobutamine stress may be required.

Emergency

Admit the patient if there is heart failure and treat with diuretics with a view to early inpatient valve replacement. Try to avoid inotropes. Exercise great caution with angiotensin-converting enzyme inhibitors and other vasodilators, and never use them if the patient is hypotensive.

Long term

Follow moderate disease with repeat echocardiography at yearly intervals. Severe stenosis requires closer supervision to detect onset of symptoms. Antibiotic prophylaxis is required for dental procedures, etc. Valve replacement should be considered in all patients with severe aortic stenosis who become symptomatic. It is also indicated in asymptomatic patients who develop LV dysfunction or prior to non-cardiac surgery.

Complications

The following are associated with aortic stenosis:

- cardiac failure and pulmonary hypertension;
- sudden death;
- infective endocarditis;
- embolic disease;
- complete heart block.

Prognosis

Symptoms occur only after the stenosis has become severe. Mild aortic stenosis progresses to severe stenosis in about 20% of cases, two-thirds remaining unchanged. On average, the valve gradient will increase by 4–8 mmHg per year. Extensive valve calcification, the presence of a bicuspid valve and coexistent coronary artery disease predispose those affected to more rapid stenosis progression. Asymptomatic patients have an excellent prognosis. In symptomatic disease, the average survival with angina or syncope is 2–3 years, and with heart failure 1 year.

FURTHER READING

Baumgartner H. Aortic stenosis: medical and surgical management. *Heart* 2005; 91: 1483–8.

- - - - - - - - - - - - - - - -

Decena BF III and Tischler MD. Stress echocardiography in valvular heart disease. *Cardiol. Clin.* 1999; 17: 555–72.

2.5.2 Aortic regurgitation

Aetiology/pathophysiology/pathology

Aortic regurgitation (AR) may result from primary disease of the valve leaflets, dilatation of the aortic root, loss of commissural support or failure of valve prosthesis, either alone or in combination. The result is the addition of a regurgitant volume to the normal inflow from the left atrium.

> **Aetiology of AR**
>
> Dilatation of the aortic root:
>
> - Degenerative (senile).
> - Cystic medial necrosis: isolated/associated with Marfan's syndrome.
> - Aortic dissection.
> - Systemic hypertension.
> - Aortitis (connective tissue disorders and syphilis).
>
> Primary disease of valve leaflets:
>
> - Rheumatic heart disease.
> - Infective endocarditis.
> - Bicuspid valve.
> - Myxomatous degeneration with prolapse.
> - Trauma.
>
> Loss of support of the aortic valve cusps:
>
> - High ventricular septal defect.
> - Fallot's tetralogy.
>
> Failure of a prosthetic valve

Clinical presentation

The patient may present with the following:

- exertional dyspnoea, orthopnoea and paroxysmal nocturnal dyspnoea;
- lethargy;
- palpitations;
- angina.

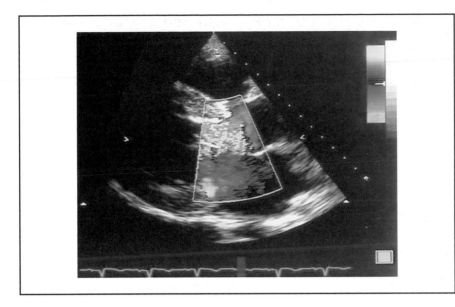

▲ **Fig. 54** Parasternal long-axis view showing severe AR with colour flow mapping. In early diastole there is a broad-based regurgitant jet (yellow–blue) filling the whole of the left ventricular outflow tract.

Investigations

ECG

Look for the following:

- normal/left ventricular (LV) hypertrophy;
- left atrial enlargement;
- prolongation of PR interval;
- non-specific ST-segment and T-wave changes.

Chest radiograph

This is normal or shows cardiomegaly, which may be gross. There is pulmonary oedema in acute cases. Look for evidence of aortic dilatation or dissection.

Echocardiography

Echocardiography may enable diagnosis of the aetiology from the anatomy of the aortic valve and root. Severity assessment is semi-quantitative and derived from colour and continous-wave Doppler (Fig. 54). LV dilatation and reduced ejection fraction occur with untreated severe disease. Transoesophageal echocardiography

may be required to exclude dissection and endocarditis.

Coronary angiography

Coronary angiography will be required before surgery to assess the coronary arteries in most cases. The AR can be assessed with an aortogram.

Differential diagnosis

Consider pulmonary regurgitation and mitral stenosis with Graham Steell murmur.

Treatment

Emergency

In patients with acute severe AR or severe decompensated chronic AR, treat heart failure aggressively with diuretics, vasodilators and inotropes. Look for the underlying cause and plan early or emergency valve replacement.

Long term

Patients with asymptomatic mild/moderate AR with normal ventricular function require annual clinical and echocardiographic

assessment. Antibiotic prophylaxis is required. All patients with severe symptomatic AR should be considered for surgery. Early surgery is indicated if there is evidence of LV dilatation or LV systolic dysfunction. Patients with coexistent aortic root dilatation >5 cm and AR of any severity should have aortic root reconstruction and valve resuspension or replacement.

Complications

Complications commonly encountered include the following:

- progressive heart failure;
- mitral regurgitation;
- atrial fibrillation;
- sudden death.

Prognosis

The risk of developing symptoms and/or LV dysfunction in severe AR with normal LV function is 4% annually. If there is LV dysfunction, the risk is >25% annually. Prognosis is excellent in mild or moderate disease. In symptomatically severe AR, the yearly mortality rate is >10%.

FURTHER READING

Bonow RO. Chronic aortic regurgitation: role of medical therapy and optimal timing for surgery. *Cardiol. Clin.* 1998; 16: 449–61.

Carabello BA and Crawford FA Jr. Valvular heart disease. *N. Engl. J. Med.* 1997; 337: 32–41.

2.5.3 Mitral stenosis

Aetiology

Most mitral stenosis (MS) is acquired through rheumatic heart disease. It is more common in women, presenting in developed countries in the fourth or fifth decades of life.

Clinical presentation

MS commonly presents with the following:

- exertional dyspnoea;
- orthopnoea;
- paroxysmal nocturnal dyspnoea;
- haemoptysis;
- palpitations;
- fatigue;
- weight loss;
- embolic phenomena in up to 15%.

Physical signs

See Section 1.2.6.

Investigations

ECG

- Normal.
- Left atrial enlargement or atrial fibrillation (AF).
- Right venricular hypertrophy.

Chest radiograph

- Normal.
- Straightening of left cardiac border as a result of dilated left atrial appendage.
- Pulmonary oedema.

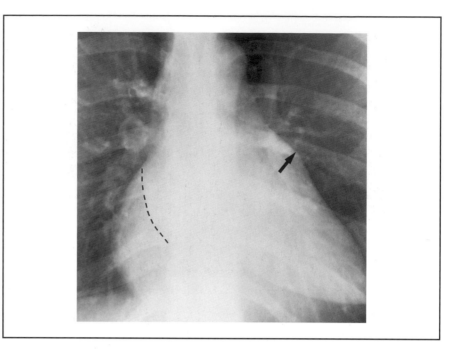

▲**Fig. 55** CXR showing left atrial enlargement in a patient with mitral valve disease: note the double atrial shadow (left atrial border indicated by broken line) and dilatation of the left atrial appendage (arrow). (Reproduced with permission from Axford JS, ed. *Medicine*. Oxford: Blackwell Science, 1996.)

- Atrial double shadow along right cardiac border (Fig. 55).

Echocardiography

This enables visualisation of leaflet mobility and calcification. Quantification of the valve area and mean gradient (Table 28) are derived from continous-wave Doppler. Left atrial size and right ventricular function should be assessed. Left ventricular size is usually small and left ventricular systolic function normal. Doppler echocardiography allows estimation of the pulmonary artery pressure (PAP). A transoesophageal study is usually required to assess suitability for valvuloplasty if this is being considered (Fig. 56).

Cardiac catheterisation

This is advisable when patient symptoms and echocardiographic findings are discordant or coexistent coronary artery disease is suspected. The mean mitral valve (MV) gradient can be calculated from the difference between left ventricular end-diastolic pressure and pulmonary artery wedge pressure recorded simultaneously.

Dynamic assessment

Some symptomatic patients may have evidence of only mild or moderate MS at rest. However, during exercise the rate of mitral inflow increases, which may cause the transvalvular gradient to increase significantly. Diastolic filling time may also be reduced, causing raised left atrial pressure. Exercise echocardiography should therefore be considered in patients who are symptomatic with apparent mild or moderate disease only, and no other

TABLE 28 **SEVERITY OF MITRAL STENOSIS ASSESSED BY MEAN GRADIENT AND MITRAL VALVE AREA**		
Severity	**Mean gradient (mmHg)**	**Mitral valve area (cm²)**
Mild	0–6	<1.5
Moderate	6–11	1.0–1.5
Severe	>12	<1.0

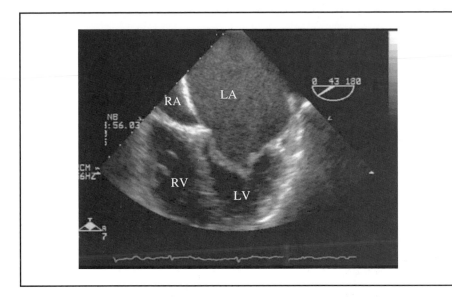

▲**Fig. 56** Rheumatic MS: note thickening of the leaflet tips and subvalvar apparatus causing marked restriction of leaflet excursion in diastole. There is marked left atrial enlargement with a relatively small left ventricular cavity. Spontaneous echo contrast (smoky appearance) can be seen in left atrium, suggestive of a prothrombotic state. LA, left atrium; LV, left ventricle; RA, right atrium; RV, right ventricle.

FURTHER READING

Bruce CJ and Nishimura RA. Newer advances in the diagnosis and treatment of mitral stenosis. *Curr. Probl. Cardiol.* 1998; 23: 125–92.

- - - - - - - - - - - - - - - - -

Lawrie GM. Mitral valve repair vs. replacement. Current recommendations and long-term results. *Cardiol Clin* 1998; 16: 437–48.

explanation for their symptoms (eg anaemia, other valvular disease or coronary artery disease). An increase in mean MV gradient to >15 mmHg or PAP to >60 mmHg with exercise is considered significant.

Differential diagnosis
Consider the following:

- Austin Flint murmur (of aortic regurgitation);
- left atrial myxoma;
- tricuspid stenosis.

Treatment

Emergency
Treat acute pulmonary oedema with diuretics.

Short term
Beta-blockers or rate-limiting calcium antagonists may help symptoms. AF may require treatment (see Section 2.2.2).

Long term
Formal anticoagulation with warfarin is required. Antibiotic prophylaxis is needed irrespective

of severity. Intervention is required if there is severe stenosis and symptoms. If the MV has minimal calcification, there is merely mild mitral regurgitation and there is no evidence of left atrial thrombus, then mitral valvuloplasty should be considered (see Section 3.8). Otherwise, open valvuloplasty or MV replacement is required.

Complications
The following are possible:

- AF;
- pulmonary hypertension or infarction;
- chest infections;
- tricuspid regurgitation;
- right ventricular failure;
- thromboembolic disease.

Prognosis
In severe MS, 5-year survival rates range from 62% with New York Heart Association class III symptoms to 15% with class IV. After surgery, 5-year survival rates are between 90 and 96%.

2.5.4 Mitral regurgitation

Aetiology/pathophysiology/pathology
Abnormalities of the mitral valve annulus, valve leaflets, chordae tendineae, papillary muscles or adjacent left ventricular (LV) wall may cause mitral regurgitation (MR).

Common causes of MR in the adult

- Idiopathic mitral valve prolapse (MVP): most common cause.
- After myocardial infarction:
  (a) Papillary muscle dysfunction (ischaemia or rupture).
  (b) Ruptured chordae tendineae.
  (c) Annular dilatation (ischaemic heart disease or dilated cardiomyopathy).
- Rheumatic heart disease.
- Infective endocarditis.
- Atrial septal defect.
- Failure of valve prosthesis/paraprosthetic leak.

Epidemiology
The prevalence of MVP varies from 1 to 6%, and is twice as common in women. After myocardial infarction, the prevalence is 20%.

Clinical presentation
Common symptoms include exertional dyspnoea, orthopnoea, fatigue and lethargy. Occasionally,

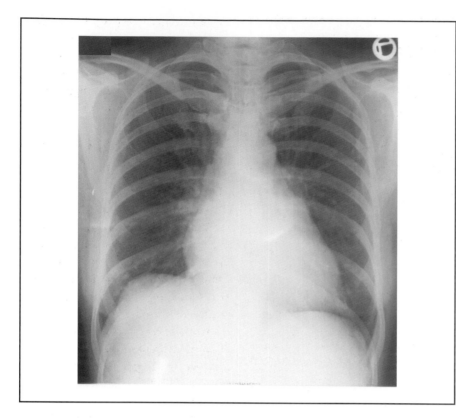

▲ **Fig. 57** Mitral annular calcification: a ring of calcification can be seen within the heart shadow.

there are palpitations and, in severe acute MR, the patient may be very unwell with severe dyspnoea.

Physical signs

In mild disease, there are few signs apart from an apical pansystolic murmur radiating to the axilla. In more haemodynamically significant regurgitation, there can be the following:

- atrial fibrillation (AF);
- laterally displaced, hyperdynamic apex beat with systolic thrill;
- left parasternal late systolic heave (atrial filling) in severe MR;
- soft first heart sound, wide splitting of the second heart sound, and a third heart sound;
- late systolic murmur in association with a systolic click suggests MVP.

In acute severe MR, there is poor perfusion with pulmonary oedema.

A murmur may not be heard due to very rapid equalisation of pressures between the left atrium and left ventricle during early diastole.

Investigations

ECG

This may be normal, but look for AF, left atrial enlargement or LV hypertrophy.

Chest radiograph

This can be normal, or may show cardiomegaly with left atrial enlargement. Mitral annular calcification may be seen (Fig. 57). There is pulmonary oedema in acute MR.

Echocardiography

The presence of excess leaflet motion, restricted leaflet motion and annular size must be carefully assessed with both transthoracic and transoesophageal echocardiography.

In the case of prolapse, a precise assessment of the scallops involved is required. Severity assessment is semi-quantitative from colour and continous-wave Doppler. Measurements of left and right ventricular size, systolic function and pulmonary artery pressure are required (Fig. 58).

Coronary angiography

Coronary angiography may be required if there is a suspicion of coronary artery disease.

Dynamic assessment

In patients with ischaemic MR, baseline MR may only be mild to moderate. However, during exercise ischaemia of the papillary muscles and adjacent myocardium may cause the MR to become severe. Exercise (stress) echocardiography should therefore be considered in patients with ischaemic heart disease and severe cardiac symptoms that cannot be explained by baseline MR or any other cause.

Treatment

Emergency

Treat acute pulmonary oedema and shock. Vasodilator therapy reduces the afterload and is of benefit. Intravenous nitroprusside may be life-saving. Urgent surgery is required.

Short term

Symptomatic patients with severe MR who are awaiting surgery should receive diuretic and vasodilator therapy. Digoxin is of particular benefit in the treatment of AF. Anticoagulation will be required.

Long term

All patients should receive antibiotic prophylaxis. Mild to moderate disease requires annual monitoring

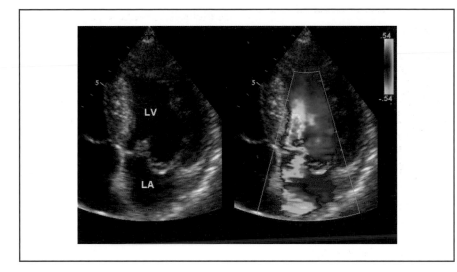

▲**Fig. 58** Apical four-chamber view of a patient with prolapse of the posterior mitral valve leaflet. An anteriorly directed jet of mitral regurgitation can be seen with colour flow mapping (coloured green).

only. All patients with symptomatic severe MR require surgery. Asymptomatic patients with severe MR should be referred once LV function starts to decline or LV dilatation occurs. Generally, surgical outcome is better with mitral valve repair than replacement.

> **Indications for surgery in severe MR**
>
> • If surgical repair is possible, it should be considered in all patients aged <75 years who have a flail leaflet or persistent AF.
> • Deteriorating ventricular function (ejection fraction <60% or end-systolic diameter >45 mm).
> • The presence of symptoms, although careful consideration of the aetiology and severity of LV dysfunction is needed in older patients.

Complications

The following are possible:

• LV failure;

• AF;

• infective endocarditis;

• pulmonary hypertension;

• right ventricular failure;

• thromboembolism (more common in MVP);

• sudden death (more common in flail leaflet).

Prognosis

Progression of MR depends on the aetiology, but it develops in 15% of patients with MVP over 10–15 years. Without surgery, patients with severe MR have a 5-year survival rate as low as 45%. After surgery, the 5-year survival rates vary from 40% in MR caused by ischaemic heart disease to over 75% in rheumatic mitral valve disease.

> **FURTHER READING**
>
> Cooper HA and Gersh BJ. Treatment of chronic mitral regurgitation. *Am. Heart J.* 1998; 135: 925–36.
>
> -------------------
>
> Quinones MA. Management of mitral regurgitation: optimal timing for surgery. *Cardiol. Clin.* 1998; 16: 421–35.

2.5.5 Tricuspid valve disease

Aetiology/pathophysiology/pathology

Tricuspid regurgitation (TR) is usually secondary to a combination of right ventricular (RV) dilatation and high pressure resulting from severe pulmonary hypertension. Tricuspid stenosis (TS) is almost invariably rheumatic in origin, and accompanies mitral stenosis. In both, right atrial enlargement and hypertrophy occur with the risk of atrial fibrillation.

Clinical presentation

This is usually asymptomatic, and in the case of TR is usually discovered secondary to other more significant cardiac pathology. TR and TS may cause a sensation of neck pulsation, right upper quadrant discomfort and peripheral oedema. Occasionally, a low cardiac output syndrome comprising fatigue, weight loss and syncope may be present.

Physical signs

TR causes prominent *v* waves in the JVP, whereas TS causes prominent *a* waves in sinus rhythm. In more severe cases, both cause pulsatile hepatomegaly, ascites and peripheral oedema. In TR, a pansystolic murmur that increases on inspiration and is heard best at the lower left sternal edge is usual. The corresponding murmur in TS is a presystolic murmur in sinus rhythm with a mid-diastolic murmur.

Investigations

ECG

This is usually normal, but right atrial enlargement is a feature of tricuspid valve disease. There is evidence of RV hypertrophy in TR.

Chest radiograph

• Often normal, but there may be an enlarged right atrium and superior vena cava in both TR and TS.

• RV enlargement may be evident in TR.

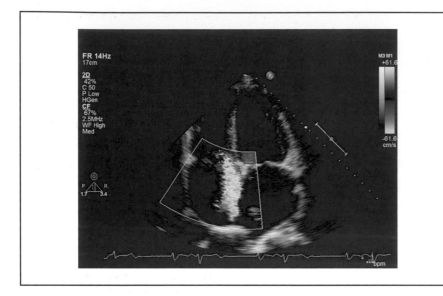

▲**Fig. 59** TR: a broad band seen mainly as blue extends back into the right atrium. (Courtesy of Dr J. Chambers.)

Echocardiography

This gauges the severity (from colour and continuous-wave Doppler) and enables calculation of pulmonary artery pressure from a TR jet (Fig. 59).

Treatment

Both TR and TS are usually well tolerated irrespective of their severity. When TR is the result of a correctable left-sided cause, eg mitral valve disease, annuloplasty at the time of surgery is corrective. TS rarely requires valvotomy.

FURTHER READING

Kratz J. Evaluation and management of tricuspid valve disease. *Cardiol. Clin.* 1991; 9: 397–407.

2.5.6 Pulmonary valve disease

Aetiology/pathophysiology/ pathology

Pulmonary stenosis (PS) is usually congenital in origin, and may form part of Fallot's tetralogy. Rarely, it may be the result of rheumatic fever or the carcinoid syndrome. Pulmonary regurgitation (PR) invariably results from dilatation of the pulmonary annulus, which may occur with pulmonary hypertension, leading to right ventricular hypertrophy (RVH) and right atrial hypertrophy (RAH).

Clinical presentation

Both PR and mild PS are asymptomatic. More severe disease presents with a low cardiac output syndrome and right heart failure.

Physical signs

There is a characteristic harsh ejection systolic murmur at the left sternal edge in the second intercostal space, which is louder on inspiration. Other signs include the following:

- prominent *a* wave in JVP;

- thrill over pulmonary area, right ventricular heave;

- soft pulmonary second heart sound;

- right ventricular fourth heart sound.

PR is characterised by a decrescendo early-diastolic murmur heard in the pulmonary area (Graham Steell murmur).

Investigations

ECG

This is normal, or there is RAH and RVH.

Chest radiograph

This is normal, or shows right atrial and ventricular enlargement.

Treatment

Pulmonary valvotomy may be necessary in severe PS. Severe PR may require surgery if the patient is symptomatic.

FURTHER READING

Waller BF, Howard J and Fess S. Pathology of pulmonic valve stenosis and pure regurgitation. *Clin. Cardiol.* 1995; 18: 45–50.

2.6 Pericardial disease

2.6.1 Acute pericarditis

Aetiology/pathophysiology/ pathology

There are many causes of acute pericarditis (Table 29). In the developed world the cause of many cases is never established (idiopathic) but a viral cause is often suspected, coxsackievirus B being most often incriminated. Tuberculosis is a major cause in the developing world.

There is inflammation of the pericardium with infiltration of polymorphonuclear leucocytes, increased pericardial vascularity and deposition of fibrin. Inflammation can involve the superficial myocardium and fibrinous adhesions may form between the pericardium and epicardium, and between the pericardium, adjacent sternum and pleura. The visceral pleura may exude fluid, leading to pericardial effusion.

TABLE 29 CAUSES OF ACUTE PERICARDITIS

Pathogenesis	Cause
Acute idiopathic pericarditis	Unknown
Infectious	Viral
	TB
	Other bacteria
	Fungi
Inflammatory	Post myocardial infarction/cardiotomy
	Autoimmune rheumatic disorder
Other	Neoplastic
	Uraemia
	Trauma
	Aortic dissection
	Hypothyroidism
	Irradiation
	Drugs, eg hydralazine

Clinical presentation

Common

- Chest pain: usually retrosternal or left precordial in location, radiating to the neck. The pain is aggravated by supine posture, coughing, deep inspiration and swallowing; it is eased by sitting up and leaning forward. It may be preceded by a few days of malaise.

- Fever.

Uncommon

- Dyspnoea.

- Symptoms of any underlying cause.

- Acute epigastric pain mimicking an acute abdomen.

- Anginal type pain.

- Cardiac tamponade.

Physical signs
The patient may present with the following:

- pericardial friction rub;

- fever;

- atrial fibrillation;

- evidence of an underlying disease;

- signs associated with tamponade.

Investigations

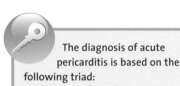

The diagnosis of acute pericarditis is based on the following triad:

- typical chest pain;
- pericardial friction rub;
- classical ECG changes.

ECG
The ECG may be normal. There is an initial, widespread (not V1 or aVR), upwardly concave ST elevation, followed by return of the ST segments to baseline and flattened T waves. T waves then become inverted before returning to normal over 1 week. It is necessary to distinguish these changes from those of acute myocardial infarction, in which ST elevation is convex and regional, R waves are lost, Q waves form and conduction abnormalities may develop (Fig. 60). Acute pericarditis generally affects the ECG more extensively, with little in the way of the 'reciprocal changes'

seen with ST-elevation myocardial infarction.

Blood tests
Look for the following:

- elevated white cell count, erythrocyte sedimentation rate and C-reactive protein;

- blood culture, atypical bacterial antibody and viral titres;

- renal function to exclude uraemia;

- serial cardiac enzymes, which may show a modest rise;

- as directed by suspicion of underlying cause (Table 29).

Chest radiograph
This is often normal, but look for evidence of pericardial effusion, malignancy, tuberculosis or aortic dissection.

Echocardiography
Echocardiography is useful to exclude pericardial effusion or suspicion of aortic dissection.

Differential diagnosis
Consider the following:

- acute coronary syndrome;

- aortic dissection;

- pulmonary embolism;

- musculoskeletal pain.

Treatment

Emergency
Pericardiocentesis if there is cardiac tamponade.

Short term
Admit if there is severe pain or large effusion, or for treatment of underlying condition. Treatment should include bed-rest with oral NSAIDs given for symptomatic relief. Consider corticosteroids if there is severe pain not responding to NSAIDs after 48 hours.

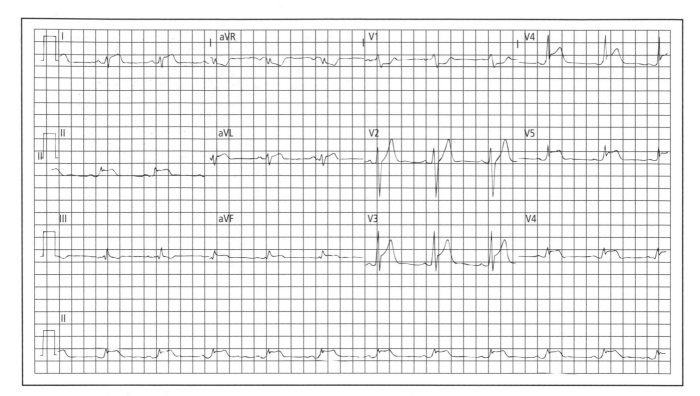

▲ **Fig. 60** ECG showing changes of acute pericarditis.

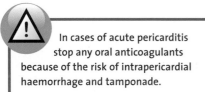 In cases of acute pericarditis stop any oral anticoagulants because of the risk of intrapericardial haemorrhage and tamponade.

Long term
If idiopathic relapsing pericarditis develops, corticosteroids or colchicine may be effective.

Complications
Beware of the following:

- pericardial effusion;
- idiopathic relapsing pericarditis;
- cardiac tamponade;
- constrictive pericarditis.

Prognosis
There is complete resolution within 3 months in 80% of patients, although 20% develop idiopathic relapsing pericarditis with chronic symptoms of pericardial inflammation. Cardiac tamponade may cause death if untreated, as may some of the precipitating conditions.

> ### FURTHER READING
>
> Maisch B. Pericardial diseases, with a focus on aetiology, pathogenesis, pathophysiology, new diagnostic imaging methods, and treatment. *Curr. Opin. Cardiol.* 1994; 9: 379–88.
>
> – – – – – – – – – – – – – – –
>
> Soler-Soler J, Sagrista-Sauleda J and Peranyer-Miralda G. Relapsing pericarditis. *Heart* 2004; 90: 1364–8.

2.6.2 Pericardial effusion

Aetiology/pathophysiology/pathology
Pericardial effusion may develop in cases of acute pericarditis from any cause. The normal pericardial space contains 15–50 mL fluid and can only accommodate a rapid increase in pericardial volume to 150–200 mL before the intrapericardial pressure starts to rise. Once intrapericardial pressure exceeds intracardiac pressure, left ventricular filling and cardiac output decline. With a gradual accumulation of fluid, volumes of up to 2 L may be present before left ventricular filling becomes compromised.

Acute cardiac tamponade typically follows cardiac trauma (which may be iatrogenic), aortic dissection, spontaneous bleeding or cardiac rupture after a myocardial infarction. Chronic tamponade usually results from malignancy, idiopathic pericarditis or uraemia, although almost any cause of acute pericarditis may be responsible.

Clinical presentation

Common
In chronic cases the patient may be asymptomatic despite a large effusion. Typical symptoms include shortness of breath and and mild chest discomfort.

Uncommon

In a large pericardial effusion without tamponade, compression of adjacent structures may lead to the following:

- dysphagia (oesophagus);
- cough (bronchus/trachea);
- hiccups (phrenic nerve);
- hoarseness (laryngeal nerve);
- abdominal bloating and nausea (abdominal viscera).

Physical signs

In most patients, the examination will be normal. In large effusions without tamponade, there may be muffled heart sounds, crackles (compression of lung parenchyma) or Ewart's sign (patch of dullness below the angle of the left scapula caused by compression of the base of the left lung). There may also be pericardial friction rub or signs of cardiac tamponade. Cardiac tamponade should be suspected in a shocked patient with apparent clear lung fields and elevated JVP.

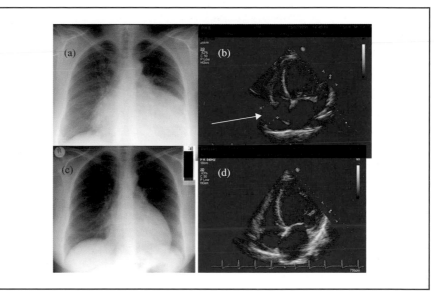

▲ **Fig. 61** (**a**) CXR demonstrating enlarged globular-shaped heart. (**b**) Transthoracic echocardiography confirmed this was due to a large pericardial effusion, seen as an echo-free space around the heart (arrow) in apical four-chamber view. After drainage of the effusion, cardiomegaly resolved on CXR (**c**) and an effusion can no longer be seen around the heart at echocardiography (**d**).

> **Cardiac tamponade may present in three ways:**
>
> 1. cardiac arrest;
> 2. a severely ill patient who is stuporous or agitated and restless (survivor of acute tamponade);
> 3. with dyspnoea, chest pain, weight loss, anorexia and weakness (more slowly developing tamponade).
>
> Rapid recognition of the clinical signs of tamponade is essential.
>
> - Tachypnoea and tachycardia.
> - Pulsus paradoxus (pulse becomes impalpable on inspiration in severe cases).
> - Elevated JVP with prominent systolic *x* descent and absence of diastolic *y* descent.
> - Rarely, normal JVP in severe dehydration.
>
> If you suspect the diagnosis, organise an urgent echocardiogram.

Investigations

ECG

This is usually normal, although changes of acute pericarditis may be present. There may be a non-specific reduction in QRS voltage and T-wave flattening. Electrical alternans is suggestive of a large effusion.

Chest radiograph

This is often normal, although a large effusion may cause an enlarged globular cardiac silhouette with clear lung fields. Look for separation of the pericardial fat lines and a left-sided pleural effusion (Fig. 61).

Echocardiography

Echocardiography is the most sensitive test for detection of pericardial fluid (as little as 20 mL). This appears as an echo-free space around the heart (Fig. 61b). Diastolic left and right heart collapse, marked decrease in mitral inflow with inspiration and a dilated inferior vena cava that fails to collapse with inspiration suggest tamponade.

Differential diagnosis

In chronic cases consider the following:

- constrictive pericarditis;
- restrictive cardiomyopathy.

In those with tamponade consider causes of circulatory collapse (see *Acute Medicine*, Section 1.2.2), in particular massive pulmonary embolus and severe asthma.

Treatment

Consider the following.

- Urgent pericardiocentesis is essential in cardiac tamponade. It is also needed for diagnosis if there is suspicion of purulent or tuberculous pericarditis, or prolonged and otherwise unexplained illness.
- Symptom relief as for acute pericarditis (see Section 2.6.1).
- Recurrent or persistent symptomatic effusions may require balloon pericardiostomy or surgical pericardiectomy.

Complications

Common

Complications arise more commonly from the underlying condition than from the effusion, although chronic pericardial effusion lasting more than 6 months may be seen. This is more likely after idiopathic, uraemic, myxoedematous or malignant pericarditis.

Uncommon

Uncommon complications are cardiac tamponade and constrictive pericarditis.

FURTHER READING

Chong HH and Plotnick GD. Pericardial effusion and tamponade: evaluation, imaging modalities, and management. *Compr. Ther.* 1995; 21: 378–85.

Devlin GP, Smyth D, Charleson HA, *et al.* Balloon pericardiostomy: a new therapeutic option for malignant pericardial effusion. *Aust. NZ J. Med.* 1996; 26: 556–8.

Tsang TS, Oh JK and Seward JB. Diagnosis and management of cardiac tamponade in the era of echocardiography. *Clin. Cardiol.* 1999; 22: 446–52.

2.6.3 Constrictive pericarditis

Aetiology/pathophysiology/ pathology

Constrictive pericarditis is characterised by an abnormally thickened and non-compliant pericardium, which abruptly limits ventricular filling in mid to late diastole. This results in elevated end-diastolic cardiac filling pressures and the equalisation of pressure in all four chambers at end diastole. As cardiac filling is compromised, cardiac output is reduced. The clinical features are secondary to systemic venous congestion.

Before the 1960s, tuberculous constrictive pericarditis was the most common cause of pericardial constriction worldwide. In the developed world its importance has declined, and the aetiology is usually idiopathic, post radiotherapy or post surgery.

Clinical presentation

Common

Oedema, abdominal swelling and discomfort caused by ascites or hepatic congestion are most frequent. Vague abdominal symptoms such as postprandial fullness, dyspepsia, flatulence and anorexia may also be present. Cachexia and fatigue suggest a reduced cardiac output.

Uncommon

Exertional dyspnoea and orthopnoea may occur when ventricular pressures become severely elevated, as may platypnoea (dyspnoea in upright position).

Physical signs

Common

Elevation of the JVP with prominent x and y descents is the most important clinical sign, plus the following:

- atrial fibrillation;

- Kussmaul's sign (inspiratory rise in JVP);

- pericardial knock (third heart sound);

- hepatosplenomegaly, ascites and peripheral oedema;

- cachexia.

Uncommon

Pulsus paradoxus and signs of severe liver failure.

Investigations

ECG

This may be normal or show non-specific generalised T-wave changes, low-voltage complexes or atrial fibrillation.

Chest radiograph

This is usually normal, but the cardiac silhouette may be either reduced or enlarged. Left atrial enlargement, pleural effusions and pericardial calcification are non-specific findings.

Echocardiography

Echocardiography shows pericardial thickening. Septal motion is abnormal and the left ventricular posterior wall flattens abruptly in early diastole due to rapid equalisation of left and right ventricular pressures. During inspiration there is a marked reduction in diastolic mitral inflow (Fig. 62).

Cardiac catheterisation

This is usually needed to confirm the diagnosis, with characteristic equalisation of end-diastolic pressures in the two ventricles, persisting with respiration and fluid challenge (Fig. 63).

CT/MRI

These imaging techniques may be used to demonstrate the extent and distribution of pericardial thickening (Fig. 64).

Differential diagnosis
Consider the following:

- chronic pericardial effusion;

- restrictive cardiomyopathy (see Section 2.4.3);

- superior vena cava obstruction (excluded if there is a pulsatile waveform in JVP);

- congestive cardiac failure;

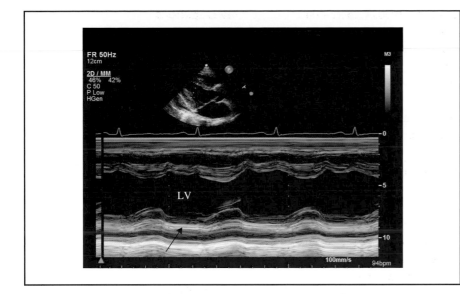

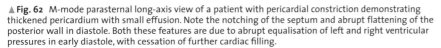

▲ **Fig. 62** M-mode parasternal long-axis view of a patient with pericardial constriction demonstrating thickened pericardium with small effusion. Note the notching of the septum and abrupt flattening of the posterior wall in diastole. Both these features are due to abrupt equalisation of left and right ventricular pressures in early diastole, with cessation of further cardiac filling.

- nephrotic syndrome (see *Nephrology*, Section 2.1.4);

- malignant hepatic or intra-abdominal disease.

Treatment

A minority of patients may be managed medically with diet and diuretic therapy. Most will require pericardiectomy: an early operation is recommended.

Complications

Severe venous congestion with chronic hepatic impairment is common. Death results from the consequences of an inadequate cardiac output.

Prognosis

Morbidity

Without treatment, most patients deteriorate progressively with severely limiting symptoms. With pericardiectomy, 90% improve and 50% may gain complete relief of symptoms.

Mortality

The outlook in untreated cases is poor. Hospital mortality rate after pericardiectomy is 5–16%, and 5-year survival rate after surgery is 74–87%.

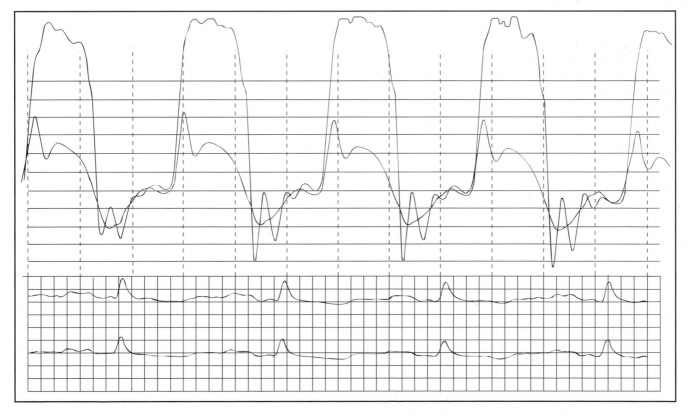

▲ **Fig. 63** Pericardial constriction: the top section of the image shows pressure tracings from catheters placed simultaneously in the left and right ventricles. The pressures from the two chambers are seen to equalise at the end of diastole. (Courtesy of E. Tomsett.)

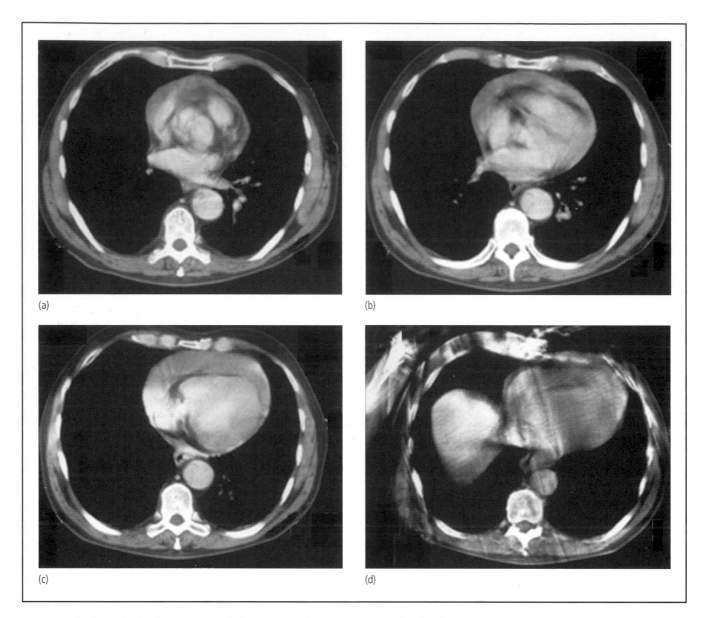

▲ **Fig. 64** Pericardial thickening: these sections (**a–d**) through the heart show a markedly thickened pericardium.

FURTHER READING

Mehta A, Mehta M and Jain AC. Constrictive pericarditis. *Clin. Cardiol.* 1999; 22: 334–44.

Tuna IC and Danielson GK. Surgical management of pericardial diseases. *Cardiol. Clin.* 1990; 8: 683–96.

Vaitkus PT and Kussmaul WG. Constrictive pericarditis vs. restrictive cardiomyopathy: a reappraisal and updpate of diagnostic criteria. *Am. Heart J.* 1991; 122: 1431–41.

2.7 Congenital heart disease

Advances in paediatric cardiology over the past three decades have resulted in the survival of a large number of individuals with congenital heart disorders into adulthood. Management of these patients is a challenging area of cardiology, with over 100 separate diagnostic conditions. Congenital cardiac abnormalities can be associated with genetic syndromes or other diseases (Table 30). Abnormalities are divided into cyanotic and acyanotic conditions. The most common conditions are reviewed in this section (Table 31). Diagnosis of these conditions depends on accurate imaging of underlying cardiac abnormalities. This is increasingly performed using non-invasive techniques such as echocardiography and cardiac MRI. Both of these diagnostic methods

TABLE 30 EXAMPLES OF GENETIC DISEASES AFFECTING THE CARDIOVASCULAR SYSTEM

Syndrome	Inheritance	Cardiac manifestations	Management
Marfan's	AD	Aortic root dilatation/rupture	Echo surveillance, beta-blockade and elective aortic root repair when >5.5 cm in diameter
Turner's		Coarctation of aorta and bicuspid aortic valve	Echo surveillance of valve and surgery for coarctation
Noonan's	AD	Pulmonary stenosis most common	
Down's		Atrioventricular canal defects	Surgical
DiGeorge's	AD or sporadic	Conotruncal	Surgical
Williams'		Supravalvar aortic stenosis	Echo surveillance
Holt–Oram	AD	Septal defects (hand–heart)	See Sections 2.7.1.1 and 2.7.1.2
Muscular dystrophies	Various	Conduction defects. Cardiomyopathy may also be seen in female carriers of X-linked dystrophies	Pacing for heart block, standard treatment for left ventricular dysfunction, echocardiography and ECG screening of carriers

See also cardiomyopathy (Section 2.4) and muscular dystrophies (*Neurology*, Section 2.2.3). AD, autosomal dominant.

TABLE 31 COMMON CONGENITAL HEART DISORDERS

Cyanotic	Acyanotic
Tetralogy of Fallot	Atrial septal defect
Complete transposition of the great arteries	Ventricular septal defect
Ebstein's anomaly	Patent ductus arteriosus
	Coarctation of the aorta

can also be used to calculate intracardiac shunts, which play an important part in determining treatment. As a consequence cardiac catheterisation is performed less frequently.

In congenital heart disease particular care should be taken to prevent infective endocarditis associated with dental or surgical procedures by using appropriate prophylactic antibiotics. The highest risk is associated with high-pressure jets of blood:

- tetralogy of Fallot;
- Ebstein's anomaly;
- ventricular septal defect;
- patent ductus arteriosus;
- coarctation of the aorta.

2.7.1 Acyanotic congenital heart disease

2.7.1.1 Atrial septal defect

Anatomy/pathophysiology/ pathology

An atrial septal defect (ASD) may be ostium primum, secundum or sinus venosus in type (Fig. 65). The haemodynamic consequences depend on the size of the defect. In larger defects blood can shunt from the left atrium to the right because the right ventricle (RV) is more compliant than the left. As a result, over time the RV may dilate and fail leading to the development of pulmonary hypertension and possibly Eisenmenger's syndrome (see Section 2.7.3).

A patent foramen ovale is common in young people. It does not permit left-to-right shunting but allows right-to-left shunting when right atrial pressure exceeds left (eg Valsalva manoeuvre). This can result in an increased risk of stroke as a result of paradoxical embolism.

Epidemiology

ASDs are the most common congenital heart abnormality and account for around 30% of all congenital heart defects in adults (female/male ratio 2:1 and 75% are ostium secundum).

Clinical presentation

In most adults ASDs are asymptomatic and discovered incidentally as a result of other investigations. Symptoms are more likely if there is a left-to-right shunt and include:

- atrial arrhythmias (including atrial fibrillation, atrial flutter and sick sinus syndrome);

- exertional fatigue or dyspnoea;

- right heart failure;

- stroke/other arterial territory infarcts (eg lower limbs) secondary to paradoxical embolism.

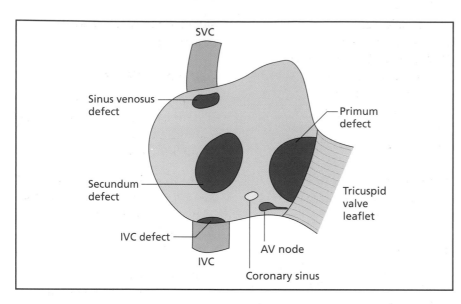

▲ Fig. 65 Sites of defects in the atrial septum seen from the right atrium. AV, atrioventricular; IVC, inferior vena cava; SVC, superior vena cava.

Physical signs

- Along with increasing flow through the right heart, an ejection systolic pulmonary flow murmur and wide fixed splitting of S2 (equalisation of right and left ventricular stroke volumes throughout the respiratory cycle) can be heard.

- RV heave with large shunts.

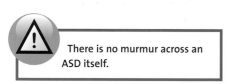

There is no murmur across an ASD itself.

Investigations

ECG

Look for the following:

- right-axis deviation and right bundle-branch block;

- left-axis deviation in ostium primum defects;

- atrial arrhythmias.

Chest radiograph

Look for cardiomegaly (from right atrial and RV enlargement), dilated pulmonary arteries and pulmonary plethora indicating increasing pulmonary blood flow.

Echocardiography

Transthoracic and transoesophageal echocardiography can be used for confirmation of diagnosis.

Transoesophageal echocardiography with microbubble contrast study is ideal for visualising shunts (Fig. 66).

Treatment

Surgical and percutaneous closure are both possible. Haemodynamically non-significant ASDs do not require closure unless to prevent paradoxical emboli. In asymptomatic patients with a pulmonary/systemic flow ratio (shunt) in excess of 1.5:1 or mild to moderate pulmonary hypertension, closure should be considered.

Prognosis

- Shunt <1.5:1 has an excellent long-term outcome.

- Shunt >1.5:1, if untreated, restricts life expectancy to fifth decade (RV failure, rarely Eisenmenger's syndrome). Good long-term outcome if ASD is closed before development of pulmonary hypertension.

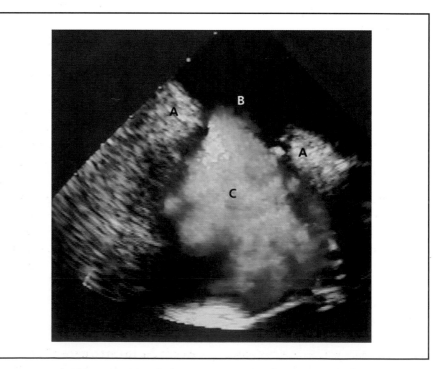

▲ Fig. 66 Transoesophageal echocardiographic image of left-to-right flow across a large atrial septal defect. A, atrial septum; B, left atrium; C, flow into right atrium. (Courtesy of Dr L.M. Shapiro.)

2.7.1.2 Isolated ventricular septal defect

Anatomy/pathophysiology/ pathology

Defects can occur at any level in the ventricular septum. A small defect causes a high-pressure left-to-right jet but no haemodynamic abnormality. Large defects with a shunt can eventually result in Eisenmenger's syndrome (see Section 2.7.3). Small defects in the membranous part of the septum noted during childhood often close by the age of 2 years.

Epidemiology

Ventricular septal defect (VSD) is the second most common congenital malformation of the heart, accounting for 20% of all congenital malformations.

Clinical presentation

Small defects with no shunt are usually asymptomatic and detected incidentally, secondary to the identification of a cardiac murmur. Defects with a significant shunt present with progressive dyspnoea, reduced exercise tolerance and eventually cyanosis in adult life.

Physical signs

- Pansystolic murmur and thrill at the lower left sternal edge.

- Signs of pulmonary hypertension.

- Clubbing and cyanosis of Eisenmenger's syndrome.

Investigations

ECG

In a small VSD it is often normal. However, with progressive worsening of the shunt there may be atrial arrhythmias (eg atrial fibrillation), right-axis deviation and right ventricular hypertrophy.

Chest radiograph

Normal in small defects. With progressive shunts there are radiographic signs of pulmonary hypertension, including cardiomegaly, enlarged pulmonary trunk and reduced lung markings in the periphery.

Echocardiography

Used to confirm diagnosis and calculate shunt.

Treatment

Surgical closure of the defect should be considered. Small VSDs without a shunt do not need closure. VSDs with a haemodynamically significant shunt should be closed if pulmonary hypertension is not severe and/or reversible.

Prognosis

Long-term outcome in patients who have successful closure of their VSD prior to development of pulmonary hypertension is excellent.

2.7.1.3 Patent ductus arteriosus

Anatomy/pathophysiology/ pathology

The ductus arteriosus is part of the lung bypass circuit in the fetal circulation (connecting the left pulmonary artery to the descending aorta) that ensures oxygenated blood from the right heart is delivered directly to the systemic circulation. The ductus normally closes soon after birth. However, in a small number of people it can remain patent, resulting in a left-to-right shunt that leads to left ventricular enlargement and eventually pulmonary hypertension.

Epidemiology

Patent ductus arteriosus (PDA) accounts for 10% of all congenital heart cases. The incidence is higher with maternal rubella and in preterm infants.

Clinical presentation

- Small PDA: patients are asymptomatic and PDA is detected incidentally from murmur or cardiac imaging for other causes.

- PDA with moderate or large shunt: patients present with progressive fatigue, dyspnoea, palpitations or eventually Eisenmenger's syndrome.

- Infective endocarditis is a risk and may be the first presentation.

Physical signs

- Continuous machinery murmur in the second left intercostal space.

- Significant shunt: wide pulse pressure, hyperdynamic apex and signs of left ventricular failure (in large shunts).

- Pulmonary hypertension: machinery murmur shortens (as proportion of cardiac cycle during which pulmonary pressure is lower than systemic pressure reduces) and eventually disappears.

Investigations

ECG

Normal in small PDA. With large shunts there is evidence of left atrial and left ventricular hypertrophy.

Chest radiograph

Normal in small PDA. With large shunts there is initially left-sided and then right-sided cardiomegaly, prominent proximal pulmonary arteries/ascending aorta and pulmonary plethora.

Echocardiography

Can be used to identify defect, calcuate extent of the shunt and estimate pulmonary arterial pressures.

Treatment

Both surgical (very low mortality of <0.5%, as does not require cardiopulmonary bypass) and percutaneous closure (suitable anatomy) of PDA are possible. Closure of all clinically detectable PDA (in the absence of irreversible pulmonary hypertension) is recommended.

Prognosis

Excellent outcome if PDA closed before development of any complications. Without closure, one-third of patients will be dead by the age of 40 years and two-thirds by 60 years. Potential complications include:

- infective pulmonary artery endarteritis and consequent septic pulmonary emboli;
- ductal aneurysm and calcification can also occur with risk of rupture.

2.7.1.4 Coarctation of the aorta

Anatomy/pathophysiology/ pathology

Aortic coarctation is the result of a flow-limiting narrowing in the aorta at the site of the fetal ductus arteriosus (see Section 2.7.1.3), most commonly just distal to the left subclavian artery (may also be positioned more proximally in the aortic arch; Fig. 67). With time an arterial supply to the lower body is achieved by extensive collateralisation. Often hypertension develops during childhood. Most patients have other abnormalities, including bicuspid aortic valve (50–80% of cases) and intracranial aneurysms of the circle of Willis.

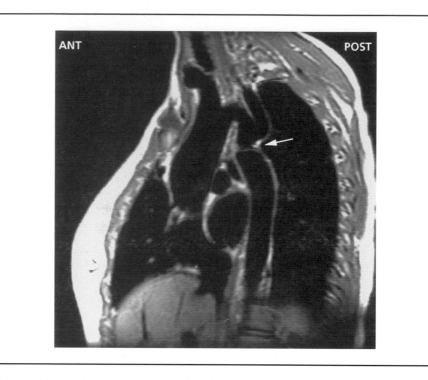

▲ **Fig. 67**   MRI scan of coarctation of the aorta (arrow).

Epidemiology

This condition is more common in males than in females (3:1).

Clinical presentation

Common

- Asymptomatic: incidental finding of murmur or systolic hypertension in the upper limbs.

Uncommon

- Symptoms of hypertension (epistaxis, headache and haemorrhagic stroke).
- Palpitations.
- Claudication in the legs.
- Heart failure.

Physical signs

- Systolic BP is usually greater in the arms than in the legs.
- Radiofemoral delay.

- Left sternal edge and/or interscapular systolic murmur emanating from the coarctation.

Investigations

ECG

Often normal, but there may be evidence of left ventricular hypertrophy.

Chest radiograph

Rib notching of posterior third to eighth ribs (from enlarged intercostal arteries because of collateral flow; Fig. 13). Prestenotic and poststenotic dilatation of the aorta can give rise to a '3' sign appearance.

Echocardiography

Can be used for diagnosis of coarctation and calculation of gradient acoss stenosis.

MRI and CT

Both can be used for accurate diagnosis.

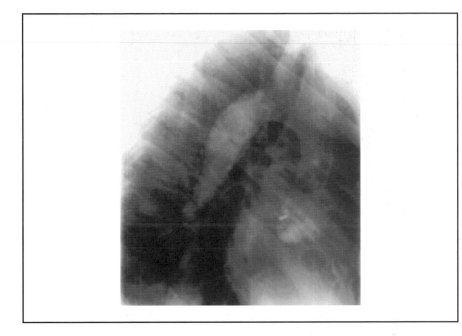

▲**Fig. 68** Angiogram showing coarctation of aorta, which can be seen to taper just after the arch. On a plain radiograph the feature to look for is rib notching produced by collateral vessels (Fig. 13).

Angiography

May aid in diagnosis, although MRI and CT may preclude the need (Fig. 68).

Treatment

- Surgical repair is often the first-line treatment if gradient across the coarctation is >30 mmHg.

- Percutaneous dilatation with or without stent deployment is also possible. However, routine current use is confined to treatment of paediatric or adolescent cases, and for the dilatation of repeat coarctation. Percutaneous treatment in adults remains experimental.

Complications

These may include the following:

- left ventricular failure;
- aortic dissection;
- premature coronary disease.

Prognosis

- Uncorrected: mean survival is around 35 years and 75% will die by the age of 50 years.

- Corrected: survival depends on the age at surgery, the younger the better.

Disease associations

- Turner's syndrome.
- Bicuspid aortic valve.
- Circle of Willis aneurysms.

2.7.2 Cyanotic congenital heart disease

Patients with cyanotic congenital heart disease are chronically hypoxaemic. This causes a number of adaptive physiological changes leading to complications. These adaptive changes are common to all patients in this group with significant cyanosis regardless of the underlying anatomical abnormality. These changes must be treated accordingly as detailed below.

Polycythaemia and hyperviscosity syndrome

Polycythaemia increases oxygen delivery but the resultant hyperviscocity can result in multiple symptoms including headaches, altered mental activity, fatigue, myalgia and visual problems. Dehydration can worsen the situation. Recurrent venesection is one possible treatment.

Iron-deficiency anaemia

This is often a result of excessive venesection, but can also occur secondary to haemoptysis and epistaxis.

Stroke

Arterial thrombosis may be associated with polycythaemia. Alternatively, thrombotic strokes may occur secondary to paradoxical emboli. Haemorrhagic strokes are also possible as coagulation pathways may be deranged, thereby increasing the risk of bleeding.

Bleeding abnormalities

There is a range of presentations, ranging from easy bruising to epistaxis and haemoptysis. Bleeding can be catastrophic.

Renal impairment

Overt renal failure is rare and often associated with increased uric acid absorption from excessive erythrocyte degradation.

2.7.2.1 Tetralogy of Fallot

Anatomy/pathophysiology/pathology

Four anatomical defects contribute to this abnormality (Fig. 69):

1. large ventricular septal defect (VSD);

2. overriding of the aorta;

3. right ventricular outflow tract obstruction (RVOTO);

4. compensatory right ventricular hypertrophy (RVH).

The large VSD results in equal left and right ventricular pressures.

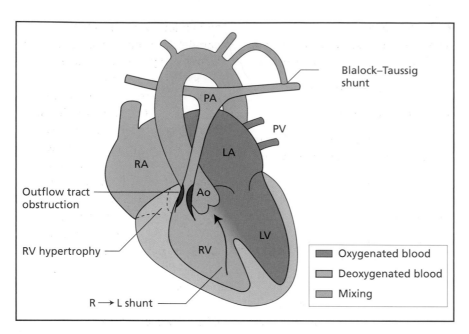

▲ **Fig. 69** Tetralogy of Fallot with left Blalock–Taussig shunt. Ao, aorta; LA, left atrium; LV, left ventricle; PA, pulmonary artery; PV, pulmonary veins; RA, right atrium; RV, right ventricle.

However, there is right-to-left shunting (cyanosis) as result of RVOTO. Shunting (and hence level of cyanosis) increases with any decrease in systemic vascular resistance. Most patients require some form of partial or complete surgical correction to ensure their survival into adult life. Partial surgical correction involves a surgical shunt to increase pulmonary flow and reduce cyanosis, commonly achieved by a Blalock–Taussig shunt (Fig. 69), which connects the subclavian artery to the pulmonary artery.

Epidemiology

This is the most common cyanotic congenital heart defect to occur after infancy and accounts for around 10% of all cogenital heart abnormalities.

Clinical presentation

- Patients who have had no correction present with cyanosis from birth or early infancy and become progressively more short of breath on exertion as their age increases.

- Patients with partial correction develop increasing cyanosis in adult life as RVOTO increases.

- Patients who have had total correction can present later in life with palpitations and syncope (from atrial and ventricular arrhythmias) as well as heart failure as pulmonary and/or aortic valve regurgitation develops.

- All patients have complications of cyanosis.

Physical signs

- Cyanosis.

- Clubbing (Fig. 70).

- There may be unequal upper limb pulses in patients with Blalock–Taussig shunts.

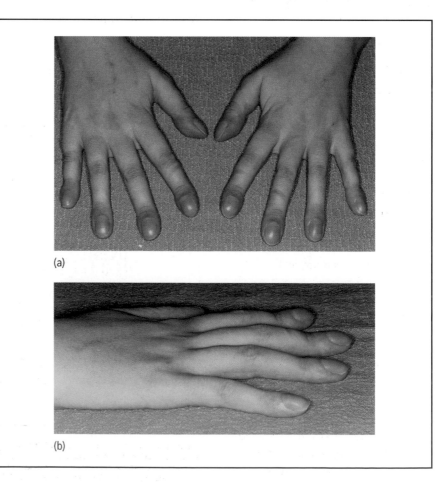

(a)

(b)

▲ **Fig. 70** Example of digital clubbing in a patient with cyanotic heart disease.

- Right ventricular heave and right ventricular outflow tract thrill.

- Normal S1, inaudible P2.

- Right ventricular outflow tract ejection systolic murmur.

Investigations

ECG
Can illustrate right-axis deviation, RVH and right bundle-branch block.

Chest radiograph
Will detect boot-shaped heart.

Echocardiography
Demonstrates all anatomical features which constitue the condition.

Cardiac MRI
As with echocardiography, cardiac MRI can be used to identify anatomical abnormalities, but has the added advantage of identifying other thoracic (pulmonary vascular and aortic) abnormalities.

Cardiac catheterisation
Useful preoperatively for identifying coronary arterial abnormalities.

Treatment
Most patients now undergo complete repair during infancy. In adulthood most of these individuals will require repeat surgical procedures for repair of recurrent VSDs and regurgitation in the right ventricular outflow tract/pulmonary valve and/or aortic valve. Adults who have had partial repair (eg Blalock–Taussig shunt) should be considered for complete repair in adult life as cyanosis worsens or other complications develop. Surgical repair is still recommended for adults who have had no form of correction. This is now extremely rare in the developed world.

Complications
These are often seen in patients who have complete correction as a child:

- ventricular arrhythmias;

- atrial fibrillaton and/or flutter;

- pulmonary regurgitation with right ventricular dilatation and failure;

- recurrent RVOTO.

Prognosis

- Without surgical repair, the survival rate is 66% at age 1 and 10% at age 20 years.

- With complete surgical correction outcomes are excellent, with over 94% of patients surviving at least 25 years.

2.7.2.2 Complete transposition of great arteries

Anatomy/pathophysiology/pathology
In patients with complete transposition of the great arteries (TGA) the pulmonary and systemic circulations are connected in parallel. The aorta arises anteriorly from the right ventricle (RV), the systemic ventricle, and the pulmonary artery (PA) from the left ventricle (LV). As a result the two circulations are completely separate. A communication such as a patent foramen ovale, patent ductus arteriosus or atrial septal defect/ventricular septal defect between the two circulations is necessary for survival (Fig. 71). Other anatomical variants, such as congenitally corrected TGA, also exist.

Clinical presentation
The majority of patients who survive to adulthood will have had a surgical corrective procedure soon after birth.

- Cyanosis is present from birth.

- Heart failure and valvular regurgitation (secondary to degenerative changes) are commonly seen in adults who have had corrective surgery.

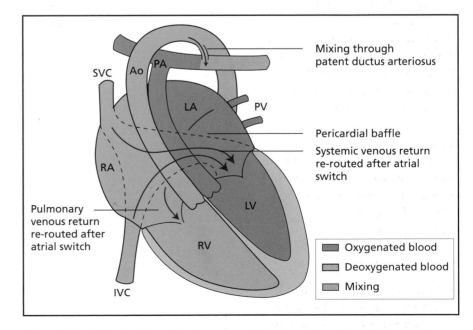

▲ **Fig. 71** TGA with the circulations mixing through a patent ductus arteriosus. The effect of an atrial switch operation is shown in dashed lines, re-routing the venous return to the correct great vessel. In the arterial switch, the great vessels are transected above the valves and switched, with reimplantation of the coronaries. Ao, aorta; IVC, inferior vena cava; LA, left atrium; LV, left ventricle; PA, pulmonary artery; PV, pulmonary veins; RA, right atrium; RV, right ventricle; SVC, superior vena cava.

Physical signs

- Cyanosis.

- Signs of heart failure.

- Single loud S2 (anterior aorta).

Investigations

ECG

Findings are variable and depend on exact anatomy and type of surgical correction. These include normal traces, atrial arrhythmias, RV hypertrophy and right bundle-branch block.

Chest radiograph

Narrow vascular pedicle and cardiomegaly.

Echocardiography

Demonstrates anatomical changes, calculates shunts and shows valvular abnormalities post repair.

Cardiac MRI

Very effective at demonstrating anatomical abnormalities and useful in monitoring patients postoperatively.

Treatment

Emergency

Mixing of blood between the pulmonary and systemic circulation is vital for survival at birth. This can be achieved with prostaglandin E to maintain a patent ductus arteriosus and/or atrial septostomy.

Surgery

A number of complex surgical procedures have been developed.

Atrial switch procedures (Mustard or Senning procedures) Blood is redirected at the level of the atria using a baffle made from either Terylene (Dacron)/pericardium (Mustard procedure) or atrial flaps (Senning procedure) in order to restore physiological circulation. Blood from the pulmonary veins is directed through the mitral valve and blood from the systemic venous return through the tricuspid valve. However, the RV remains the systemic ventricle and commonly fails in adult life (Fig. 71).

Arterial switch procedures Blood is redirected at the arterial level by switching the position of the aorta and the PA. Therefore, the LV is connected to the aorta and the RV to the PA.

Heart transplantation Potential option for patients with significant heart failure subsequent to corrective surgery.

Prognosis

- Without intervention the mortality rate is around 90% by 6 months.

- Life expectancy is shortened in most patients even if they do have surgical correction. Only 70% of patients survive more than 20–30 years after corrective surgery.

2.7.2.3 Ebstein's anomaly

Anatomy/pathophysiology/ pathology

An abnormal tricuspid valve (regurgitant or stenotic) is displaced down into the right ventricle, leaving a small functional right ventricle. A majority of patients (80%) have other associated cardiac abnormalities, including atrial septal defect or patent foramen ovale (most common, seen in 50% of cases), aberrant conduction pathways, ventricular septal defect, coarctation of the aorta, patent ductus arteriosus and, on rare occasions, other more complex abnormalities. If the abnormality is mild, most patients remain asymptomatic well into adult life. Right-to-left shunting secondary to rising right atrial pressure (Fig. 72) leads to symptoms.

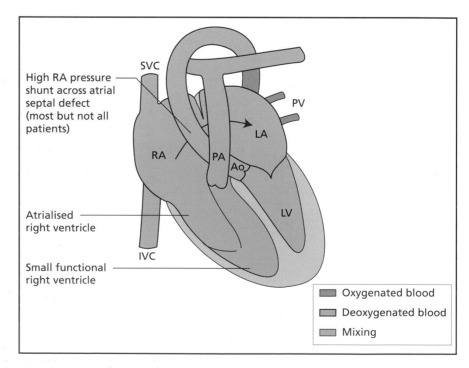

▲ **Fig. 72** Ebstein's anomaly with shunting across an associated atrial septal defect. Ao, aorta; IVC, inferior vena cava; LA, left atrium; LV, left ventricle; PA, pulmonary artery; PV, pulmonary veins; RA, right atrium; SVC, superior vena cava.

Clinical presentation

There is a wide spectrum of presentation.

- In mild disease patients remain entirely asymptomatic well into adult life and diagnosis is made incidentally.

- Progressive dyspnoea, reduced exercise tolerance and palpitations can occur in the event of a worsening shunt.

- In rare instances sudden death can occur as a result of conduction abnormalities.

Physical signs

- Low JVP secondary to a large compliant right atrium.

- Pansystolic murmur of tricuspid regurgitation.

- Hepatomegaly.

- Cyanosis depending on the extent of the right-to-left shunt.

Investigations

ECG

An ECG may be normal, but common abnormalities include tall/broad P waves, right bundle-branch block, first-degree heart block, delta waves if abnormal conduction pathways present and atrial arrhythmias (atrial fibrillation and flutter).

Chest radiograph

Convex right heart border secondary to right atrial enlargement. Cardiomegaly is also a possibility.

Echocardiography and cardiac MRI

Both can be used to make the diagnosis and outline other associated cardiac abnormalities.

Treatment

- Repair of the anatomical abnormality should be

considered if there is progressive symptoms, cyanosis or heart failure. Multiple surgical procedures are available depending on the exact anatomy, including tricuspid valve repair/replacement and more complex surgical corrective procedures.

- Complications (such as heart failure and arrhythmias) should be treated conventionally.

Complications

Common complications include arrhythmias arising from the atria, often from aberrant conduction pathways (eg Wolff–Parkinson–White syndrome).

Prognosis

Patients with no symptoms have a good prognosis without surgical correction and can survive well into adult life. The medium-term prognosis of patients who have undergone successful surgery is good, but they require long-term

follow-up to ensure symptoms do not recur.

2.7.3 Eisenmenger's syndrome

Aetiology/pathophysiology/pathology

A large left-to-right shunt causes increased pulmonary blood flow. Over time this can result in vascular obstructive disease leading to pulmonary hypertension and right ventricular hypertrophy. As the pulmonary arterial pressures approach and exceed systemic pressures, the original left-to-right shunt becomes bidirectional and then reverses (right to left). This shunt reversal results in cyanosis. These changes and their associated complications are known as Eisenmenger's syndrome and can complicate both 'simple' (eg atrial septal defect and ventricular septal defect) as well as more 'complex' congenital cardiac abnormalities. Shunt reversal often takes many years and typically occurs in the third decade (Fig. 73).

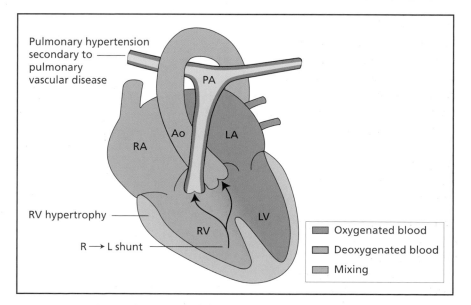

▲ **Fig. 73** Eisenmenger's syndrome secondary to ventricular septal defect. Ao, aorta; LA, left atrium; LV, left ventricle; PA, pulmonary artery; RA, right atrium; RV, right ventricle.

Clinical presentation

- Cyanosis.

- Limiting exertional dyspnoea.

- Palpitations secondary to atrial arrhythmias (atrial fibrillation and flutter) and ventricular arrhythmias (ventricular tachycardia).

- Haemoptysis.

- Syncope and sudden death.

- Congestive heart failure.

Physical signs

- Cyanosis.

- Clubbing.

- Signs of pulmonary hypertension: right ventricular heave, right ventricular outflow tract thrill, loud P2, pulmonary ejection flow murmur and high-pitched early diastolic murmur of pulmonary regurgitation (Graham Steell murmur).

- Signs of tricuspid regurgitation (elevated JVP and pansystolic murmur).

⚠ In Eisenmenger's syndrome, the murmur of the original shunt will have disappeared.

Investigations

ECG
Peaked P waves (right atrial enlargement), right ventricular hypertrophy and atrial arrhythmias.

Chest radiograph
Prominent central pulmonary arteries and 'pruning' of peripheral pulmonary vessels.

Echocardiography
Can be used to identify the anatomic site and direction of the shunt. The shunt can also be quantified.

Cardiac catheterisation
Pulmonary pressure and saturation can be measured directly. It also allows assessment of pulmonary vascular reactivity, which may determine the succes of future surgical procedure.

Treatment
The main management principle in this group of patients is to avoid any factors that may destabilise the circulation and to treat any complications. In those with reactive pulmonary vessels, surgical correction of the underlying shunt may be of value. In the remaining patients, a combination of oxygen therapy, prostacyclin and/or calcium channel blockers may provide variable levels of disease stability and marginal symptom improvement. Lung and/or heart transplantation may be required (see Section 2.12.1).

Prognosis
After diagnosis, the 10-year survival is 80% and the 25-year survival 40%. A poor prognosis is associated with the following:

- syncope.

- signs of right ventricular failure;

- low cardiac output;

- severe hypoxaemia.

Prevention
Early closure of haemodynamically significant left-to-right shunts and/or protective pulmonary artery banding will reduce pulmonary flow and avoid development of pulmonary vascular disease.

2.8 Infective diseases of the heart

2.8.1 Infective endocarditis

Aetiology/pathophysiology/pathology
Microbial infection of the endocardium develops as a result of a two-stage process.

1. Non-bacterial thrombotic endocarditis (NBTE): a sterile mass arises from the deposition of platelets and fibrin on areas of endocardium injured from exposure to high-velocity jets, flow from high- to low-pressure chambers, and flow across a narrow orifice.

2. Bacteraemia with organisms that have the capacity to adhere to NBTE result in the formation of infected vegetation. Bacteraemia rates are higher in the presence of diseased mucosa, especially if infected.

The consequences of infective endocarditis (IE) vary from trivial to catastrophic valvular and paravalvular tissue destruction. Risk factors for IE are classified as cardiac or non-cardiac and are summarised in Table 32.

Epidemiology
The incidence of IE in North America and Western Europe remains unchanged at around 1.7–6.2 per 100,000 person-years. The risk of IE increases with age and it is more common in men. However, the risk profile of IE patients has changed over the past decade. Rheumatic heart disease is no longer the leading cause of IE and has been replaced by increasing cases of IE ocurring secondary to intravenous drug abuse,

TABLE 32 RISK FACTORS FOR IE

System	Level of Risk	Cause
Cardiac	*High*	Prosthetic heart valves Aortic and mitral (especially regurgitation) valve disease Cyanotic congenital heart disease Uncorrected left-to-right shunts (except atrial septal defect)
	Moderate	Mitral valve prolapse/isolated mitral stenosis Tricuspid and pulmonary valve disease Hypertrophic cardiomyopathy
	Low	Isolated ASD MVP with no regurgitation Corrected left-to-right shunt Atrial myxoma Cardiac pacemakers
Non-cardiac		Recurrent bacteraemia (intravenous drug abuse and periodontal disease) Medical conditions increasing risk of infection (eg diabetes, renal failure and immunosuppression)

ASD, atrial septal defect; IE, infective endocarditis; MVP, mitral value prolapse.

- pulmonary, causing lung abscess or pneumonia;
- other arterial territories including joints and soft-tissue infections.

> IE must always be considered in a patient presenting with chronic fever, weight loss and malaise, irrespective of the presence of a murmur. Elderly patients may present with little apart from confusion. The absence of the much over-emphasised 'classic' signs of Janeway's lesions, Osler's nodes, etc does not exclude the diagnosis.

implantation of intracardiac devices, haemodialysis and increasing age.

Clinical presentation and physical signs

IE can present rapidly (acute IE) or insidiously (subacute IE) over a number of days to weeks. Clinical features of IE are varied and at times it can be difficult to initially differentiate from other chronic medical conditions (Fig. 74).

Features of systemic sepsis

Fever and rigors, sweats, general malaise, anorexia and weight loss.

Local cardiac manifestations

New cardiac murmur, heart failure, pericarditis and conduction abnormalities.

Features of immune complex deposition

- Dermatological: petechiae (most common), splinter haemorrhages, Osler's nodes and Janeway lesions.
- Ophthalmological: Roth spots, conjunctival and retinal haemorrhage.

- Renal: features of glomerulonephritis and renal impairment.

Embolic events

Septic emboli seen in 20–40% of cases including:

- cerebral, leading to abscess formation and focal neurological abnormalities;
- spleen, leading to pain secondary to infarction;
- renal, resulting in renal failure;

Investigations

A definite pathological diagnosis can be achieved only via isolation or culture of the bacteria from material obtained from a vegetation or abscess. This is not possible in most patients, and diagnosis depends on a combination of clinical criteria. The modified Duke Criteria (Table 33) based on a number of major and minor clinical and microbiological features are designed to assist diagnosis of IE. Cases are defined as follows.

- Definite IE: presence of two major criteria, one major and three minor criteria or five minor criteria.

TABLE 33 DUKE CRITERIA FOR THE DIAGNOSIS OF IE

Criteria Grade	Clinical Evidence
Major	Microbiological: typical microorganism isolated from two separate blood cultures or persistently positive blood cultures Evidence of cardiac involvement: echocardiographic evidence of new native or prosthetic valve regurgitation, vegetation and/or intracardiac abscess
Minor	Presence of risk factor predisposing to IE (see Table 32) Fever >38°C Vascular complications Immune complications Microbiological findings that do not meet major criteria

IE, infective endocarditis.

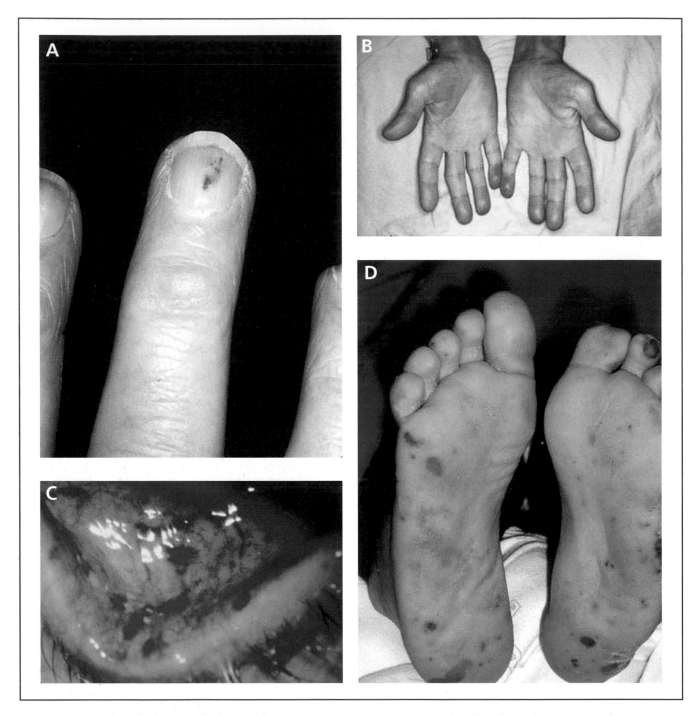

▲ **Fig. 74** Peripheral manifestations of IE including: (**a**) finger splinter haemorrhage; (**b**) Osler's nodes; (**c**) Conjunctival petechiae; (**d**) Janeway's lesions.

- Possible IE: presence of one major and one minor criteria or three minor criteria.

- Unlikely diagnosis: presence of firm alternative diagnosis, or sustained resolution of clinical features with less than 4 days of antibiotic therapy.

Blood tests

FBC:

- Mild-to-moderate normochromic/ normocytic anaemia.

- Neutrophil leucocytosis is usual in acute IE.

- Thrombocytopenia in chronic infections.

Biochemical profile:

- Renal function (urea and creatinine) may be deranged.

- Liver function tests may be abnormal, especially alkaline phosphatase and γ-glutamyl transpeptidase.

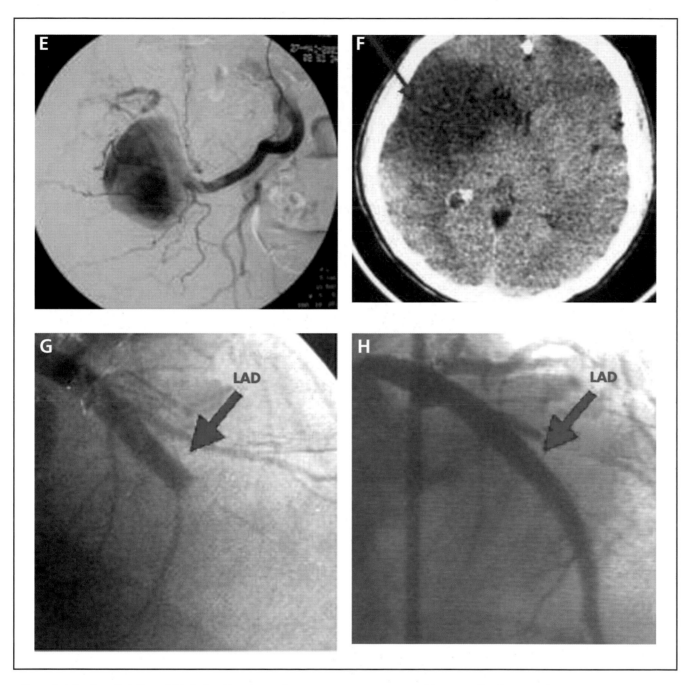

▲ **Fig. 74** Peripheral manifestations of IE including: (**e**) angiogram demonstrating mycotic aneurysm of iliac artery; (**f**) CT brain scan showing cerebral infarction in a patient with staphylococcal endocarditis; (**g**) coronary angiogram showing embolic obstraction of the left anterior descending artery in a parent with streptococcus bovis endocarditis; and (**h**) the same patient as in panel (**g**) after angioplasty. (Adapted and with permission from BMJ Publishing Group; from Habib G. Management of infective endocarditis. *Heart* 2006; 92: 124–30.)

Acute-phase markers:

- C-reactive protein (CRP) and erythrocyte sedimentation rate (ESR) are typically elevated.

Immunology:

- Polyclonal increase in serum immunoglobulins.

- Reduced complement levels.

- Positive rheumatoid factor.

Microbiology
Blood culture:

- Take at least three to four sets of blood cultures from different sites, leaving around 60 minutes between each puncture.

- Discuss cultures with microbiologist to ascertain if there is a need for prolonged cultures and the use of specific culture media for infections caused by fastidious organisms and fungi.

TABLE 34 INFECTIVE ORGANISMS ISOLATED IN MICROBIOLOGICAL INVESTIGATIONS

Infective organisms	Frequency (%)
Streptococci (especially *Streptococcus viridans* group)	50–60
Staphylococci (coagulase-positive *Staphylococcus aureus*, coagulase-negative *Staphylococcus epidermidis*)	25
Enterococci	10

Culture-negative organisms
    Fastidious organisms (Mycobacteria, *Brucella*, *Neisseria*, *Legionella* and the HACEK group of oropharyngeal organisms)
    Previous antibiotic therapy
    Chlamydia
    Rickettsiae (eg *Coxiella*)
	5–10

Gram-negative bacteria, mixed organisms and fungi	<1

HACEK, *Haemophilus, Actinobacillus, Cardiobacterium, Eikinella, Kingella.*

 A normal echocardiogram does not exclude a diagnosis of IE.

Serum:

• Take a sample of serum for immunological tests of atypical organisms, including *Aspergillus* precipitins, *Candida* antibodies, rising *Brucella* agglutinins (two samples required) and *Chlamydia* complement fixation tests.

See Table 34.

Chest radiograph
This is usually normal. There may be evidence of pulmonary oedema and areas of infarction or consolidation from septic emboli (often associated with involvement of the right-sided heart valves).

ECG
Important to look for prolongation of the PR interval or higher levels of atrioventricular (AV) block, indicating involvement of the conduction system (commonly associated with aortic root abscess).

Urinalysis
Microscopic haematuria with or without proteinuria is common. Heavy proteinuria and red cell casts indicate glomerulonephritis.

Echocardiography
Transthoracic echocardiography is the first-line investigation for native valve IE, looking for evidence of new valve regurgitation and/or vegetations. If inadequate, negative or non-diagnostic in a patient with high suspicion of IE, transoesophageal echocardiography (TOE) should be performed. TOE is more sensitive for imaging of the aortic root (especially detection of an abscess) and the mitral valve (Fig. 75). TOE is the investigation of choice in suspected prosthetic valve IE.

Treatment

Medical treatment
Antibiotics are the main therapy. 'Blind' treatment (Table 35 shows a sample protocol) should be started as soon as a clinical diagnosis of IE is suspected (after multiple blood cultures have been taken). Early disscussion with microbiology and cardiothoracic teams is important. Identification of the infective organism is invaluable and antibiotic treatment should be modified according to sensitivities. Duration of therapy varies according to the severity of infection and organism. Often a total antibiotic course of around 4–6 weeks is required, with intravenous administration during the first 2 weeks.

All patients must be closely monitored to chart their response to treatment.

• Daily monitoring for clinical signs of ongoing infection, such as persistent fever, changing and/or new cardiac murmurs, and embolic signs.

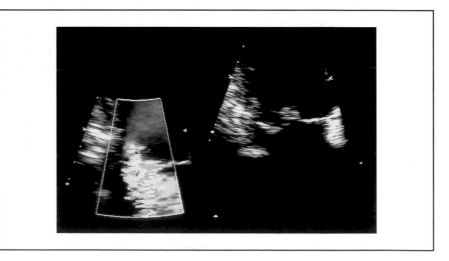

▲ **Fig. 75** Transoesophageal echocardiogram showing (on right) a vegetation on the atrial side of a native mitral valve and (on left) assounted mitral regurgitation.

TABLE 35 'BLIND' ANTIBIOTIC TREATMENT FOR INFECTIVE ENDOCARDITIS. MODIFY WHEN MICROBIOLOGICAL SENSITIVITIES ARE KNOWN

Presentation	Antibiotic regimen
Gradual onset	Benzylpenicillin 2.4 g iv 4-hourly + gentamicin 3 mg/kg daily in one to three divided doses guided by levels
Acute onset	Flucloxacillin 2 g iv 6-hourly + gentamicin 3 mg/kg daily in one to three divided doses guided by levels
Recent prosthetic valve	Vancomycin 15 mg/kg iv 12-hourly infused over 60 minutes guided by levels + gentamicin 3 mg/kg daily in one to three divided doses guided by levels + rifampicin 300 mg po 12-hourly
Intravenous drug abuser	Vancomycin 15 mg/kg iv 12-hourly infused over 60 minutes guided by levels + flucloxacillin 2 g iv 6-hourly

- Regular monitoring of changes in acute-phase markers (CRP and ESR).

- Regular urinalysis.

- Twice-weekly ECG looking for conduction abnormalities.

- Weekly echocardiogram.

- Monitoring of antibiotic levels (especially for aminoglycoside antibiotics and vancomycin).

Surgical treatment
Surgical treatment should be considered in the following scenarios:

- haemodynamic compromise secondary to valve destruction;

- inadequate response to medical treatment and/or relapsing infection (consider early surgery for fungal and prosthetic valve endocarditis);

- complications including formation of intracardiac abscess, high-degree AV block, recurrent septic emboli, perforation of intracardiac structures (eg interventricular septum and chordae) and unstable prosthetic valves.

Prognosis
Endocarditis is a serious medical condition with a high mortality rate. Prognosis is variable and depends on the infective organism and clinical scenario. In an uncomplicated streptococcal native valve endocarditis, the mortality rate is <10%, whereas *Aspergillus* prosthetic valve endocarditis is associated with virtually a 100% mortality rate.

FURTHER READING

Habib G. Management of infective endocarditis. *Heart* 2006; 92: 124–30.

Melikian N. Infective endocarditis in cardiovascular emergencies. In: Ramrakha P and Moore K, eds. *Oxford Handbook of Acute Medicine*, 2nd edn. Oxford: Oxford University Press, 2004: 120–30.

Mylonakis E and Calderwood SB. Infective endocarditis in adults. *N. Eng. J. Med.* 2001; 345: 1318–30.

2.8.2 Rheumatic fever

Aetiology/pathophysiology/pathology
Rheumatic fever results from an abnormal immune response to pharyngeal infection with group A β-haemolytic streptococci. There is evidence of a genetic predisposition with specific B-cell antibody D8/17 in over 90% of patients, and linkage with HLA-DR1, -DR2, -DR3 and -DR4.

Characteristic perivascular Aschoff's nodules have a widespread distribution in the connective tissues of joints, tendons and blood vessels. A pancarditis may develop, with endocardial inflammation affecting valve leaflets, chordae tendineae and papillary muscles. Fusion of leaflets and chordae leads most commonly to mitral stenosis, which is worsened further by the progressive fibrosis and eventual calcification that occur after the acute episode (Fig. 76). Mitral regurgitation may occur and tricuspid involvement is seen in 10% of rheumatic fever cases. Aortic valve involvement more commonly leads to aortic regurgitation.

Epidemiology
Rheumatic fever is rare in developed countries, with an incidence of <5 per 100,000 per year, usually between the ages of 4 and 18.

Clinical presentation/physical signs/investigations
See Table 36.

Blood cultures
These help to exclude infective endocarditis (IE).

Blood tests
Look for the following:

- anaemia and leucocytosis;

- elevated ESR and CRP;

- streptococcal serology.

ECG

- Normal.

- May show prolonged PR interval.

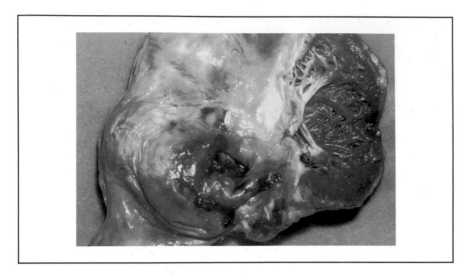

▲ **Fig. 76** Rheumatic mitral valve disease. The thickened and contracted mitral valve leaflets with the fish-mouth valve orifice can be seen in this post-mortem specimen.

TABLE 36 DUCKETT–JONES CRITERIA FOR DIAGNOSIS OF RHEUMATIC FEVER

Major	Minor
Carditis	Fever
Migrating polyarthritis	Previous rheumatic fever
Chorea	Raised CRP or ESR
Erythema marginatum	Arthralgia
Subcutaneous nodules	Long PR interval

Diagnosis is based on evidence of antecedent streptococcal infection – eg positive throat swab for group A β-haemolytic streptococci, (GAS), elevated streptococcal antibodies or a history of recent scarlet fever – together with either two or more major criteria, or one major plus two minor criteria.

CRP, C-reactive protein; ESR, erythrocyte sedimentation rate.

Chest radiograph

This is either normal or shows cardiomegaly, pericardial effusion, pulmonary oedema or increased pulmonary vascularity.

Echocardiography

Echocardiography helps to exclude IE, valvular abnormalities, myocardial dysfunction, pericarditis and pericardial effusion.

Consider the following in your differential diagnosis:

- IE;
- viral infection with or without congenital cardiac abnormality;
- non-rheumatic acute streptococcal infections;
- juvenile chronic arthritis;
- systemic lupus erythematosus;
- traumatic or septic arthritis;
- gout.

Treatment

Emergency

Treat heart failure (see Section 2.3). Severe valve lesions with deteriorating cardiac function may require valve replacement in rare instances.

Short term

Bed-rest eases joint pains. A 10-day course of oral/intramuscular penicillin (erythromycin in allergic patients) will eradicate the organism. Treatment with salicylates or steroids is symptomatic and does not affect the outcome.

Long term

Duration of anti-inflammatory therapy varies from 1 month in mild cases to 2–3 months in more severe ones. Taper steroid therapy at the end of the course with the substitution of aspirin to reduce rebound inflammation.

Prognosis

Joint pain and fever usually settle within 2 weeks. The risk of residual heart disease increases with the severity of the initial carditis, as does the risk of further damage during any rheumatic recurrence.

FURTHER READING

da Silva NA and Pereira BA. Acute rheumatic fever. Still a challenge. *Rheum. Dis. Clin. North Am.* 1997; 23: 545–68.

2.9 Cardiac tumours

Aetiology/pathophysiology/pathology

Most cardiac tumours are secondary deposits. Cardiac metastasis occurs most commonly with lung and breast carcinomas and melanosarcomas. The most common primary cardiac tumour is a myxoma; 75% of myxomas occur in the left atrium, the remainder in the right atrium and ventricle. Myxomas usually arise from the endocardium at the border of the fossa ovalis as a pedunculated mass. This may prolapse through the mitral valve (MV) mimicking mitral stenosis.

Renal cell carcinoma may invade the inferior vena cava (IVC) into the right heart, resulting in signs of right heart failure. Carcinoid tumours may embolise to the tricuspid valve, resulting in regurgitation.

Epidemiology
The prevalence of myxoma is estimated at 2 per 100,000, most commonly in those aged 30–60 years. The female to male ratio is 2:1.

Clinical presentation
Myxomas are discovered when individuals present with constitutional upset or the effects of MV obstruction, or the tumour is an incidental finding. Symptoms include fever, malaise, exertional dyspnoea and weight loss. Transient pulmonary oedema, paroxysmal nocturnal dyspnoea, haemoptysis, dizziness and syncope may occur. The first presentation may be due to an embolic phenomenon.

Malignant tumours usually present acutely with haemorrhagic pericardial effusions or heart block. Renal cell cancer invading the IVC may present with signs of right heart failure and a renal mass. Carcinoid metastasis to the tricuspid valve may present with facial flushing and bronchospasm.

Physical signs
Fever, finger clubbing and anaemia of chronic disease reflect the chronic nature of myxomas. A tumour 'plop' may be heard, or auscultatory

findings of mitral stenosis with or without regurgitation may be present. The murmur varies with posture, unlike in cases of valvular disease.

Investigations

Blood tests
In myxomas these typically show the anaemia of chronic disease, raised inflammatory markers (erythrocyte

sedimentation rate and C-reactive protein) and gamma-globulins.

Chest radiograph
The tumour may distort the cardiac silhouette. Sudden cardiac or pericardial enlargement, mediastinal lymphadenopathy or an irregular/ indistinct cardiac border may be seen. Intracardiac calcification may occur in myxomas (Fig. 77).

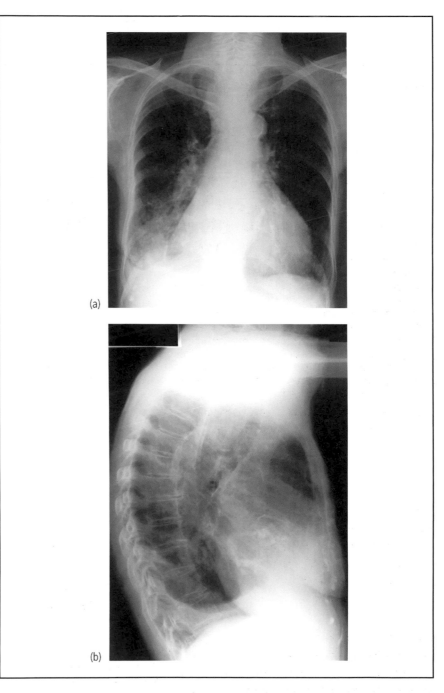

▲ **Fig. 77** Intracardiac calcification: **(a)** posteroanterior and **(b)** lateral views illustrating visible deposition of calcium within the heart.

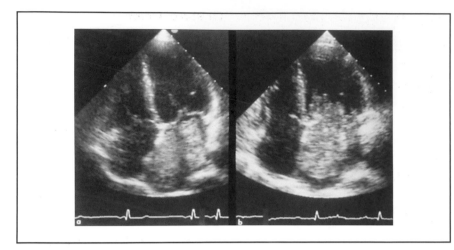

▲ Fig. 78 Echocardiography: left atrial myxoma. (Courtesy of Dr J. Chambers.)

Echocardiography

This is usually visible on ransthoracic echo, but transoesophageal echocardiography may be required in some cases (Fig. 78).

Differential diagnosis

Consider endocarditis and MV disease.

Treatment

Urgent surgical resection of myxomas is required: delay risks embolisation ('never let the sun go down on a myxoma'). Most malignant tumours are treated palliatively, although renal cell tumours invading the IVC may be excised. Palliative chemotherapy may be appropriate for certain tumour types.

Complications

Myxomas may embolise or cause pulmonary oedema due to MV obstruction. Malignant disease may cause tamponade, heart block, arrhythmias and heart failure. Recurrent pericardial effusions are treated with a pericardial window.

Prognosis

Once removed, the prognosis for patients with myxoma is a normal lifespan.

Disease associations

Myxomas can be familial (Carney's syndrome or 'syndrome myxoma'), with autosomal dominant transmission in 10% of cases. This is associated with endocrine hyperactivity, lentigines and myxomas elsewhere in the body. Multiple tumours occur in approximately 50% of familial cases, and are more common in the ventricle. The mean age of presentation of familial cases is 25 years, and for sporadic cases 56 years.

2.10 Traumatic heart disease

Traumatic heart disease is often fatal. Rapid diagnosis and intervention are vital to reduce both mortality and morbidity.

Aetiology

- Road traffic accident.

- Assault (non-penetrating or penetrating, including stab and gunshot wounds).

- Sports injuries.

- Falls.

- Iatrogenic (catheter, pacing/ implantable cardioverter defibrillator lead or pericardiocentesis induced, or post cardiopulmonary resuscitation).

Pathophysiology/pathology

Virtually all cardiac components may be affected by thoracic trauma.

- Myocardium: contusion (approximately 20% of patients after blunt trauma) and laceration/ pericardial tamponade or rupture (ventricles more than atria, and interventricular septum); 80% of stab wounds will present with tamponade. In the acute situation as little as 100 mL of blood is required to cause tamponade.

- Pericardium: pericarditis, laceration or post-pericardiotomy syndrome.

- Endocardium: ruptured chordae/ papillary muscles or valve leaflets/cusps.

- Coronary arteries: injury/rupture/ thrombosis (left anterior descending artery most commonly).

- Conduction system: bundle-branch block, atrioventricular (AV) block or atrial/ventricular arrhythmias.

- Thoracic vessels: trauma to the aorta carries a very high mortality (Table 37).

Clinical presentation

The initial insult is usually obvious and leads directly to presentation. Occasionally, apparent minor trauma causes significant mediastinal injury, leading to a more insidious presentation:

- chest pain (including angina);

- presyncope/syncope.

TABLE 37 KEY FEATURES OF AORTIC TRAUMA

Prognosis	80% will die at scene, and of those that survive >50% die within 48 hours
Site of injury	80–90% between left subclavian and ligamentum arteriosum
Mechanism of injury	Usually blunt trauma with severe deceleration, eg road traffic accident
Symptoms	Retrosternal or interscapular pain
Signs	Hypotension, decreased pulses and systolic murmur
CXR	Widened mediastinum (>8 cm) and oesophageal/tracheal deviation
Treatment	Maintain systolic BP <120 mmHg but may require volume if hypotensive Consider intravenous beta-blockers if hypertensive Urgent cardiothoracic surgical input
Complications	Paraplegia and renal failure

Physical signs

Look for the following:

- hypotension;

- pulsus paradoxus;

- 'muffled' heart sounds;

- pulmonary oedema;

- murmur/thrill of mitral regurgitation;

- diastolic murmur of aortic regurgitation if ascending aorta involved;

- absent or abnormal peripheral pulses.

Investigations

ECG

Look specifically for the following:

- ST/T changes (may be non-specific, ST elevation secondary to pericarditis or acute myocardial infarction);

- conduction abnormlaties (bundle-branch block or any degree of AV block);

- arrhythmias (sinus tachycardia, atrial fibrillation, ectopic beats or ventricular arrhythmias).

Cardiac enzymes

Commonly raised following cardiac trauma but only have prognostic relevance if related to coronary artery trauma.

- Elevated creatine kinase-myocardial bound fraction (may be elevated if there has been huge musculoskeletal trauma).

- Elevated troponin (see Section 3.7).

Chest radiograph

- Widened mediastinum (Fig. 79).

- Ribs/sternal fracture.

- Haemothorax.

Echocardiography (transthoracic and transoesophageal)

- Pericardial effusion.

- Abnormal wall motion (coronary artery involvement).

Transoesophageal echocardiography is best for identifying myocardial injury and valvular involvement. It is contraindicated in the following circumstances:

- severe facial trauma;

- cervical spinal injury;

- possible oesophageal injury.

Aortography

Aortography is usually considered the gold standard for diagnosing aortic trauma (Fig. 80). Damage is most commonly seen in the upper descending aorta, at the site of the ligamentum arteriosum.

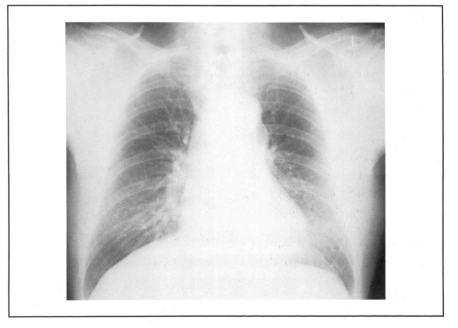

▲ **Fig. 79** CXR of patient with traumatic aortic rupture. Note the widened mediastinum and abnormal descending aortic outline.

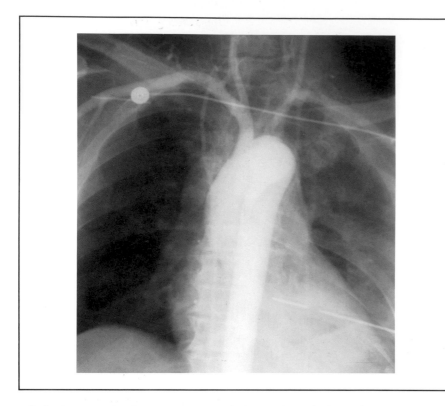

▲ **Fig. 80** Aortogram of aortic rupture/transection. The aortic outline is clearly irregular, representing aortic rupture.

Cross-sectional imaging is helpful in identifying surrounding haematoma. CT is generally performed as the scan is quicker than MRI.

Radionuclide imaging
Reduced myocardial perfusion with contusion or ischaemia secondary to coronary thrombosis may be demonstrated.

Treatment
Each patient must be individually assessed. Patients can be broadly separated as follows.

- Low risk: minor trauma and normal/abnormal ECG.

- High risk: major trauma with associated thoracic or extrathoracic injuries and normal/abnormal ECG.

Emergency
If there is haemodynamic compromise, consider urgent

pericardiocentesis/operative intervention for pericardial tamponade. If there is any doubt, seek immediate contact with a cardiothoracic surgical centre.

If all investigations demonstrate no need for surgical intervention, then gentle mobilisation is encouraged. If there is evidence of possible coronary artery/conduction system injury, then these will need evaluating further.

FURTHER READING

Banning AP and Pillai R. Non-penetrating cardiac and aortic trauma. *Heart* 1997; 78: 226–9.

- - - - - - - - - - - - - - - - -

Olsovsky MR, Wechsler AS and Topaz O. Cardiac trauma diagnosis, management, and current therapy. *Angiology* 1997; 48: 423–32.

- - - - - - - - - - - - - - - - -

Pretre R and Chilcott M. Blunt trauma to the heart and great vessels. *N. Engl. J. Med.* 1997; 336: 626–32.

2.11 Disease of systemic arteries

2.11.1 Aortic dissection

Aetiology/pathophysiology/pathology
The aortic intima tears, exposing a diseased media that is split in two longitudinally by the force of the blood flow. This dissection usually progresses distally for a variable distance. Medial degeneration is often idiopathic but may be the result of cystic medial necrosis, especially in Marfan's syndrome. There is also an association with the following:

- hypertension (history of hypertension in 80% of cases);

- pregnancy;

- trauma.

Aortic dissection is classified according to whether there is involvement of the ascending aorta (Stanford classification, see Fig. 81). This has practical and prognostic implications.

Epidemiology
- Peak age 60 years

- Male/female ratio 2:1.

Clinical presentation

Common
There is central chest pain in 90% of cases, classically a 'tearing' pain that migrates to the back (interscapular) as dissection proceeds. A dissected aorta found incidentally in a patient without pain is usually chronic and therefore low risk. Thoracic back pain of sudden onset is also common.

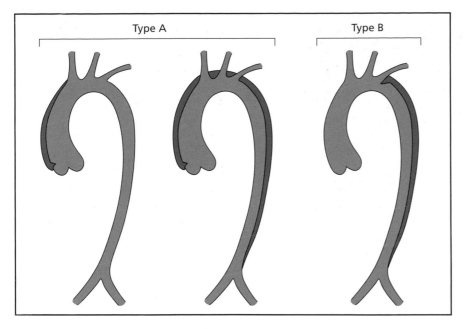

▲ Fig. 81 Stanford classification of aortic dissection. Type A refers to dissection of the ascending aorta, with or without involvement of the descending aorta. In type B, dissection is confined to the descending aorta. This classification has implications for prognosis and treatment.

Uncommon

- Syncope.
- Stroke.
- Acute pulmonary oedema.
- Pulseless electrical activity arrest.

Physical signs

Common

- Hypotension.
- Unequal radial pulses or brachial BPs (found in 50% of proximal dissections).
- Aortic regurgitation.
- Pericardial rub.
- Pleural effusion.
- Tamponade (see Section 2.6.2).
- Hemiplegia.

Investigations

ECG

The ECG may reveal inferior myocardial infarction, if dissection extends to the right coronary artery. Anterior infarction is rarely seen, perhaps because occlusion of the left main coronary artery results in such a big infarct that the patient does not reach hospital alive.

Chest radiograph

This may show widened mediastinum (Fig. 82), but an absence of this does not rule out aortic dissection. Blood in the pleural space from a leaking aorta may show as an effusion.

Echocardiography

The diagnosis is suggested by:

- dilated aortic root;
- aortic regurgitation;
- pericardial effusion;
- dissection flap in the ascending aorta (unusual).

Other investigations

Consider the following:

- CT scan of the chest with contrast;
- aortography;
- MRI;
- transoesophageal echocardiography (Fig. 83).

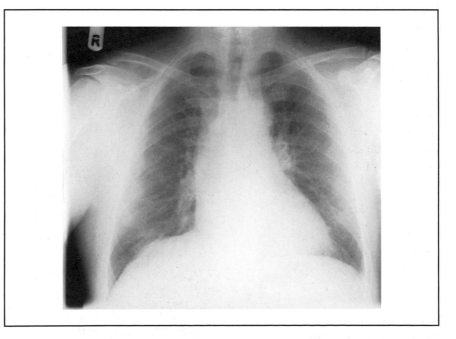

▲ Fig. 82 Chest radiograph showing widened mediastinum. Blood in the pleural space from a leaking aorta may show as an effusion.

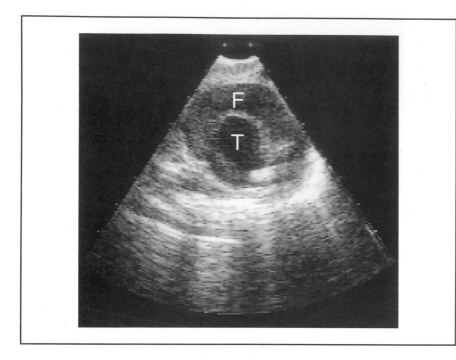

▲ **Fig. 83** Transoesophageal echocardiogram of aortic dissection demonstrating the true (T) and false (F) lumina in the descending aorta. (From Armstrong P and Wastie ML. *Diagnostic Imaging* (4th edn). Oxford: Blackwell Science, 1998.)

> The differential diagnosis of aortic dissection should include the following:
>
> - myocardial infarction/unstable angina;
> - thoracic vertebral pathology, eg fracture and discitis;
> - pulmonary embolism.

Treatment

Emergency

- Do not await confirmation of diagnosis before starting medical treatment.

- Transfer to the coronary care unit.

- Lower systolic BP to <120 mmHg with intravenous labetalol or sodium nitroprusside.

- If confirmatory imaging cannot be obtained quickly, arrange urgent transfer to cardiothoracic centre.

- Type A dissection requires emergency repair unless chronic (>2 weeks).

- Type B dissection is generally managed medically because the risks of surgery outweigh the benefits. Consider surgery if there is a rupture or vital organ/limb ischaemia. More recently, endovascular stenting has been used with some success in selected patients who were poor candidates for surgery.

Short term

After 24 hours, begin transfer of BP control to an oral agent, eg beta-blocker, angiotensin-converting enzyme inhibitor or calcium antagonist.

Complications

Death caused by aortic rupture or tamponade is common. Occlusion of any of the major aortic branches may occur, producing the following:

- hemiplegia;

- acute renal failure;

- mesenteric ischaemia;

- lower limb ischaemia.

Prognosis

There is an early mortality rate of 1% per hour if left untreated. The mortality rate in the first 2 weeks is about 80%, after which a dissection would be classed as chronic.

FURTHER READING

Treasure T and Raphael MJ. Investigation of suspected dissection of the thoracic aorta. *Lancet* 1991; 338: 490–5.

2.12 Diseases of pulmonary arteries

2.12.1 Primary pulmonary hypertension

Primary pulmonary hypertension (PPH) is defined as a sustained elevation of pulmonary artery pressure (PAP) to a mean of more than 25 mmHg at rest or 30 mmHg with exercise, in the absence of a demonstrable cause. Recent developments have highlighted that there is some overlap between primary and secondary pulmonary hypertension in their histological features and response to treatment. The latest WHO classification uses five groups defined by their mechanism (Table 38).

Aetiology/pathophysiology/pathology

The aetiology is unknown but the following have been suggested.

- Genetic: 10% of cases are familial (localised to chromosome 2) with autosomal dominant inheritance.

- Autoimmune: associated with a number of collagen vascular disorders.

- Infection: human herpesvirus 8 causes Kaposi's sarcoma.

TABLE 38 CLASSIFICATION OF PULMONARY HYPERTENSION

Classification	Subgroups
Pulmonary arterial hypertension	Idiopathic Familial Associated (collagen, congenital shunt, portal hypertension, HIV, drugs and others)
Pulmonary hypertension with left heart disease	Atrial/ventricular Valvular
Pulmonary hypertension with lung disease	Chronic obstructive pulmonary disease Interstitial Sleep disorder Alveolar hypoventilation High altitude Developmental
Pulmonary hypertension due to thromboembolism	Proximal pulmonary arteries Distal pulmonary arteries Non-thrombotic embolism
Miscellaneous	Sarcoid, tumour, compression, etc

> Clubbing is not a feature of PPH and, if present, may indicate lung disease or cyanotic congenital heart disease as the underlying cause of the pulmonary hypertension.

- Pulmonary vascular endothelial dysfunction.

Increased pulmonary vascular resistance is produced by:

- vasoconstriction;

- vascular wall remodelling (medial hypertrophy and smooth muscle);

- thrombosis *in situ*.

This results in right ventricular hypertrophy and then failure, as a result of the increased afterload.

Epidemiology
Incidence is about 1 per million per year, but the use of appetite suppressants is associated with a greater than 20-fold increased risk. The female/male ratio is 2:1, with most diagnoses made in the fourth decade.

Clinical presentation
Early symptoms of PPH are non-specific.

Common
- Exertional dyspnoea.

- Fatigue.

- Angina (right ventricular ischaemia).

- Syncope/presyncope, especially exertional.

Uncommon
- Peripheral oedema.

- Raynaud's phenomenon (mostly in women).

- Haemoptysis.

Physical signs
- Left parasternal heave.

- Loud P2 (pulmonary component of second heart sound).

- S4 originating from the right ventricle (pressure overload).

- Pansystolic murmur, prominent jugular *v* waves and pulsatile liver of tricuspid regurgitation.

- Peripheral oedema and elevated JVP of right ventricular failure.

Investigations
The following investigations are used to confirm pulmonary hypertension, determine prognosis and guide therapy.

Echocardiography
- Demonstration of dilated and/or hypertrophied right heart (Fig. 84).

- Measurement of PAP.

- Exclusion of shunts and valvular and left ventricular abnormalities.

- A transoesophageal study may be necessary to distinguish an atrial septal defect.

ECG
Look for (Fig. 85):

- tall P waves;

- right-axis deviation;

- right ventricular hypertrophy.

Chest radiograph
Look for prominent pulmonary arteries with peripheral pruning, and for features of underlying lung disease (Fig. 86).

Cardiac catheterisation
Measures pressures and saturations (prognosis and shunt calculation) and assesses response to acute vasodilators such as prostacyclin, adenosine or inhaled nitric oxide.

Investigations to exclude secondary causes
- Blood: FBC (for secondary polycythaemia), liver function

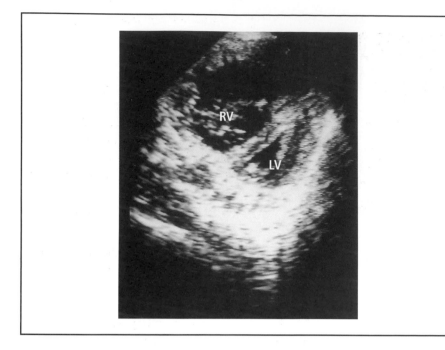

▲ **Fig. 84** Short-axis echocardiographic view of a patient with PPH showing the high-pressure dilated right ventricle (RV) compressing the left ventricle (LV) into a characteristic 'D' shape. (Courtesy of Dr L.M. Shapiro.)

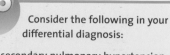

Consider the following in your differential diagnosis:

- secondary pulmonary hypertension;
- left ventricular outflow tract obstruction;
- ischaemic heart disease.

Treatment

- Anticoagulation.

- Diuretics with daily weight checks to avoid excessive fluid depletion.

- Oxygen for hypoxaemia.

- High-dose calcium channel blockers in those patients who have a significant fall in pulmonary vascular resistance on acute vasodilator testing.

In patients who fail to respond to acute vasodilator therapy and have a poor functional class, the following should be considered.

- Endothelin antagonists: bosentan (monitoring of liver function tests is needed).

tests, erythrocyte sedimentation rate, rheumatoid factor and autoantibody screen, and consider an HIV test.

- Pulmonary function tests to exclude obstructive or restrictive lung disease.

- Sleep study if there is suspicion of obstructive sleep apnoea.

- Exclusion of pulmonary thromboembolism by ventilation–perfusion scan, spiral CT scan of the chest with contrast, or pulmonary angiography (Fig. 87).

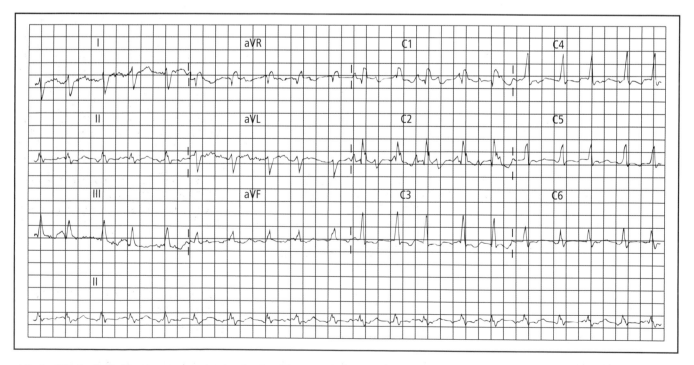

▲ **Fig. 85** ECG of patient with pulmonary hypertension showing right ventricular hypertrophy and right-axis deviation. The patient is also in atrial fibrillation. (Courtesy of the Pulmonary Vascular Disease Unit at Papworth Hospital.)

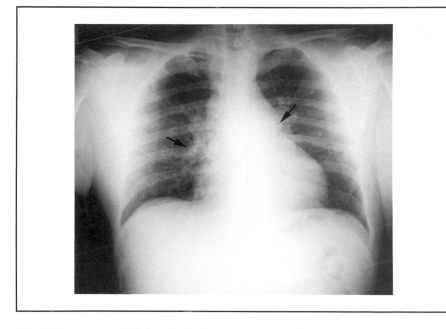

▲ **Fig. 86** Posteroanterior CXR of a patient with pulmonary hypertension showing prominent pulmonary arteries (arrows) and cardiomegaly. (Courtesy of the Pulmonary Vascular Disease Unit at Papworth Hospital.)

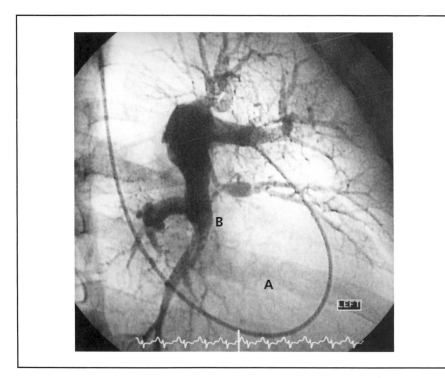

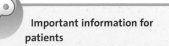

▲ **Fig. 87** Left pulmonary angiogram of a patient with thromboembolic pulmonary hypertension showing (B) the characteristic bands and cut-offs of vessel occlusion and (A) lack of perfusion in the left lower lobe. (Courtesy of the Pulmonary Vascular Disease Unit at Papworth Hospital.)

- Prostacyclin analogues: intravenous/nebulised prostacyclin therapy.

- Phosphodiesterase type 5 antagonists: sildenafil.

- Atrial septostomy to decompress the right ventricle and improve left-sided filling pressures.

- Lung or heart–lung transplantation in those

who fail to respond to any other treatment.

Prognosis

Survival depends on right ventricular function. Overall the 5-year survival rate is 20%, but the subgroup with adverse haemodynamics has a 20% 3-year survival rate. Responders to chronic calcium channel blocker therapy have a 95% 5-year survival rate.

Anticoagulation, prostacyclin and heart–lung transplantation (5-year survival rate of 50–60%) all confer a survival benefit. Bosentan and sildenafil have been shown to improve haemodynamics and exercise capacity.

> **Important information for patients**
>
> Strongly advise against pregnancy. Avoid the oral contraceptive pill if possible – it may exacerbate pulmonary hypertension.

FURTHER READING

Farber HW and Loscalzo J. Pulmonary arterial hypertension. *N. Engl. J. Med.* 2004; 351: 1655–65.

Gaine SP and Rubin LJ. Primary pulmonary hypertension. *Lancet* 1998; 352: 719–25.

Humbert M, Sitbon O and Simonneau G. Treatment of pulmonary arterial hypertension. *N. Engl. J. Med.* 2004; 351: 1425–36.

2.12.2 Secondary pulmonary hypertension

Secondary pulmonary hypertension is defined as sustained elevation of the mean pulmonary artery pressure (PAP) to >25 mmHg at rest or 30 mmHg on exercise, with an identified cause.

Aetiology/pathophysiology
Causes of secondary pulmonary hypertension are shown in Table 39.

Clinical presentation

- Ankle oedema.

- Dyspnoea (may be associated with the underlying primary condition).

- The primary condition.

Physical signs
These include signs of the primary condition, including cyanosis if present, and then of pulmonary hypertension, right ventricular hypertrophy, dilatation and failure:

- left parasternal heave;

- loud P2;

- elevated JVP with prominent *v* wave;

- pansystolic murmur of tricuspid regurgitation;

- pulsatile liver;

- ankle oedema.

Investigations
See Section 2.12.

Differential diagnosis
Consider left ventricular dysfunction and primary pulmonary hypertension.

Treatment

General

- Optimise treatment of the underlying condition.

- Diuretics.

- Calcium channel blockers.

- Consideration of prostacyclin therapy, bosentan and phosphodiesterase type 5 inhibitors.

- Lung or heart–lung transplantation.

Specific
Shunts Consider defect closure or pulmonary artery banding (some protection of pulmonary vasculature against high right-sided flow), if the pulmonary hypertension is not already too severe.

Chronic obstructive pulmonary disease Long-term oxygen therapy benefits selected patients with chronic obstructive pulmonary disease (see *Respiratory Medicine*, Section 2.12.1).

Thromboembolism Anticoagulation and consider inferior vena cava filter or pulmonary thromboendarterectomy.

Ventilatory disorders Consider nocturnal continuous positive airway pressure or nasal positive-pressure ventilation (see *Respiratory Medicine*, Sections 2.12.2 and 2.12.3).

Prognosis
The prognosis is related to the underlying condition and the severity of the pulmonary hypertension. The 5-year survival rate of chronic obstructive pulmonary disease with oedema is 30%.

FURTHER READING

Ricciardi MJ and Rubenfire M. How to manage secondary pulmonary hypertension. *Postgrad. Med.* 1999; 105: 183–90.

TABLE 39 CAUSES OF SECONDARY PULMONARY HYPERTENSION

Mechanism	Cause
Increased left atrial pressure	Aortic/mitral valve disease Left ventricular dysfunction
Left-to-right shunts	Atrial septal defect, ventricular septal defect and patent ductus arteriosus
Chronic pulmonary disease	Chronic obstructive pulmonary disease Bronchiectasis Pulmonary fibrosis
Chronic venous thromboembolism	
Chronic hypoventilation/hypoxia	Kyphoscoliosis Respiratory muscle weakness Obstructive sleep apnoea

Vascular wall remodelling and vasoconstriction increase pulmonary vascular resistance and therefore PAP, with resulting right ventricular hypertrophy and right ventricular failure. When the primary cause is respiratory, this is known as cor pulmonale.

2.13 Cardiac complications of systemic disease

2.13.1 Thyroid disease

Clinical presentation

Hyperthyroidism
A patient with hyperthyroidism may have:

- sinus tachycardia;

- sustained or paroxysmal atrial fibrillation (AF) (5–15% of cases);

- hyperdynamic left ventricle.

Hypothyroidism

A patient with hypothyroidism may have:

- bradycardia with prolonged QT interval;

- cardiac enlargement;

- pericardial effusion;

- associated hypercholesterolaemia.

Treatment

Hyperthyroidism

Short term Beta-blockers for symptomatic relief until rendered euthyroid; AF generally reverts to sinus rhythm with treatment of thyroid disease.

Long term Cardioversion after anticoagulation if AF persists.

Hypothyroidism

Treat with thyroxine, starting in very small doses to avoid precipitation of myocardial ischaemia in patients with cardiovascular disease. Effusions generally resolve and drainage is hardly ever required.

Amiodarone and thyroid dysfunction

Amiodarone is rich in iodine and maintenance therapy is commonly associated with abnormal thyroid function tests. Thyrotoxicosis may occur and is confirmed by elevated levels of T_4 and T_3 with suppressed thyroid-stimulating hormone. Hypothyroidism is treated with discontinuation of drugs (where possible) and thyroxine replacement.

2.13.2 Diabetes

Aetiology/pathophysiology

Accelerated atherogenesis
This is the result of the following.

- Dyslipidaemia: increased low-density lipoprotein and triglyceride and decreased high-density lipoprotein.

- Hypercoagulable state and increased platelet aggregation.

- Hyperinsulinaemia (in type 2 diabetes) promoting vascular smooth muscle proliferation.

- Glycosylated proteins promoting the production of oxidants.

- Hypertension is very common in type 2 diabetes and leads to a disproportionate rise in risk of cardiovascular event.

- Endothelial dysfunction is the likely common final pathway resulting in macrovascular disease.

Autonomic neuropathy
This causes impairment of the protective sensation of angina (silent ischaemia) and may lead to prolonged ischaemia, arrhythmias and sudden death.

Diabetic cardiomyopathy
Impairment of systolic and diastolic function independent of macroscopic coronary artery disease, possibly secondary to microvascular disease.

Epidemiology
In people with diabetes the risk of acute myocardial infarction is increased by 50% for a man and 150% for a woman. The rate of major complications is increased and associated with higher mortality rates.

Clinical presentation
Silent ischaemia may lead to atypical presentations, eg acute myocardial infarction as ketoacidosis.

Treatment

Acute myocardial infarction
Standard treatment plus an insulin infusion ('sliding scale'). The absolute benefit of all standard interventions is greater in people with diabetes.

Coronary revascularisation
Diabetic coronary disease is generally more diffuse and distal, so that both coronary artery bypass grafting and angioplasty have poorer outcomes than in people without diabetes (appreciating that their untreated risk is greater). However, recent work suggests that coronary stenting (particularly drug-eluting stents) plus the use of a glycoprotein IIb/IIIa receptor blocker (antiplatelet) may improve results.

Prevention

Primary
Good glycaemic and BP control (<130/80 mmHg), and avoidance of smoking.

Secondary
Treatment with a statin and an angiotensin-converting enzyme inhibitor, though most of this high-risk group should now be on these drugs as primary prevention.

2.13.3 Autoimmune rheumatic diseases

Clinical presentation
The autoimmune rheumatic diseases have the following cardiac associations.

Systemic lupus erythematosus

- Premature atherosclerosis: important to differentiate from coronary vasculitis, which is also present in systemic lupus erythematosus (SLE), because the latter requires steroids.

- Pericarditis and effusion: clinically in 30%; at post-mortem examination in 60%.

- Sterile valvular vegetations (Libman–Sachs) in 60%, rarely clinically significant.

- Myocarditis.

- Conduction defects.

Primary antiphospholipid syndrome

- Pulmonary thromboembolism (also in SLE if anticardiolipin antibody positive).

- Degenerative mitral valve disease.

Rheumatoid arthritis

- Increasingly recognised as a potent risk factor for atherosclerotic vascular disease (inflammatory state).

- Pericarditis: often clinically silent but may lead to symptomatic effusion or constriction.

- Rheumatoid nodules causing valvular regurgitation and atrioventricular block.

- Coronary vasculitis (rare).

Systemic sclerosis

- Pulmonary hypertension: the major cause of death in systemic sclerosis.

- Pericarditis and chronic effusions.

- Myocardial fibrosis causing ventricular dysfunction and conduction abnormalities.

Investigations

Coronary angiography

Coronary angiography may help to distinguish between vasculitis and atheromatous disease.

Echocardiography

Transoesophageal echocardiography should be used if necessary for close inspection of valve abnormalities.

Treatment

Pericarditis

NSAIDs and steroids are used if necessary for symptomatic relief. Tamponade requires immediate pericardiocentesis followed by steroids.

Myocarditis

Standard management of left ventricular dysfunction (see Section 2.3).

Pulmonary hypertension

Standard management (see Section 2.12).

2.13.4 Renal disease

Aetiology/pathophysiology

Features of end-stage renal failure/renal replacement include:

- hypertension;

- elevated serum calcium and calcium phosphate product;

- anaemia;

- dyslipidaemia;

- uraemia;

- electrolyte imbalance;

- amyloidosis (β_2-microglobulin).

These result in the following cardiovascular complications via the mechanisms shown in Fig. 88:

- left ventricular hypertrophy;

- myocardial ischaemia;

- impaired ventricular function;

- ventricular arrhythmias and sudden death;

- valvular calcification (aortic more than mitral), with rapidly progressive stenosis in a small proportion of cases, and the risk of endocarditis.

The heart in renal failure

Abnormal cardiac structure is virtually uniform in patients with end-stage renal disease. Left ventricular hypertrophy is present in 70–80% of patients approaching dialysis, and is linked to anaemia and hypertension. Left ventricular dilatation and impairment of systolic and diastolic function are common. These are of course influenced by fluid loading and change, at least partly, following dialysis. Cardiovascular disease is also the major cause of late mortality in renal transplant recipients.

Epidemiology

Cardiovascular disease is much commoner in patients receiving renal replacement than the general population and is the most common cause of death in this group (>50%). Those whose renal failure is associated with diabetes and atherosclerotic renovascular disease are at particularly high risk.

Investigations

- Myocardial ischaemia: coronary angiography if intervention or renal transplantation is being considered. Exercise testing (abnormal ECG) and nuclear perfusion imaging have reduced predictive value in these patients. Stress echocardiography may be of value.

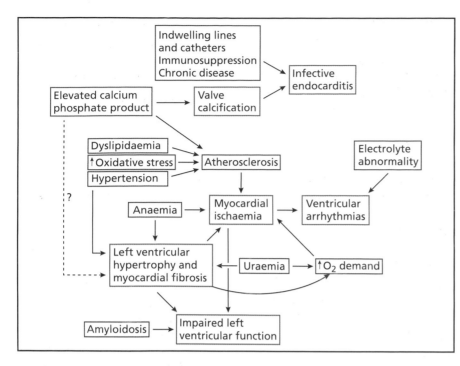

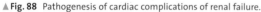

▲ **Fig. 88** Pathogenesis of cardiac complications of renal failure.

FURTHER READING

Fisher M. Diabetes and atherogenesis. *Heart* 2004; 90: 336–40.

Hussain S and Isenberg DA. Autoimmune rheumatic diseases and the heart. *Hosp. Med.* 1999; 60: 95–9.

Shurrab E and Kalra PA. Cardiovascular co-morbidity with renal disease. In: Purcell HJ and Kalra PR, eds. *Specialist Training in Cardiology.* London: Elsevier Mosby, 2005: 305–21.

Staffeld CG and Pastan SO. Cardiac disease in patients with end-stage renal disease. *Cardiol. Clin.* 1995; 13: 209–23.

Yerkey MW, Kernis SJ, Franklin BA, *et al.* Renal dysfunction and acceleration of coronary disease. *Heart* 2004; 90: 961–6.

- Echocardiography for assessment of valves, left ventricular function and pericardial effusion.

- Be aware that a patient on dialysis may have large fluctuations in serum potassium, with effects on antiarrhythmic therapy.

Treatment

Optimise haemoglobin and BP. If symptomatic coronary artery disease is present, bypass grafting is the treatment of choice as the restenosis and coronary event rates post angioplasty are very high. The indications for surgery in calcific valve disease and endocarditis are the same as in a patient without renal disease. Uraemic pericarditis is an indication for dialysis. Cardiac tamponade (of any cause) requires immediate pericardiocentesis. Recurrent effusions may warrant pericardiectomy (a 'window' to enable drainage into the pleural space).

- Prescribing in renal failure: see *Clinical Pharmacology,* Section 4.6.

Prognosis

The presence of left ventricular dysfunction in a dialysis patient reduces the 2-year survival rate from 80 to 33%. Acute myocardial infarction and cardiac surgery have a higher mortality than in the general population, but when indicated coronary artery bypass grafting and valve surgery still have an acceptable risk.

Prevention

Careful control of phosphate and calcium phosphate product reduces valve calcification. Good aseptic technique is essential when inserting and using dialysis catheters to minimise the risk of infective endocarditis. Aim for good control of BP and serum cholesterol, and maintenance of haematocrit. It is important that the patient stops smoking.

2.14 Systemic complications of cardiac disease

2.14.1 Stroke

Aetiology

Up to 20% of all ischaemic strokes are cardiogenic in cause. Cardiac causes can be divided into a direct source of embolus or a substrate for embolus formation. Direct sources of embolus include:

- left ventricular apical thrombus after myocardial infarction;

- left atrial appendage thrombus in patients with atrial fibrillation (AF);

- prosthetic valve thrombus in a patient with inadequate anticoagulation;

- valve vegetations;

- aortic dissection;

- cardiac tumours (especially atrial myxoma).

Cardiac substrates for embolus formation include patent foramen ovale (PFO), aortic arch atheroma, left ventricular non-compaction, dilated left atrium or dilated cardiomyopathy.

Physical signs

Common

- AF (in up to 25% of patients who have a cerebrovascular accident).

- Murmurs (particularly mitral).

Uncommon

- Pulmonary oedema.

- Added heart sounds.

Investigations

ECG

There is a significant chance that if there is underlying cardiac pathology resulting in thromboembolism, the ECG will be abnormal.

When examining an ECG for a cardiac cause of stroke look for:

- AF;
- previous myocardial infarction (in 90% of cases it is anterior);
- persistent ST elevation suggestive of left ventricular aneurysm;
- left ventricular hypertrophy suggestive of hypertension or aortic stenosis.

Chest radiograph

Look for abnormal cardiac shape/size, pulmonary oedema and wide mediastinum suggestive of enlarged aorta.

Echocardiography

If any possible cardiac cause has been identified from the history, examination or ECG/CXR, it is reasonable to examine the structure and function of the heart with echocardiography. Contrast aids in the diagnosis of left ventricular thrombus. Transoesophageal echocardiography should be used to search for aortic arch atheroma, left atrial appendage thrombus and function, and the presence of a PFO. For the diagnosis of a PFO, the patient is asked to perform a Valsalva manoeuvre and agitated colloid is injected peripherally. On release of the Valsalva manoeuvre, immediate passage of bubbles from right atrium to left atrium suggests a PFO.

Treatment

Correct the underlying abnormality and aim for restoration of sinus rhythm where possible (see Section 2.2.2). Percutaneous closure of a PFO is recommended in young patients with any of the following:

- stroke/transient ischaemic attack (TIA) where no other cause can be found;

- recurrent embolic events despite medical treatment;

- cerebral embolic events in more than one carotid territory.

Complication

The risk of haemorrhage into an ischaemic stroke if anticoagulated usually outweighs the benefit of secondary prevention.

Prevention

Anticoagulation in AF/atrial flutter: indications for warfarin (target INR 2.0–3.0)

- Previous cardiovascular accident/TIA.
- Age >65 years.
- Diabetes.
- Hypertension.
- Structural abnormality on echocardiography.

For all other patients, consider aspirin 300 mg once daily.

FURTHER READING

Barnett HJM, Eliasziw M and Meldrum HE. Evidence based cardiology: prevention of ischaemic stroke. *BMJ* 1999; 318: 1539–43.

2.15 Pregnancy and the heart

Aetiology

Normal physiological changes in pregnancy include:

- decrease in systemic and pulmonary vascular resistance;

- increase in heart rate, blood volume (large shifts after delivery) and cardiac output;

- no significant change in BP;

- anaemia (caused by increased blood volume and/or haematinic deficiency).

These can all cause problems in women with cardiovascular disease.

Clinical presentation

Fatigue, mild dyspnoea, ankle oedema, palpitations (usually ectopics) and postural dizziness are all common in normal pregnancy, but likely to be more severe in those with cardiac disease.

Physical signs

The following are common in a normal pregnancy:

- third heart sound;

- soft systolic flow murmur at the lower left sternal edge;

- mild ankle oedema.

Look for signs of worsening cardiac failure and/or exacerbation of the physical signs of particular cardiac lesions.

Investigations

To exclude cardiac disease conduct the following:

- echocardiography to check for ventricular function and valvular abnormalities;

- ECG/24-hour tape to check for arrhythmias;

- CXR is rarely clinically indicated, but should be performed if it is because the dose to a screened fetus is negligible.

In a pregnant woman a 12-lead ECG may show a minor axis shift or non-specific ST changes in the left-sided precordial leads. These usually resolve after pregnancy, but may recur in subsequent pregnacies.

Prognosis/treatment

In a patient with pre-existing cardiac disease the ability to tolerate pregnancy is related to the following:

- cyanosis;

- pulmonary hypertension;

- haemodynamic significance of the lesion;

- pre-pregnancy functional status.

High risk

Primary pulmonary hypertension/ Eisenmenger's syndrome There is a 50% maternal mortality rate and patients should be strongly advised to consider sterilisation.

Mitral stenosis This may present for the first time in pregnancy with pulmonary oedema secondary to increased cardiac output or an episode of atrial fibrillation. Treatment consists of diuretics to clear the pulmonary oedema, and digoxin or beta-blockers to control heart rate and thereby improve atrial emptying. Mitral valvuloplasty may be necessary during pregnancy in rare occasions.

Aortic/pulmonary stenosis Gradients are exacerbated by decreased vascular resistance. There is no effective medical therapy other than supportive.

Marfan's syndrome There is an increased risk of aortic dissection; those who already have echocardiographic evidence of aortic root dilatation >4.5 cm should be advised against pregnancy.

Intermediate risk

- Coarctation of the aorta (risk of aortic dissection).

- Hypertrophic cardiomyopathy.

- Cyanotic congenital heart disease without pulmonary hypertension; note increased risk (40%) of fetal death if mother is cyanotic.

Low risk

- Well-tolerated valvular regurgitation.

- Septal defects without pulmonary hypertension.

- Totally corrected congenital heart disease.

- Prosthetic valves: bioprostheses do not require anticoagulation, but pregnancy reduces their lifespan. There is no consensus on the optimum management of anticoagulation in pregnant women with mechanical valves. In addition to the issues discussed in *Clinical Pharmacology*, Section 4.3, there is the concern that heparin is not as effective as warfarin in preventing valve thrombosis.

Antibiotic prophylaxis is recommended for vaginal delivery in cases at high risk of endocarditis (prosthetic valves, prior episode of infective endocarditis, complex cyanotic congenital heart disease and surgical shunts) and for instrumented delivery in any cardiac lesion, but not for Caesarean section.

New cardiac disease in pregnancy

Thromboembolic disease

Thrombolysis should be used for a massive life-threatening pulmonary embolus, as in the non-pregnant patient.

Myocardial infarction

This is rare in pregnancy but is associated with considerable mortality. Atheroma is responsible for less than half of instances and coronary artery dissection is more common than in the normal population. Ideally the treatment should be urgent coronary angiography and intervention if needed. Aspirin, nitrates and beta-blockers may be used. Angiotensin-converting enzyme inhibitors and statins should be avoided.

Peripartum cardiomyopathy

This presents as dilated cardiomyopathy in the third trimester or in the first 6 months postpartum.

Hypertension

Hypertension may be chronic (ie pre-dates the pregnancy or develops before 20 weeks) or pregnancy induced (part of a spectrum that includes pre-eclampsia).

> **Important information for patients**
>
> Recurrence risk of non-syndromic congenital heart disease in the baby is 3–5%.

FURTHER READING

Magee LA, Ornstein MP and von Dadelszen P. Management of hypertension in pregnancy. *BMJ* 1999; 318: 1332–6.

– – – – – – – – – – – – – – – – –

Oakley GDG. Pregnancy and heart disease. In: Julian DG and Camm AJ, eds. *Diseases of the Heart*, 2nd edn. Philadelphia: WB Saunders, 1996: 1331–7.

– – – – – – – – – – – – – – – – –

Thorne SA. Pregnancy in heart disease. *Heart* 2004; 90: 450–6.

2.16 General anaesthesia in heart disease

Pathophysiology

Assessment of fitness for anaesthesia involves understanding the effects it has on cardiovascular physiology, the direct effects of anaesthetic agents and the effects of artificial ventilation as well as the effect of surgery. Anaesthesia tends to cause:

- hypotension;
- reduced preload;
- hypoxaemia;

- hypercapnia;
- acidosis.

Patients with congenital cyanotic heart disease or pulmonary hypertension are at particularly high risk from general anaesthesia. These patients cannot adapt to reduced preload and develop severe systemic hypotension.

Epidemiology

The risk of reinfarction during anaesthesia after a myocardial infarction is:

- 6% within 3 months;
- 2% between 3 and 6 months.

Clinical presentation

The key to assessing fitness for anaesthesia is exercise ability. Good exercise performance suggests anaesthesia will be well tolerated. Patients with unstable symptoms are likely to be at risk.

Investigation

The following may help determine suitability for anaesthesia.

Exercise testing

Objective evidence of exercise ability and ischaemia is obtained.

Echocardiography

This is unlikely to be of routine help. Patients with severe left ventricular impairment and good exercise tolerance are likely to have a good outcome from anaesthesia. Patients with suspected aortic stenosis should have echocardiography, as the risk of complication with general anaesthesia is high.

ECG

A history of syncope and evidence of trifascicular block indicates the need for permanent pacing. Generally, asymptomatic bifascicular and trifascicular block do not require temporary transvenous pacing prior to general anaesthesia.

Coronary angiography

Generally, patients with ischaemic heart disease who require urgent/emergency surgery should be treated medically with beta-blockers, which may be given intravenously if required. Revascularisation prior to non-cardiac surgery has been shown to carry a higher risk than medical treatment with beta-blockade. There is a high risk of fatal stent thrombosis within the first 4 weeks after percutaneous coronary intervention (PCI). Patients undergoing emergency surgery soon after PCI should continue antiplatelet therapy.

> **The following identify patients at high risk when undergoing surgery under general anaesthesia:**
>
> - myocardial infarction within the last 6 months;
> - congestive cardiac failure;
> - aortic stenosis;
> - age >70 years;
> - undergoing emergency operation;
> - metabolic abnormality;
> - congenital cyanotic heart disease;
> - pulmonary hypertension.
>
> These patients should be managed postoperatively in a high-dependency unit with invasive haemodynamic monitoring. Close liaison between surgeon, anaesthetist and cardiologist is vital.

2.17 Hypertension

Aetiology/pathophysiology/pathology

Over 90% of all cases of hypertension are of unknown aetiology (essential hypertension), reflecting deranged interaction between multiple genetic and environmental factors on the homeostatic mechanisms of the

TABLE 40 SECONDARY CAUSES OF HYPERTENSION

Presentation	Cause
Commonly with hypertension	Renal disease Renal artery stenosis: atherosclerotic or fibromuscular dysplasia Coarctation of the aorta Phaeochromocytoma Primary hyperaldosteronism (Conn's syndrome)
Rarely present with hypertension as the dominant feature, but may be associated with it	Cushing's syndrome Exogenous steroids Hyperthyroidism Myxoedema Acromegaly Excessive liquorice consumption

body (including abnormalities of the renin–angiotensin and autonomic nervous systems, endothelial dysfunction and sodium intake). Secondary causes of hypertension are much more uncommon (Table 40). However, treatment of the underlying cause can often cure the resultant high BP.

Epidemiology

BP is a continuous variable, so hypertension is difficult to define. Up to one-quarter of adults in Western populations are found to have a BP in excess of 140/90 mmHg at screening. This proportion increases with age, rising from 4% in those aged 18–29 years to 65% in those >80 years. However, despite recognition of the high prevalence of hypertension and its dangers it remains inadequately treated, with estimates that <30% of recognised hypertensive patients have adequate BP control.

Clinical presentation

Common

Essential hypertension is usually asymptomatic until complications (eg cardiac failure) arise. Hypertension is commonly detected 'opportunistically' when a patient attends with some complaint and the doctor or nurse takes the opportunity to measure the BP. It may also be detected at a routine health screening, or as part of a deliberate assessment of a patient's cardiovascular risk (eg when presenting with symptoms that might indicate cardiovascular disease such as ischaemic heart disease, stroke/transient ischaemic attack or peripheral vascular disease). A number of complaints are commonly associated with hypertension, but are non-specific:

- headache (occipital and present on waking, settling gradually during the day);

- epistaxis;

- nocturia.

Uncommon

Presentation with symptoms suggestive of a secondary cause apart from those attributable to hypertension.

- Phaeochromocytoma: anxiety, diaphoresis, tremor, epigastric and chest pain, and dyspnoea.

- Primary hyperaldosteronism: symptoms suggestive of marked hypokalaemia (cramps, muscle weakness, polydipsia, polyuria and/or nocturia).

- Cushing's syndrome: weight gain, characteristic facial appearance, easy bruising, thinning of hair and skin, striae and muscle weakness.

- Other less common features include symptoms suggestive of thyroid disease (see *Endocrinology*, Section 2.3) and acromegaly (see *Endocrinology*, Section 2.1.2).

Physical signs

Apart from elevated BP, commonly there are no other abnormal signs. In moderate or severe hypertension, a loud aortic second sound may be heard. Look for evidence of the following.

1. Left ventricular hypertrophy (LVH).

2. Hypertensive retinopathy (Fig. 89):

    (a) Grade I: light reflex from the arterial wall is increased as a result of thickening.

    (b) Grade II: the arterial light reflex is wider, giving rise to a 'silver wire' appearance. Nipping of the veins is an optical illusion caused by the inability to see the blood within the vein through the thickened arterial wall. There is a generalised reduction in the diameter of arteries compared with veins.

    (c) Grades III and IV: associated with accelerated hypertension (see Section 2.17.1).

3. Signs of associated vascular disease: vascular bruits and absent pulses.

Investigations

The following should be considered.

Blood tests

FBC, electrolytes, renal function, fasting glucose and lipids.

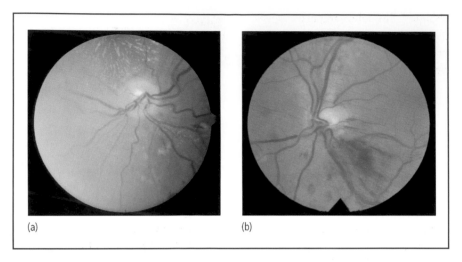

(a)　　　　　　　　　　　(b)

▲**Fig. 89** Hypertensive retinopathy: (**a**) grade IV showing mild papilloedema, hard exudates (12 o'clock), cotton-wool spots and flame haemorrhages (4 o'clock); (**b**) grade III showing extensive flame-shaped haemorrhages. (Courtesy of Professor J. Ritter.)

Urine

A clean midstream urine should be tested for blood, protein and glucose. In the presence of haematuria or proteinuria, the sample should be sent for microscopy and culture.

ECG

The ECG may be normal. Look for signs of LVH and/or coronary artery disease.

Chest radiograph

This may be normal. Look for cardiomegaly, pulmonary oedema and coarctation (Fig. 90).

Other baseline investigations

Other tests may be required in some cases.

- To determine whether hypertension is present in patients with no evidence of end-organ damage: arrange 24-hour ambulatory BP measurement for a better understanding of the pattern of changes and its control in the patient's normal environment (at home and work). This will also be useful for excluding isolated clinic ('white coat') hypertension.

- To assess end-organ damage secondary to hypertensive retinopathy: conduct transthoracic echocardiography and look for LVH and systolic or diastolic failure.

Investigations for secondary hypertension

In suspected cases of secondary hypertension, further investigations led by clinical suspicion will be required. Indications for investigating secondary causes of hypertension include:

- any evidence of underlying cause in history or examination (see Table 40);

- accelerated (malignant) hypertension;

- hypokalaemia (not diuretic induced);

- young age (<35 years);

- resistant hypertension (uncontrolled by three drugs).

Possible investigations include the following.

- A 24-hour urine collection: measure catecholamine levels and look for features of renal disease (eg creatinine clearance and urinary protein excretion).

- Renal ultrasound and Doppler: the presence of two small kidneys indicates chronic renal disease. Marked asymmetry of renal size (>2 cm difference in length) increases the probability of renal artery stenosis. Doppler

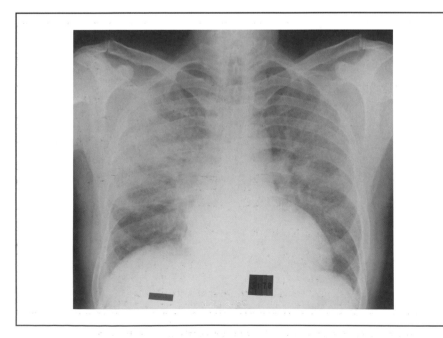

▲**Fig. 90** CXR demonstrating pulmonary oedema.

ultrasound of the renal arteries can accurately diagnose renal artery stenosis.

- MRI of the renal arteries: an alternative accurate method of diagnosis for renal artery stenosis.

- Test of plasma renin and aldosterone.

Differential diagnosis

Consider the following:

- essential hypertension;

- secondary hypertension;

- erroneous reading of elevated BP as a result of inadequate cuff size;

- isolated clinic hypertension ('white coat' hypertension).

Treatment

Essential hypertension

Treatment of both systolic and diastolic blood pressure is equally important across all age groups. Having diagnosed hypertension, pharmacological therapy should be combined with advice on lifestyle changes. The following are considered recommendations for pharmacological treatment of hypertension:

- patients with a persistently high BP of 160/100 mmHg or more;

- patients with raised cardiovascular risk (10-year risk of coronary heart disease 15% and of cardiovascular disease 20%, existing cardiovascular disease or evidence of target organ damage) with a persistent BP of 140/90 mmHg or more.

The choice of antihypertensive therapy should be tailored to the patient's medical requirements. In patients who do not respond to single- or dual-agent therapy, low-dose combination therapy must be considered. A recommended treatment algorithm is outlined in Fig. 91.

Secondary hypertension

Treatment should be directed towards management of the underlying cause.

Advice regarding lifestyle modifications for patients with hypertension

- Stop smoking.
- Lose weight as appropriate.
- Moderate alcohol intake (<14 units/week for women and <21 units/week for men).
- Dietary changes: consume a lower amount of saturated fat, and increase oily fish, fruit and vegetable intake.
- Limit salt intake.
- Sensible regular exercise.

Complications

These are often seen if BP remains untreated or poorly managed:

- retinopathy and retinal haemorrhages;

- renal impairement;

- left ventricular hypertrophy and cardiac failure (both systolic and diastolic);

- vascular events (stroke, myocardial infarction and peripheral arterial disease);

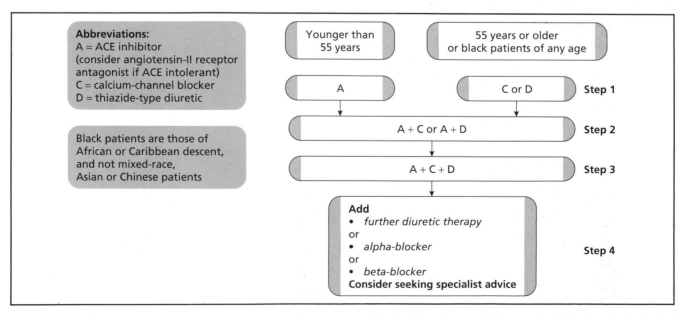

Abbreviations:
A = ACE inhibitor
(consider angiotensin-II receptor antagonist if ACE intolerant)
C = calcium-channel blocker
D = thiazide-type diuretic

Black patients are those of African or Caribbean descent, and not mixed-race, Asian or Chinese patients

Younger than 55 years

55 years or older or black patients of any age

| A | C or D | Step 1 |

A + C or A + D — Step 2

A + C + D — Step 3

Add
- *further diuretic therapy*
or
- *alpha-blocker*
or
- *beta-blocker*
Consider seeking specialist advice

Step 4

▲ **Fig. 91** Treatment algorithm for essential hypertension recommended by NICE. (Adapted with permission from National Institute for Health and Clinical Excellence. *Quick Reference Guide. Hypertension: Management of Hypertension in Adults in Primary Care. Guideline 34*, June 2006.)

- worsening hypertension (especially if poorly treated).

Prognosis

Morbidity

Essential hypertension increases the risk of stroke six-fold, of coronary artery disease and heart failure three-fold, and doubles the risk of peripheral vascular disease. Renal failure usually occurs only in cases of malignant hypertension, but elevated BP increases the progression of renal failure from other causes. It is well established that treatment of hypertension reduces the incidence of cardiovascular disease.

Mortality

- Age <50 years: both diastolic and systolic hypertension are risk factors for cardiovascular death. A reduction of 5–6 mmHg in diastolic pressure is associated with a 12% reduction in mortality rate over 5 years.

- Age >50 years: evidence suggests that systolic BP is the important determinant of risk and that it has an inverse relationship with diastolic blood pressure, ie the greater the pulse pressure for a given value of systolic pressure, the higher the risk.

FURTHER READING

Franklin SS, Khan SA, Wong ND, *et al.* Is pulse pressure useful in predicting risk for coronary heart disease? The Framingham Heart Study. *Circulation* 1999; 100: 354–60.

Hansson L, Zanchetti A, Carruthers SG, *et al.* Effects of intensive blood-pressure lowering and low-dose aspirin in patients with hypertension: principal results of the hypertension optimal treatment (HOT) randomised trial. HOT Study Group. *Lancet* 1998; 351: 1755–62.

National Institute for Health and Clinical Excellence. *Quick Reference Guide. Hypertension: Management of Hypertension in Adults in Primary Care.* Guideline 34, June 2006. Available at www.nice.org.uk

Ramsay LE, Williams B, Johnston GD, *et al.* British Hypertension Society guidelines for hypertension management 1999: summary. *BMJ* 1999; 319: 630–5.

UK Prospective Diabetes Study Group. Tight blood pressure control and risk of macrovascular and microvascular complications in type 2 diabetes: UKPDS 38. *BMJ* 1998; 317: 703–13.

2.17.1 Hypertensive emergencies

Aetiology/pathology

A hypertensive crisis is defined as a severe elevation in BP (systolic BP >200 mmHg, diastolic BP >120 mmHg). Rate of change in BP is important. A rapid rise is poorly tolerated and leads to end-organ damage, whereas a gradual rise in a patient with existing poor BP control is tolerated better.

Conditions that can cause hypertensive emergencies include the following.

- Essential hypertension.

- Renovascular hypertension: atheroma, fibromuscular dysplasia and acute renal occlusion.

- Renal parenchymal disease: acute glomerulonephritis, vasculitis and scleroderma.

- Endocrine disorders: phaeochromocytoma, Cushing's syndrome, primary hyperaldosteronism, thyrotoxicosis, hyperparathyroidism, acromegaly and adrenal carcinoma.

- Eclampsia and pre-eclampsia.

- Vasculitis.

- Drugs: cocaine, amphetamines, monoamine oxidase inhibitor interactions, ciclosporin, beta-blockers and clonidine withdrawal.

- Autonomic hyperactivity in presence of spinal cord injury.

- Coarctation of the aorta.

Epidemiology

The incidence is around 1–2 per 100,000 per year.

Clinical presentation

Hypertensive emergencies can present in a number of ways.

- Hypertensive emergency with retinopathy (previously known as accelerated hypertension): patients suffering from this often have visual disturbances and retinal haemorrhages.

- Hypertensive emergency with papilloedema (previously called malignant hypertension).

- Hypertensive emergency with encephalopathy: patients present with headaches, drowsiness and epileptic fits. Other ocular complications are also often present.

Physical signs

Common

The diagnosis of a hypertensive emergency cannot be made without high BP and evidence of fibrinoid necrosis of vessels, which can be viewed directly only in the fundi.

- Grade III retinopathy: flame-shaped superficial haemorrhages or 'dot-and-blot' haemorrhages deeper within the retina, cotton-wool spots (retinal microinfarcts) and hard exudates (see Fig. 89).

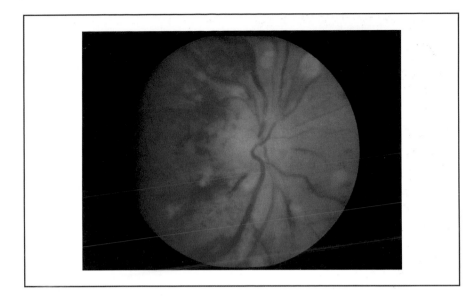

▲**Fig. 92** Hypertensive retinopathy: grade IV showing florid papilloedema, haemorrhages and cotton-wool spots. (Courtesy of Mr H. Towler.)

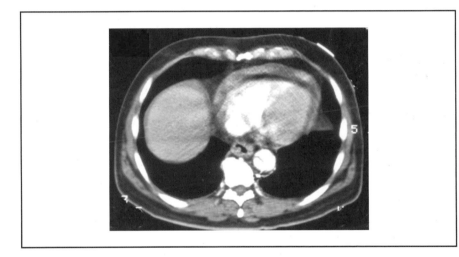

▲**Fig. 93** CT scan of aortic dissection. The descending aorta is enlarged and contrast shows a double lumen.

- Grade IV retinopathy: haemorrhages and exudates with papilloedema (Fig. 92).

Uncommon
Drowsiness, coma, epileptic fitting, stroke, pulmonary oedema and aortic dissection.

Investigations

Immediate
Check urine for blood, protein and red-cell casts. Perform ECG, CXR, FBC, electrolytes, coagulation profile, and renal and liver function tests. If there is clinical suspicion of aortic dissection, an urgent CT scan of the chest or transoesophageal echocardiography is needed (Fig. 93). If there is clinical suspicion of a renal inflammatory condition (eg systemic lupus erythematosus, vasculitis or scleroderma), then specific serological tests will be needed.

Elective
When BP has been controlled, all patients with accelerated-phase hypertension require a thorough work-up for secondary causes of hypertension. Renal biopsy may be required.

Differential diagnosis
The differential diagnosis is of acute glomerulonephritis or renal vasculitis, or scleroderma renal crisis.

Treatment
All patients with accelerated-phase hypertension should be admitted to hospital for BP control with appropriate drugs and treatment of any complications or secondary cause.

Complications
Stroke, aortic dissection and chronic renal failure.

Prognosis
If untreated, 80% of sufferers will die within 2 years. One recent series reported a 69% survival rate at 12 years.

FURTHER READING

Ahmed MEK, Walker JM, Beevers DG, *et al*. Lack of difference between malignant and accelerated hypertension. *BMJ* 1986; 292: 235–7.

McGregor E, Isles CG, Jay JL, *et al*. Retinal changes in malignant hypertension. *BMJ* 1986; 292: 233–4.

Webster J, Petrie JC, Jeffers TA, *et al*. Accelerated hypertension: patterns of mortality and clinical factors affecting outcome in treated patients. *Q. J. Med.* 1993; 86: 485–93.

2.18 Venous thromboembolism

2.18.1 Pulmonary embolism
Embolism can be from any source (eg tumour, air or amniotic fluid), but this section considers

TABLE 41 RISK FACTORS FOR PE

Hypercoagulable states	Acquired conditions
Factor V Leiden mutation Protein C abnormalities (mutations and/or resistance) Protein S deficiency Antithrombin III deficiency Hyperhomocysteinaemia Antiphospholipid antibodies (including lupus anticoagulant and anticardiolipin antibodies)	Surgery/trauma/fractures Immobilisation of any cause Obesity Hypertension Increasing age Pregnancy/postpartum Malignancy Chronic cardiorespiratory disease Stroke/spinal cord injury Indwelling central venous catheter Current (not prior) use of combined oral contraceptive pill or hormone-replacement therapy (minor risk only)

PE, pulmonary embolism.

only thrombotic venous thromboembolism.

Aetiology/pathophysiology/pathology

Virchow's triad (local trauma to the vessel wall, hypercoagulability and venous stasis) causes thrombosis in the deep veins of the legs, pelvis or (more rarely) arms, which can propagate and extend proximally. The thrombus may dislodge and embolise to the pulmonary arterial tree. This causes physical obstruction of the vasculature and release of vasoactive substances, leading to:

- elevation of pulmonary vascular resistance;

- redistribution of blood flow, causing ventilation–perfusion mismatch and impairment of gas exchange;

- increased right ventricular afterload, causing dilatation and dysfunction of the right ventricle.

Often patients have a genetic predisposition to thrombosis but require an environmental stress to elicit overt thrombus formation.

Epidemiology

The incidence of venous thromboembolism is 60–70 per 100,000 population. Despite treatment, the 3-month mortality of pulmonary embolism (PE) remains high at 17.5%. The incidence of PE doubles with each 10-year increase in age. It is estimated that PE accounts for 10% of all in-hospital deaths.

Risk factors

These are divided into hypercoagulable states associated with venous thrombosis and acquired conditions that may precipitate venous thrombosis (Table 41).

Clinical presentation

Common

- Small and moderate-sized PE:

  (a) Isolated dyspnoea.

  (b) Symptoms of pulmonary infarction: pleuritic pain, cough and/or haemoptysis.

- Massive PE: severe dyspnoea, syncope, haemodynamic collapse and cyanosis.

- Symptoms of deep venous thrombosis (DVT): swelling and tenderness in calf.

Uncommon

- Progressive ankle oedema and dyspnoea (secondary pulmonary hypertension).

- Pyrexia of unknown origin.

- Atrial fibrillation (AF).

A young woman with isolated pleuritic chest pain and no risk factors except the oral contraceptive pill is extremely unlikely to have a PE if she has a respiratory rate of <20/minute and a normal CXR. However, the risk of missing a life-threatening condition means that you should pursue the investigation unless you can make a confident alternative diagnosis.

Physical signs

Common

- Tachypnoea.

- Tachycardia.

- Crackles on auscultation.

- Pleural rub.

Uncommon

- Cyanosis suggests large PE.

- Postural hypotension in the presence of a raised JVP.

- Signs of raised right heart pressure:

  (a) Raised JVP wih prominent *a* wave.

  (b) Pansystolic murmur of tricuspid regurgitation.

  (c) Loud pulmonary valve (P2) closure sound with wide splitting of S2.

(d) Early diastolic murmur of pulmonary regurgitation.

(e) Left parasternal heave.

- Swollen firm calf suggestive of DVT.

Investigations

Investigations must be used in conjunction with an assessment of the clinical probability of PE.

ECG

Changes are often non-specific and include sinus tachycardia and anterior T-wave inversion. ECG changes of raised right heart pressure are rare and only seen with massive PE. These include right-axis deviation, S1Q3T3, new right bundle-branch block, right ventricular hypertrophy and AF.

Chest radiograph

This is often normal. Abnormal findings include pulmonary oligaemia, raised diaphragm, small pleural effusion and segmental collapse.

Arterial blood gases

Hypoxaemia (in larger PEs) and hypocapnia (associated with respiratory alkalosis secondary to hyperventilation) increase suspicion of PE. Normal arterial blood gases do not exclude a diagnosis of PE.

Venous ultrasonography

This is used if there is clinical suspicion of a current DVT, although normal results do not exclude a PE.

Echocardiography

Echocardiography identifies right ventricular pressure overload and dysfunction. In patients with non-PE-related haemodynamic collapse, it can be used to identify alternative cardiac causes for the abnormal haemodynamic state. It is useful as a quick source of information in a critically ill patient, but does not provide a diagnosis of PE.

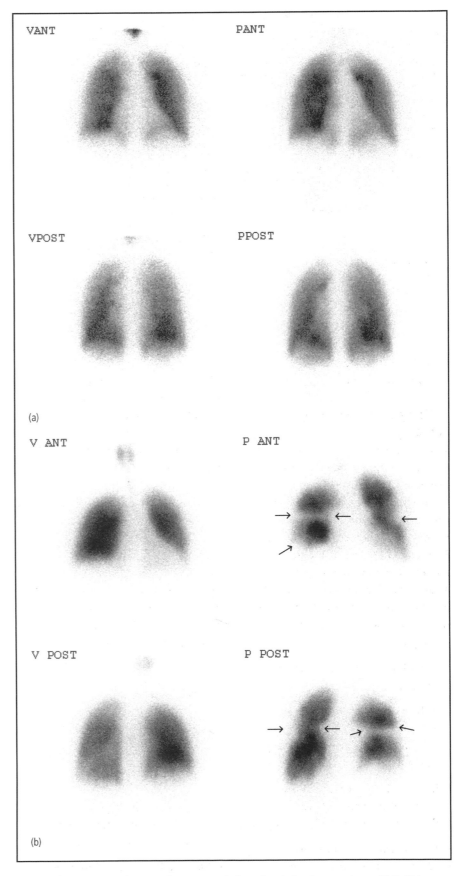

▲ **Fig. 94** (**a**) Normal ventilation–perfusion scan: anterior and posterior views are shown. (**b**) Multiple perfusion defects (arrowed) that are not matched by ventilation defects and therefore indicate a high probability of PE.

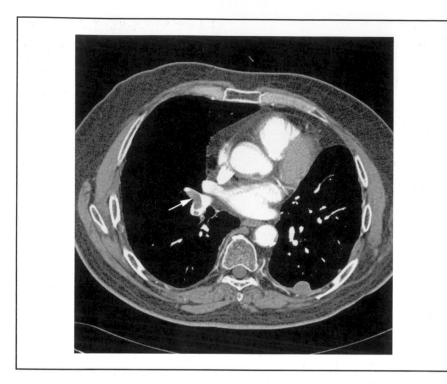

▲**Fig. 95** Contrast CT scan of a patient with a large PE visible as a grey filling defect (arrowed) against the white contrast in the pulmonary artery.

Plasma D-dimer

This test is sensitive but not specific for the presence of thrombus (ie it helps to exclude the diagnosis of a thrombus).

Ventilation-perfusion lung scan

A normal scan rules out a PE. Abnormal scans with a high probability of PE must be treated as PE. Medium or low probability scans must be interpreted in the context of the clinical scenario and may require alternative modes of imaging. Perfusion scanning alone gives comparable diagnostic yield (Fig. 94). Pre-existing lung disease makes interpretation difficult.

Spiral CT of the chest with contrast

Increasingly used in the diagnosis of PE (Fig. 95). Clearly the imaging technique of choice when there is pre-existing pulmonary disease.

Pulmonary angiography

Remains the gold-standard investigation. However, it is an invasive test and, with the increasing availability of spiral chest CT, is only used in rare cases where diagnosis remains unclear.

> **Consider the following in the differential diagnosis of PE:**
>
> • pleurisy/breathlessness;
> • pneumothorax;
> • pneumonia;
> • musculoskeletal pain;
> • rib fracture;
> • asthma/chronic airflow obstruction;
> • other causes of circulatory collapse (myocardial infarction and cardiac tamponade).

Management

Emergency

General measures are required until a definitive diagnosis is reached.

• Maximal inspired oxygen.

• Analgesia: NSAIDs are often very useful. Use opiate analgesia with caution in severe pain as this may depress respiratory efforts and/or cause hypotension secondary to vasodilation.

• Peripheral fluids.

• Give intravenous loading dose of heparin followed by infusion until a diagnosis is confirmed.

• Monitor cardiac rhythm, pulse, BP, oxygen saturation and respiration rate regularly.

The following are often required in cases of massive PE, especially if associated with hypotension.

• Thrombolysis: often recombinant tissue plasminogen activator is used, but protocol is different from that used in myocardial infarction. Can be given via a peripheral vein or pulmonary artery catheter.

• Give colloids if hypotensive and obtain central venous access for monitoring (preferably prior to anticoagulation).

• Inotropes may be required if hypotension persists.

• Discuss case with cardiothoracic team early should surgical embolectomy be required because the patient does not respond to thrombolysis and colloids and/or if thrombolysis is contraindicated.

Short term

• Analgesia.

• Heparin: unfractionated heparin (UFH) or low-molecular-weight heparin. Prevents further thrombus formation and permits endogenous fibrinolysis. If using UFH, continue until INR >2.0.

• Start warfarin once adequate anticoagulation with heparin is achieved.

> Paradoxically, warfarin without heparin may initially increase hypercoagulability.

Long term

1. Continue warfarin for between 6 weeks and 3 months if the risk factor is temporary and/or it is the patient's first PE.

2. Consider long-term anticoagulation for recurrent embolism and persisting risk factors such as thrombophilia.

3. Investigate for underlying cause if unknown. Possible investigations include:

   (a) Thrombophilia screen (see *Haematology*, Sections 1.1.4 and 3.3).

   (b) Ultrasound of deep veins in lower limbs and pelvis.

   (c) Autoimmune screen.

   (d) Biopsy of suspicious lymph nodes.

4. Consider inferior vena cava (IVC) filter for recurrent PE in the presence of adequate anticoagulation or if anticoagulation is contraindicated.

Complications

The most significant complication is secondary pulmonary hypertension.

Prognosis

This depends on the underlying cause. In general the prognosis is worse for larger PE. Poor prognostic indicators include:

- right ventricular dysfunction on echocardiography;

- hypotension;

- hypoxia;

- significant ECG changes associated with right heart strain.

Prevention

Primary

- Consider compression stockings and prophylactic heparin in hospitalised patients, especially those with trauma, the critically ill and those undergoing general and/or orthopaedic surgery.

- Discourage smoking.

- Encourage early mobilisation postoperatively.

Secondary

- Thrombophilia screening to determine whether prolonged/lifelong anticoagulation is required.

- Discourage smoking and advise alternatives to the oral contraceptive pill.

- Weight loss and BP control if necessary.

- Consider IVC filter in selected cases.

FURTHER READING

British Thoracic Society guidelines for management of suspected acute pulmonary embolism. *Thorax* 2003; 58: 470–84.

Fedullo PF and Tapson VF. The evaluation of suspected pulmonary embolism. *N. Engl. J. Med.* 2003; 349: 1247–56.

Goldhaber SZ. Pulmonary embolism. *N. Engl. J. Med.* 1998; 339: 93–104.

2.19 Driving restrictions in cardiology

Driving restrictions are under continuous review and can be seen on the DVLA (Driver and Vehicle Licensing Agency) website (http://www.dvla.gov.uk/). Many requirements for a Group 2 licence require the completion of an exercise tolerance test (ETT) to the following standards:

- off antianginal medication for 48 hours;

- complete Stage 3 of Bruce protocol without angina, syncope, ventricular tachycardia or hypotension;

- absence of signficant ST changes (>2 mm horizontal or downsloping);

- in cases of stable coronary heart disease the ETT needs to be repeated at least every 3 years.

The current guidelines for major cardiac conditions are outlined in Table 42.

TABLE 42 REGULATIONS FOR INDIVIDUALS WITH CARDIOVASCULAR DISEASE ISSUED BY THE DVLA IN THE UK

Condition		Group 1 entitlement (cars and motorcycles)	Group 2 entitlement (large lorries and buses)
Syncope	Simple faint (definite provocational factors, prodrome and unlikely to occur sitting or lying)	No restrictions	No restrictions
	No cause, normal cardiovascular system and central nervous system evaluation and low chance of recurrence	Can drive 4 weeks after event	Can drive 3 months after event
	As above but high chance of recurrence, eg abnormal ECG, echo or significant injury	Can drive 4 weeks after event if the cause is treated. If no cause is established, then no driving for 6 months	Can drive 3 months after event if the cause is treated. If no cause is established, then no driving for 1 year
	Presumed epileptic seizure	No driving for 1 year	No driving for 5 years
	Loss of consciousness with no clinical pointers	No driving for 6 months	No driving for 1 year
Angina		Permitted unless symptoms occur whilst driving	Only able to drive when free from angina for 6 weeks and meets ETT requirements
Angioplasty (elective)		Permitted after 1 week	Permitted after 6 weeks and meets ETT requirements
Coronary artery bypass grafting		Permitted after 4 weeks	Permitted after 6 weeks and meets ETT requirements
Acute coronary syndrome		Myocardial infarction: permitted after 4 weeks Non-ST-elevation myocardial infarction: permitted 1 week after succesful angioplasty	Permitted after 6 weeks if meets ETT requirements
Pacemaker/catheter ablation		Permitted after 1 week	Permitted after 6 weeks
Implantable cardioverter defibrillator (ICD)		Permitted after 6 months if there is no incapacity during anti-tachycardia pacing. There is a further 6-month restriction after each shock If the ICD is for primary prevention, the patient may drive 4 weeks after implantation	Permanent bar
Arrhythmia		Must cease driving if likely to cause incapacity whilst driving. May be permitted 4 weeks after cause identified and treated	Must cease driving if likely to cause incapacity whilst driving. May be permitted 3 months after cause identified and treated
Heart failure		Permitted provided no symptoms during driving	Permitted if ETT requirements are met and ejection fraction >40%

DVLA, Driver and Vehicle Licensing Agency; ETT, exercise tolerance test.

3.1 ECG

Principle

The ECG is a graphic representation of the electrical potentials of the heart. Each deflection represents electrical activity in the cardiac cycle.

- P wave: atrial depolarisation. A further deflection that represents atrial repolarisation is usually hidden within the QRS complex.

- PR interval: atrioventricular (AV) conduction time.

- QRS complex: ventricular depolarisation. Q is the first negative deflection, R the first positive deflection and S the first negative deflection following a positive deflection.

- ST segment: from the end of the QRS to the start of the T wave.

- T wave: ventricular repolarisation.

- U wave: after or in the end portion of the T wave. Cause unknown.

Adopting a systematic method of interpreting an ECG will enable you to approach the most complex of ECGs with confidence. If you approach all ECGs in this manner, then certain patterns will become familiar, enabling rapid diagnosis of arrhythmias and possible structural cardiac abnormalities.

An ECG interpretation scheme should include the following questions. After establishing the basic parameters, start at the P wave, progress through the QRS and finally examine the T wave.

- What is the rhythm? Is it regular or irregular?

- What is the rate? Rate = 300/number of large squares between each QRS. This will identify whether the heart rate is normal, bradycardic or tachycardic.

- What is the QRS axis?

- What is the P-wave axis?

- Is the P-wave morphology normal?

- Is the PR interval short or long?

- Are there any delta waves?

- Are there any Q waves?

- Is the QRS morphology normal? Are there any signs of right bundle-branch block or left bundle-branch block?

- Does the ST segment look normal in every lead?

- Are any T waves inverted?

- What is the QT interval?

- Are there any additional features such as U waves?

QRS axis

To establish the QRS axis you need to do the following.

- Identify the limb lead where the QRS is isoelectric: the axis will be 90° from this.

- Look at the limb lead whose axis is at 90° to the lead where the QRS is isoelectric (Fig. 96): if deflection is positive, the axis is directed towards the positive pole of that lead (and if negative, away from it).

The normal axis is from −30° to +90°. Figure 97 demonstrates examples of the normal axis and right- and left-axis deviation.

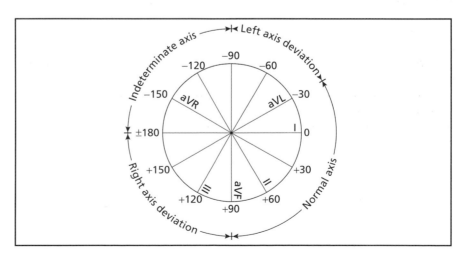

▲ **Fig. 96** Diagrammatic representation of the viewpoint of each limb lead.

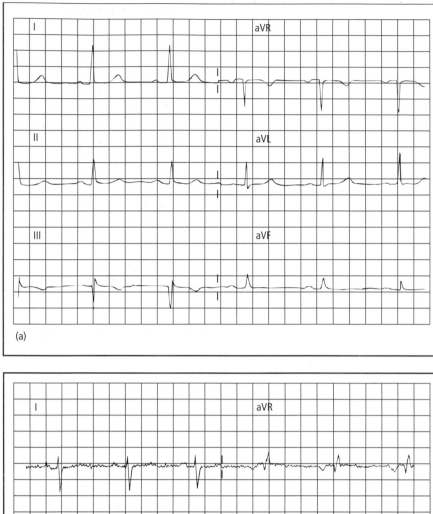

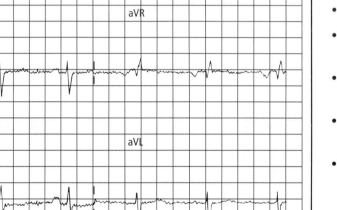

▲ **Fig. 97** Examples of (**a**) normal axis, (**b**) right-axis deviation.

Normal intervals

1 small square = 0.04 seconds.

- PR interval (onset of P wave to first deflection of QRS): 0.12–0.2 seconds.

- QRS duration: <0.12 seconds.

- QT interval (onset of QRS complex to end of T wave): 0.35–0.45 seconds.

- QTc (QT adjusted for rate) = QT/$\sqrt{(R–R\ interval)}$: 0.38–0.42 seconds.

Bradyarrhythmias/conduction disturbances

The key to identification of bradyarrhythmias is in establishing the relative relationship of the P wave and QRS complex. The following are the key features to identify:

- rate;

- whether there are irregular/regular P waves/QRS complexes;

- plot all P waves and all QRS complexes;

- no P wave before normal QRS suggests junctional rhythm;

- no P wave before wide QRS suggests ventricular escape rhythm.

Figures 98–103 illustrate varying degrees of AV block. Conduction abnormalities occur because of abnormalities in normal depolarisation from the AV node to the His bundle and bundle branches.

- Abnormalities in AV node/His bundle conduction lead to degrees of heart block, eg coronary artery disease, myocarditis, digoxin toxicity and electrolyte abnormalities.

- Abnormalities in conduction in the bundle branches leads to widened QRS complexes. Block of both bundles has the

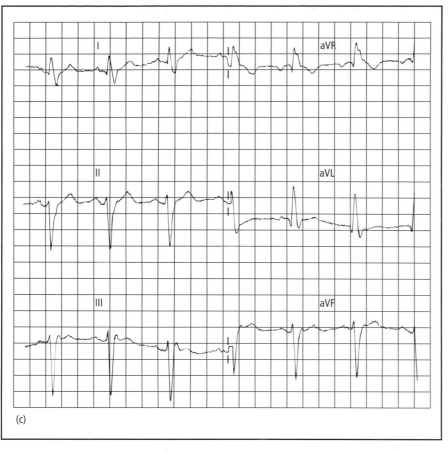

▲ **Fig. 97** (c) left-axis deviation.

- Narrow/broad complex?
- Identify whether there are irregular/regular P waves/ QRS complexes.
- 'Saw-tooth' appearance of the baseline suggests atrial flutter (ventricular rate may be irregular if there is a variable block).
- Regular narrow-complex tachycardia with no P waves seen suggests AV nodal re-entry tachycardia (see Section 2.2.2).
- Consider differential diagnosis of supraventricular tachycardia (SVT) with aberration and VT (Fig. 104) (Table 44).

Specific morphological changes in the ECG

Left ventricular hypertrophy
There are several criteria:

- usually left-axis deviation (>–30°);
- amplitude of S in V1 or V2 + R in V5 or V6 >40 mm;
- note that in young men with a thin chest wall, these criteria may be met without left ventricular hypertrophy.

same effect as block of the His bundle, causing complete heart block (Table 43).

Tachyarrhythmias
Find out whether there are any of the following.

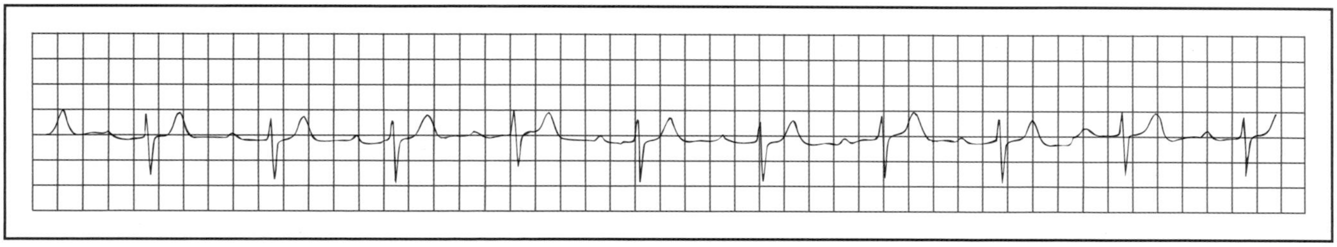

▲ **Fig. 98** Example of first-degree heart block. The PR interval is in excess of 0.20 seconds.

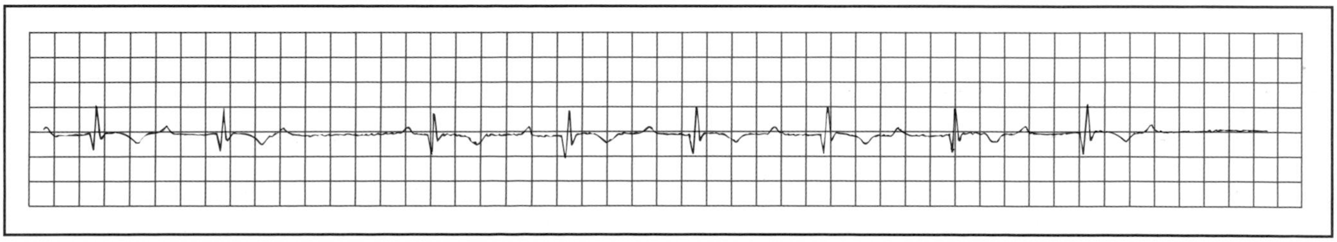

▲ **Fig. 99** Second-degree heart block (Wenckebach's or Mobitz type I) with progressively increasing PR interval prior to the failure of conduction with no QRS complex.

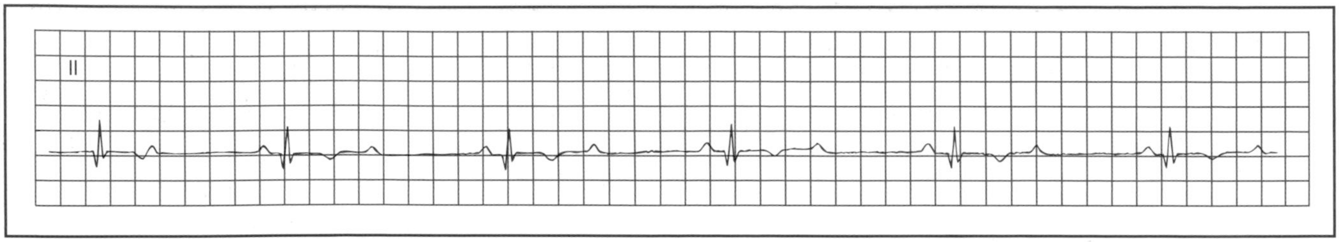

▲ **Fig. 100** Second-degree heart block (2:1): only alternate P waves are followed by a QRS complex. When there is failure of conduction without progressive increase in the PR interval, this is known as Mobitz type II.

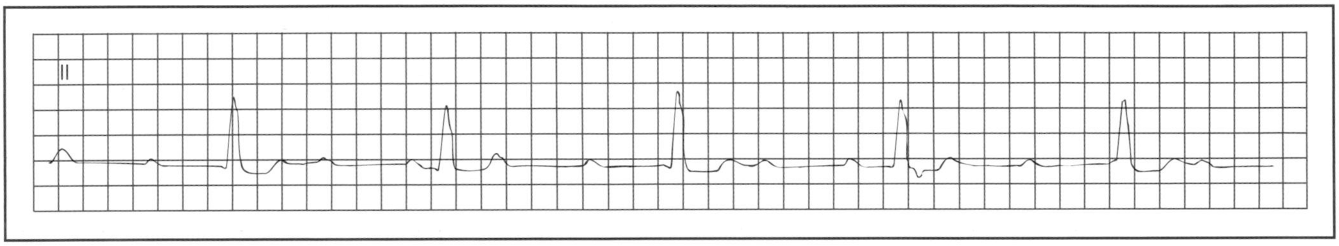

▲ **Fig. 101** Complete heart block: P waves and QRS complexes are not related. There is a slow ventricular escape rhythm (wider QRS complexes).

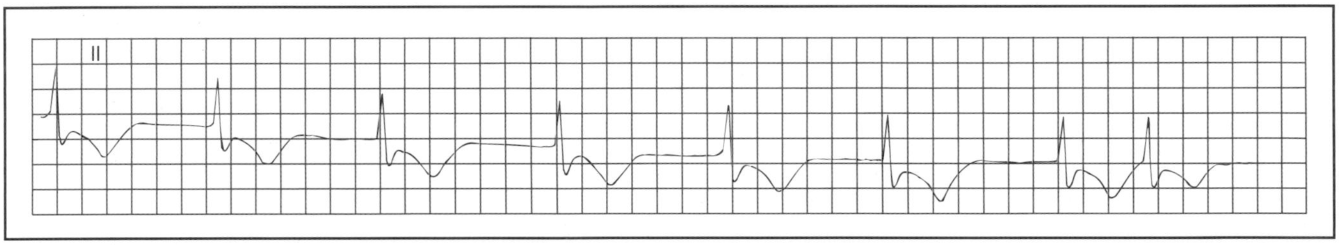

▲ **Fig. 102** Junctional bradycardia: slow ventricular rate with no discernible P waves.

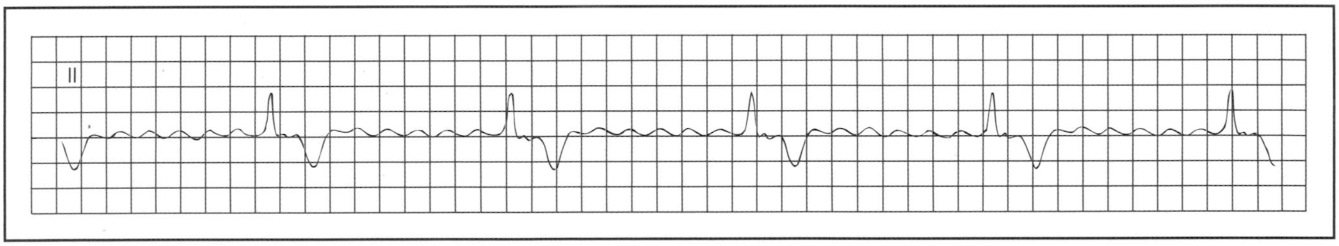

▲ **Fig. 103** Complete heart block in a patient with atrial fibrillation as the underlying atrial rhythm.

TABLE 43 SOME KEY CAUSES OF BUNDLE-BRANCH BLOCK

Right bundle-branch block	Left bundle-branch block
May be normal	Coronary artery disease
Coronary artery disease	Cardiomyopathy
Cardiomyopathy	Left ventricular hypertrophy (hypertension and
Atrial septal defect	aortic stenosis)
Ebstein's anomaly	Conduction system fibrosis
Massive pulmonary embolism	

Left bundle-branch block: wide (>0.12 seconds), notched, M- or plateau-shaped QRS complex in leads oriented to the left ventricle, ie V5, V6, aVL and I. Right bundle-branch block: M-shaped QRS complex in leads oriented to the right ventricle, ie V1 and V2.

Right ventricular hypertrophy

Criteria are the following:

- right-axis deviation (>90°);

- R V1 + S V6 >11 mm;

- R V1 or S V6 >7 mm.

Metabolic abnormalities

- Hypercalcaemia: short QT and prominent U wave.

- Hypocalcaemia: long QT.

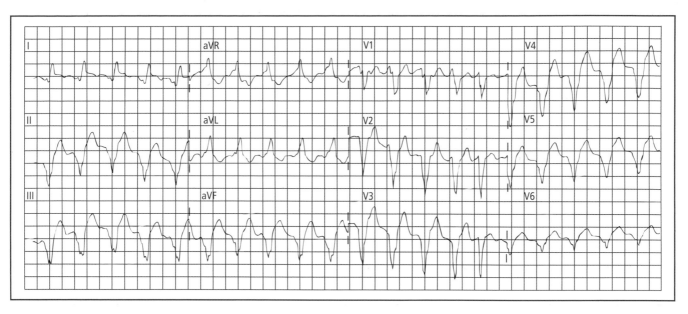

▲**Fig. 104** Twelve-lead ECG of VT with significant axis deviation, broad complexes and concordance across the chest leads.

TABLE 44 DIFFERENTIATION OF VENTRICULAR TACHYCARDIA (VT) AND SVT

Features supporting VT	Features supporting SVT
Very broad QRS complexes (>140 ms)	Termination with Valsalva manoeuvre/adenosine
Fusion beats	Association of 'p' waves and QRS complexes
Capture beats	Onset following premature atrial beat
AV dissociation	
Significant axis deviation (right or left)	
Concordance of the QRS deflections in V1–V6	
Onset following R on T	

- Hyperkalaemia: flat/lost P waves, increased PR interval, wide QRS, tented T wave and arrhythmias.

- Hypokalaemia: first-degree heart block, ST depression and U waves.

3.1.1 Exercise ECGs

Exercise ECGs are an extremely useful non-invasive investigation in appropriate clinical circumstances, but it is always important to remember that they can produce both false-negative and false-positive results. If significant diagnostic doubt remains in a patient who gives a good history of angina, further investigation should be considered (coronary angiography/myocardial perfusion imaging). Exercise testing in asymptomatic patients is of limited value.

Principle

The aim of the study is to document the electrophysiological and haemodynamic response to physical stress.

Indications

Exercise ECGs are indicated for the following:

- establishing a diagnosis of angina in a patient with chest pain;

- obtaining a measure of exercise tolerance;

- evaluating a haemodynamic response to exercise;

- evaluation of exercise-induced arrhythmias.

Contraindications

There is a very low mortality (<1 in 20,000) if the test is used in appropriate patients. The following are contraindications:

- significant aortic stenosis;

- acute pericarditis/myocarditis.

- acute myocardial infarction/unstable angina;

- acute aortic dissection;

- systemic infection;

- physical impairment that restricts patient from exercising.

Practical details

Before investigation

Omit antianginal medication if the test is for diagnostic reasons. Continue if a functional assessment on treatment is required. Note that beta-blockers and antihypertensives will mask the haemodynamic response.

The investigation

Close observation of the patient is required, with full resuscitation facilities to hand. At least two qualified people should supervise the test.

After investigation

Continue to observe the patient closely. Dramatic haemodynamic changes can occur during the recovery period. Terminate the investigation only when all the parameters have returned to normal levels.

Results

Normal ECG response to exercise

- Ventricular rate increases.

- P wave increases in amplitude.

- PR shortens.

- QRS: R-wave amplitude decreases.

- ST is sharply up-sloping.

- QT shortens.

- T wave decreases in amplitude.

Abnormal ECG response to exercise (Fig. 105)

- No increase in ventricular rate.

- ST depression >1 mm (horizontal/down-sloping): myocardial ischaemia (the greater the degree and the longer it persists into recovery, the greater the probability of coronary heart disease).

- ST elevation (horizontal/up-sloping): where previous myocardial infarction suggests dyskinetic ventricle/aneurysm.

- QRS: bundle-branch block may suggest ischaemia.

- QT: prolongation of QTc (QT adjusted for rate) may be a risk marker for torsade de pointes.

- T wave: inversion suggests ischaemia.

- Arrhythmias: ventricular arrhythmia suggests ischaemia.

FURTHER READING

Cleland JGF, Findlay IN, Gilligan D and Pennell DJ. *The Essentials of Exercise Electrocardiography*. London: Current Medical Literature Ltd, 1993.

Hampton JR. *The ECG Made Easy*. Edinburgh: Churchill Livingstone, 1997.

Xiao HB and Spicer M. How to do electrocardiography. *Br. J. Cardiol.* 1996; 3: 148–50.

3.2 Basic electrophysiology studies

Principle

Pace/sense electrodes are placed transvenously via the femoral vein and/or subclavian/internal jugular vein to various intracardiac locations. Electrograms are recorded during sinus rhythm. Arrhythmias are induced using pacing protocols with programmed extra stimuli.

Indications

Electrophysiology studies may be helpful in the following circumstances.

- Narrow complex tachyarrhythmias: assessing for radiofrequency (RF) ablation.

- Broad complex arrhythmias: assessing for RF ablation or implantation of implantable cardioverter defibrillator.

- Establishing a diagnosis in patients with palpitations/syncope.

- Assessing bradyarrhythmias (although it is of limited value for this).

Contraindications

Electrophysiology studies are not indicated for patients with the following:

- reversible aetiology for arrhythmia;

- severe electrolyte abnormality.

Practical details

Before investigation

Antiarrhythmic medication is usually stopped 48 hours before study.

The investigation

Intravenous sedative (often benzodiazepine) may be used before the procedure because some pacing protocols produce extremely rapid heart rates. Quadripolar electrodes are placed to obtain intracardiac electrograms (high right atrium, right ventricular apex/outflow tract and His–Purkinje system) (Fig. 106). A multipolar electrode placed in the coronary sinus records electrograms from the left atrium and ventricle. Arrhythmias are induced by delivering extra pacing beats after a train of paced beats in the atrium and ventricle. These extra stimuli are timed to occur during the refractory period in an attempt to establish a possible re-entry mechanism (Fig. 107). The timing of the individual electrograms will indicate whether there is a possible electrophysiological substrate for arrhythmias. Assessment of the function of the sinoatrial and atrioventricular nodes indicates whether permanent pacing might be required.

After investigation

Patients are observed for up to 24 hours. Drug therapy may be changed as a result of the study.

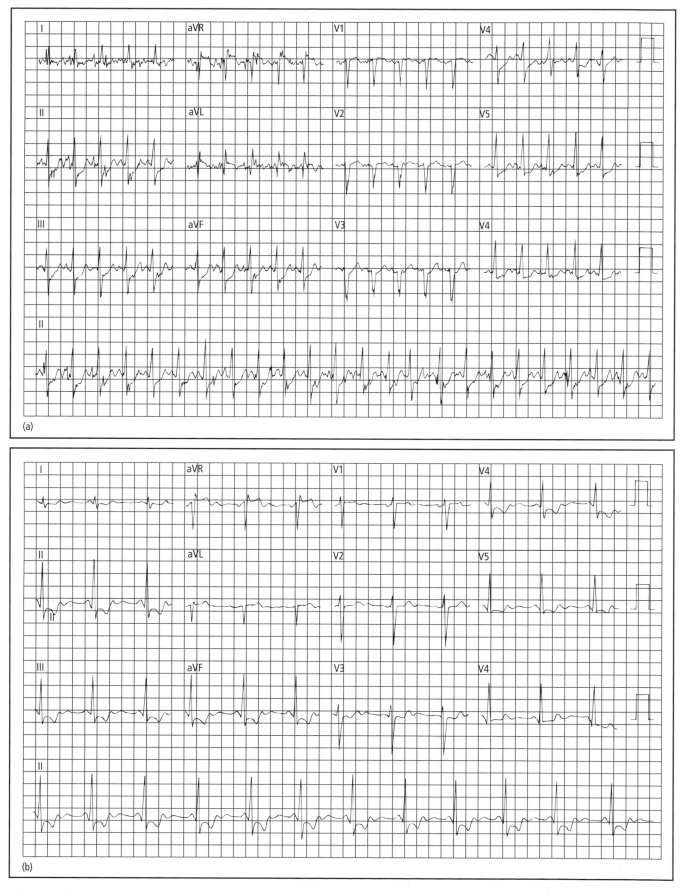

▲ **Fig. 105** Positive exercise ECGs: note the significant ST changes in the inferolateral leads (**a**) that become more marked in recovery (**b**).

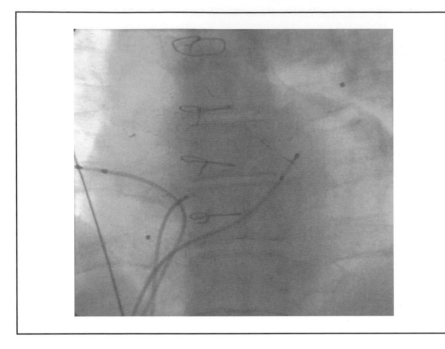

▲**Fig. 106** Radiograph demonstrating electrodes placed in the high right atrium, right ventricular outflow tract and His bundle during an electrophysiological test. Sternal wires are present from previous coronary bypass grafting.

Complications

- Femoral vein/subclavian vein (haematoma).

- Incessant arrhythmias requiring cardioversion, eg atrial fibrillation.

FURTHER READING

Fogoros RN. *Electrophysiological Testing*, 2nd edn. Oxford: Blackwell Science, 1995.

3.3 Ambulatory monitoring

Principle

Documenting a single- or dual-channel ECG over 24 hours can provide useful information in the investigation of patients with palpitations, arrhythmias and syncope. It is non-invasive and, with current analysis hardware/software, tapes can be analysed rapidly and accurately. Some devices record the ECG data on a digital card, enabling up to 10 days' continuous monitoring. It is always important when using Holter monitoring to appreciate that this provides only a brief snapshot of the patient's heart rhythm, and that a negative result does not mean that the patient's symptoms are not secondary to an arrhythmia.

Indications

Ambulatory monitoring is indicated for the following:

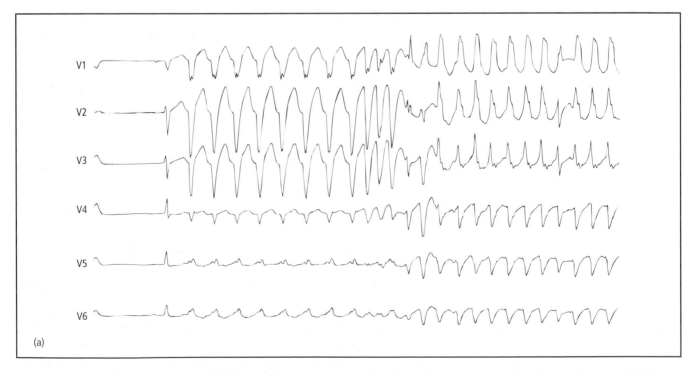

(a)

▲**Fig. 107** Induction of ventricular tachycardia (VT): **(a)** note the train of paced beats followed by earlier extra stimuli and then the onset of monomorphic VT.

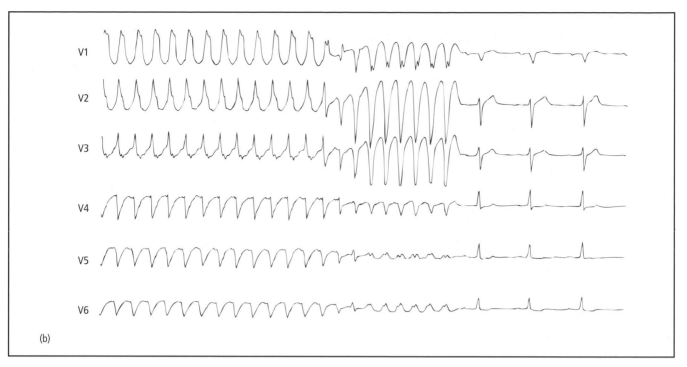

▲**Fig. 107** **(b)** VT is then terminated with nine beats of overdrive pacing.

- evaluation of patients with palpitations and syncope;

- monitoring the efficacy of antiarrhythmic therapy;

- evaluation of heart rate variability.

Practical details

There are a number of different methods by which heart rate and rhythm can be observed.

Twenty-four-hour Holter monitoring

This is used for patients with frequent symptoms. Even some patients who have infrequent symptoms may have asymptomatic arrhythmic episodes on a 24-hour recording that may provide valuable information (Fig. 108).

Patient-activated devices

These are used for less frequent symptoms, eg Cardiomemo recorder.

However, the efficacy of these devices relies on the patient activating the device, which is not always possible during or shortly after a symptomatic episode.

Implantable loop recorders

These are used for infrequent symptoms. They enable the patient to activate the device up to 40 minutes after the event and still record the heart rhythm (Figs 109 and 110).

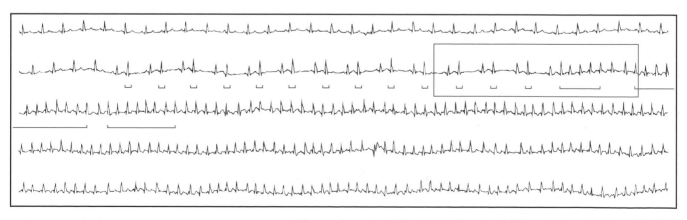

▲**Fig. 108** Holter monitor recording demonstrating atrioventricular nodal re-entry tachycardia/atrioventricular re-entry tachycardia. Note the sudden onset after a short period of ventricular bigeminy.

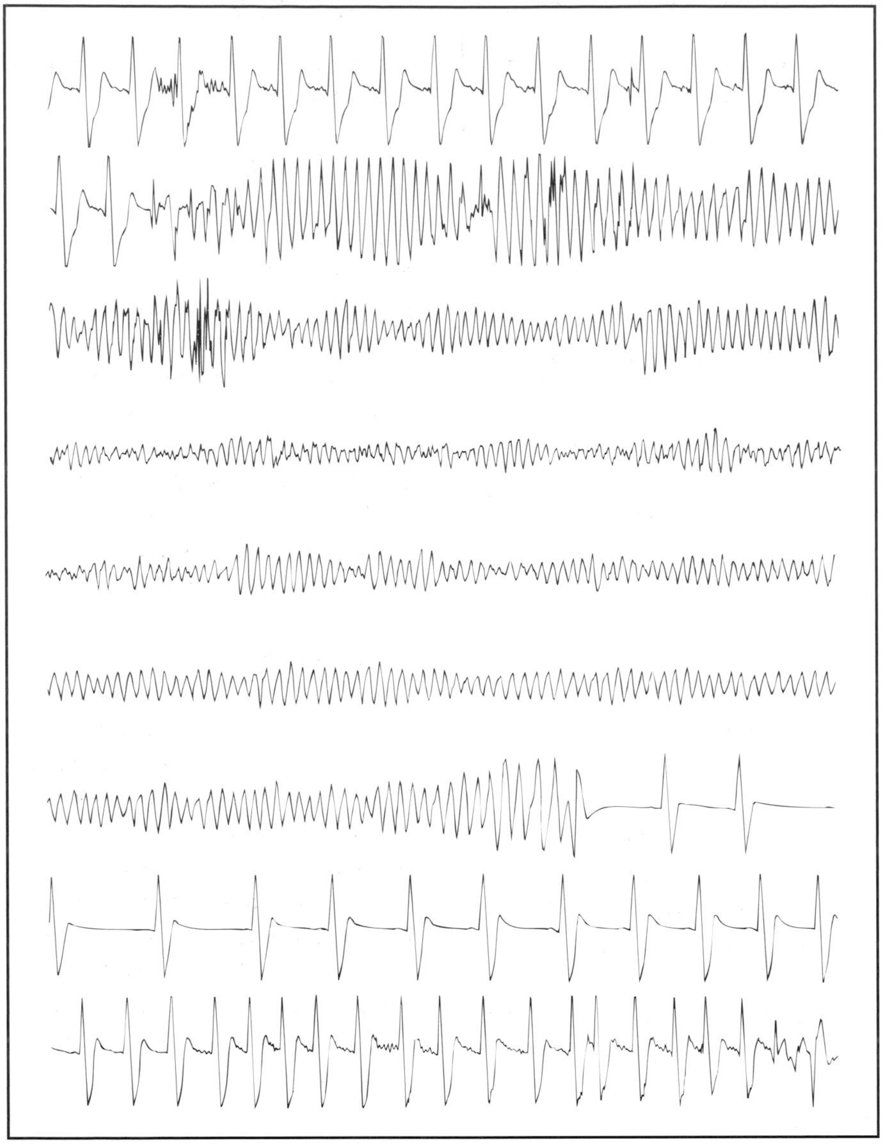

▲ **Fig. 109** Loop recording showing sinus tachycardia followed by torsade de pointes with spontaneous resolution.

3.4 Radiofrequency ablation and implantable cardioverter defibrillators

3.4.1 Radiofrequency ablation

Principle
The basic idea is to place an electrode in a specific site in the heart and then deliver energy through the electrode to produce a discrete scar. As the scar is electrically inactive, the pathways necessary for tachyarrhythmias may be disrupted. Most tachyarrhythmias can be treated with radiofrequency (RF) ablation.

- Atrioventricular (AV) nodal re-entry tachycardia.
- Wolff–Parkinson–White syndrome.
- Concealed accessory pathways (AV re-entry tachycardia).

- Ventricular tachycardia (VT).
- Focal atrial tachycardias.
- Atrial fibrillation (AF): paroxysmal/persistent AF or fast rates abolished by ablation of AV node and pacemaker implant for permanent AF.
- Most can be accessed via the right side of the heart from the femoral/subclavian veins; others (left-sided pathways/left-sided VT) have to be approached from either the femoral artery/aorta or via an atrial trans-septal approach.

Indications
Indications include those who have recurrent tachyarrhythmias despite antiarrhythmic therapy. Some patients (eg those with Wolff–Parkinson–White syndrome) who are at high risk should be considered for RF ablation even if asymptomatic.

Practical details

Before procedure
Antiarrhythmic drug therapy is usually stopped a few days before the procedure as it is usually necessary to induce the arrhythmia prior to delivering RF energy. Be careful: informed consent must be given by the patient before the procedure can go ahead.

The procedure
The treatment is usually performed under sedation.

After procedure
Most patients are discharged on the same day as the procedure or the following day.

Complications
The major complication of RF ablation procedures is the risk of unintentional damage to the AV

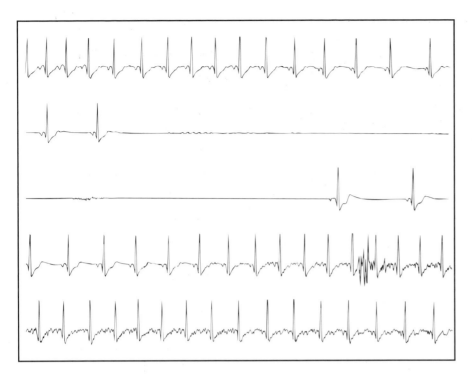

▲ **Fig. 110** Tracing from implantable loop recorder showing significant pause.

node and the need for a permanent pacemaker. This occurs in <1% of cases. A rare complication is cardiac perforation which may require pericardiocentesis or surgical repair.

Prognosis

- RF ablation is usually permanent.
- Less than 10% recurrence of the arrhythmia.

FURTHER READING

Fogoros RN. *Electrophysiological Testing*. Oxford: Blackwell Science, 1995.

3.4.2 Implantable cardioverter defibrillator

Principle

Patients who are at high risk of ventricular arrhythmias may benefit from an implantable cardioverter defibrillator (ICD). Once a ventricular arrhythmia is detected, an ICD can either deliver antitachycardia pacing or shock therapy (electrodes in the right ventricle, superior vena cava and/or casing of the ICD), or a combination of both depending on how the device is programmed.

Indications

In general, indications are becoming broader as larger prospective randomised trials are reported (eg AVID, MADIT, MUSTT, MADIT II and SCDHeFT):

- previous spontaneous ventricular tachycardia (VT)/ventricular fibrillation (VF);

- syncope of undetermined aetiology with VT inducible during electrophysiology studies (see Section 3.2).

- severely impaired left ventricular function (ejection fraction <30%).

Contraindications

- Reversible cause for VT/VF.

- Incessant VT/VF.

- Surgical, medical or psychiatric contraindication.

Practical details

Before procedure

Patients are thoroughly investigated to exclude any reversible cause of arrhythmia (undergoing echocardiography, cardiac catheterisation and CT/MRI). Some will have an electrophysiology study to confirm the diagnosis and identify whether the arrhythmia can be pace terminated (see Section 3.2).

The procedure

ICDs are implanted using local anaesthetic and sedation (e.g. midazolam), or general anaesthesia. The leads are placed transvenously via the subclavian/cephalic veins. The device is implanted either under the pectoralis major muscle or subcutaneously on the left side of the chest wall (Fig. 111). VF is produced to ensure that the device can successfully terminate it with shock therapy.

After procedure

On the following day the device is checked to ensure correct function of the pacing systems: patients often undergo a further VF induction under sedation.

Complications

Complications are similar to those associated with pacemaker implantation (see Section 3.5).

Prognosis

Most patients with ICDs die as a result of cardiac pump failure or incessant ventricular arrhythmia. ICDs last between 5 and 10 years, depending on the number of shocks delivered.

FURTHER READING

The Antiarrhythmic Versus Implantable Defibrillator (AVID) Investigators. A comparison of antiarrhythmic drug therapy with implantable defibrillators in patients resuscitated from near fatal ventricular arrhythmias. *N Engl J Med* 1997; 337: 1576–83.

Bardy GH, Lee KL, Mark DB, *et al.* Amiodarone or an implantable cardioverter-defibrillator for congestive heart failure. *N. Engl. J. Med.* 2005; 352: 225–37.

Buxton A, Lee K, Fisher J, *et al.* for the Multicenter Unsustained Tachycardia Trial (MUSTT) Investigation. A randomised study of the prevention of sudden death in patients with coronary artery disease. *N. Engl. J. Med.* 1999; 341: 1882–990.

Linde C. Implantable cardioverter-defibrillator treatment and resynchronisation in heart failure. *Heart* 2004; 90: 231–4.

Moss A, Hall J, Cannon D, *et al.* for the MADIT Investigation. Improved survival with an implanted defibrillator in patients with coronary disease at high risk of ventricular arrhythmias. *N. Engl. J. Med.* 1996; 335: 1933–40.

Moss AJ, Zareba W, Hall WJ, *et al.* Prophylactic implantation of a defibrillator in patients with myocardial infarction and reduced ejection fraction. *N. Engl. J. Med.* 2002; 346: 877–83.

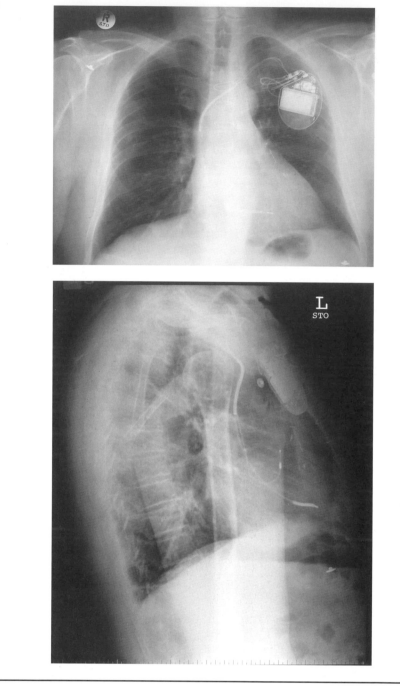

▲ **Fig. 111** CXR of patient with dual-chamber implantable cardioverter defibrillator (posteroanterior and lateral). Note electrode in right ventricle with defibrillation coil at distal end. A pace/sense electrode is positioned in the right atrial appendage.

3.4.3 Cardiac resynchronisation therapy

Some symptomatic patients who have impaired left ventricular function (ejection fraction <30%) and left bundle-branch block on their ECG will benefit from having an additional pacing lead placed on the epicardial surface of the left ventricle. This is placed through the cardiac veins, which are accessed through the coronary sinus via the right atrium. This allows the implantable cardioverter defibrillator (ICD) or pacemaker to synchronise contraction of both the right and left ventricle, leading to improved haemodynamic function. This has been shown to improve both symptoms and mortality in selected patients. Cardiac resynchronisation therapy (CRT) can be incorporated into ICDs (CRT-D) or stand-alone pacemakers (CRT-P) (Fig. 112).

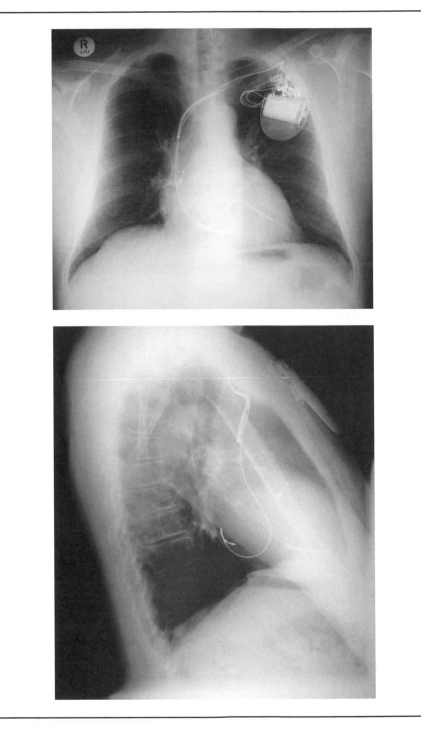

▲ **Fig. 112** Posteroanterior and lateral CXR of patient with CRT-D device. Note the additional lead positioned over the left ventricle.

3.5 Pacemakers

Pacing of patients with non-reversible significant bradyarrhythmias can restore life expectancy to close to that of the normal population. Pacemakers have improved considerably over the last two decades. Devices have increased in longevity and reduced in size. In addition, many technical innovations have resulted in pacemakers that are more physiological in their mode of action. The simplest of pacemakers consists of a single lead, with its tip in the right ventricular apex connected to the pulse generator in the subcutaneous tissue of the chest wall. Dual-chamber devices have a further lead with its tip positioned in the right atrial appendage (Fig. 113 and Fig. 114). Pacemakers have a designated terminology which describes the pacing and sensing functions of each device (Table 45).

Indications

Temporary pacemaker

Temporary pacing is useful in the following circumstances.

- As an interim measure before fitting a permanent pacemaker.

- Inferior myocardial infarction: second- or third-degree block and hypotension/heart failure.

- Anterior myocardial infarction: second- or third-degree block (usually large infarct to involve the atrioventricular node).

- Symptomatic/asymptomatic patients with trifascicular block undergoing general anaesthesia (should be assessed for a permanent pacemaker).

- Drug overdose, eg digoxin, beta-blockers or verapamil.

Temporary pacing is not indicated for asymptomatic patients with bifascicular block who are undergoing general anaesthesia.

Permanent pacemaker

The permanent pacemaker is useful for the following:

- third-degree heart block;

- symptomatic second-degree block;

- asymptomatic type II second-degree block;

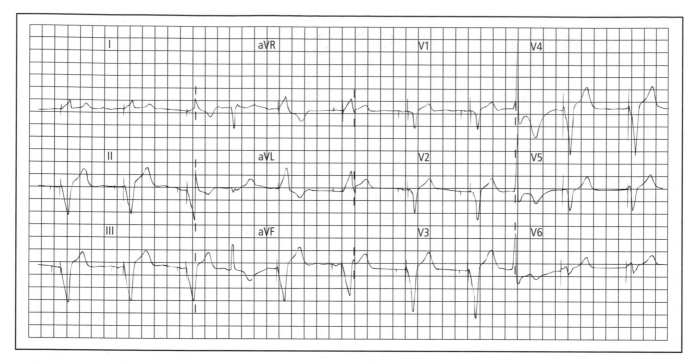

▲**Fig. 113** ECG demonstrating dual-chamber pacing. Note the pacing 'spike' before most P waves and QRS complexes.

TABLE 45 ALGORITHM FOR DESCRIBING PACEMAKER FUNCTION.

Paced chamber	Sensed chamber	Effect of sensing	Programming/rate responsiveness
0 = none	0 = none	0 = none	0 = none
A = atrium	A = atrium	T = triggered	P = simple
V = ventricle	V = ventricle	I = inhibited	M = multiprogrammable
D = dual (A + V)	D = dual (A + V)	D = dual (T + I)	C = communicating
			R = rate responsive

For example, a DDDR pacemaker both senses and paces in the atrium and ventricle, and triggers and inhibits, depending on what is or is not sensed. It also has a rate response which means that the heart will be paced faster if appropriate, eg during exercise.

- atrial fibrillation with pauses >3 seconds;
- symptomatic documented sinus node dysfunction;
- recurrent syncope associated with >3-second pause with carotid sinus stimulation.

Practical details

Before procedure
Patients should give informed consent and be fasted.

The procedure
The procedure is usually performed under local anaesthesia. The pacemaker leads are placed transvenously via the cephalic/ subclavian routes into the right ventricular apex and right atrial appendage under fluoroscopic guidance. The leads are checked to ensure correct pace/sense functions and the pulse generator is implanted subcutaneously.

After procedure
After a satisfactory pacemaker check the following day, most patients may be discharged from hospital, usually with 5 days of antibiotic therapy and after a lateral and posteroanterior CXR (Fig. 114). For driving regulations, see Section 2.19. Pacemakers can be programmed and interrogated by placing a 'wand' over the device; using electromagnetic induction, information can be received or transmitted to the pacemaker. Patients are usually seen every 6–12 months to monitor the pacemaker and re-program it if necessary. The expected life of the battery is 8–12 years.

Complications of pacemakers
Although complications are rare, the following may occur.

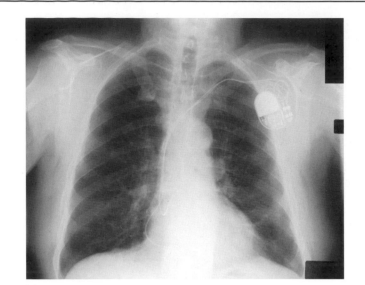

(a)

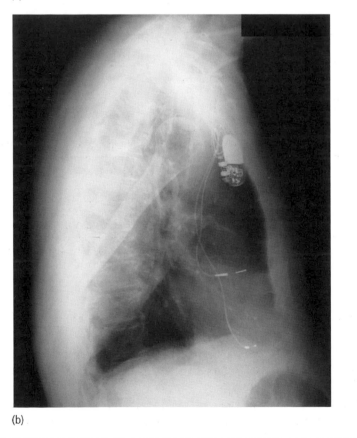

(b)

▲ **Fig. 114** CXR of dual-chamber pacemaker: (**a**) posteroanterior and (**b**) lateral.

Common

- Pneumothorax.
- Pacemaker lead displacement (Fig. 115).
- Haematoma.

Uncommon

- Local infection.
- Pericardial effusion.
- Thrombosis and thromboembolism.

- Infective endocarditis.
- Pacemaker syndrome: single-chamber pacing, leading to symptoms as a result of loss of atrioventricular synchrony.

Rare

- Twiddler's syndrome: patient consciously/subconsciously turns the pacemaker generator, leading to retraction and eventual displacement of the pacing lead.
- Component failure: lead/pulse generator.

FURTHER READING

Lamb D and Schilling R. Who's for a pacemaker? *Br. J. Cardiol.* 1999; 6: 580–2.

- - - - - - - - - - - - - - - - - -

Roberts PR. Follow up and optimisation of cardiac pacing. *Heart* 2005; 91:1229–34.

- - - - - - - - - - - - - - - - - -

Schilling R and Peters N. Insertion of permanent pacemakers. *Br. J. Cardiol.* 1999; 6: 550–6.

3.6 Chest radiograph in cardiac disease

Abnormalities of cardiac silhouette

The normal cardiac silhouette is shown in Fig. 116. Below are the most commonly encountered abnormalities.

Cardiomegaly

A cardiothoracic ratio >0.5 on posteroanterior projection is a fairly specific indicator of cardiac disease, but may be falsely increased in pes excavatum and very thin patients; the same indication cannot be assumed for anteroposterior projections of the heart. Echocardiography is much more sensitive and enables direct measurement of ventricular

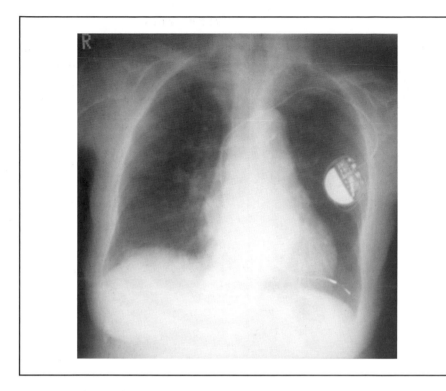

▲ **Fig. 115** CXR showing displacement of ventricular lead through ventricle to pericardial space.

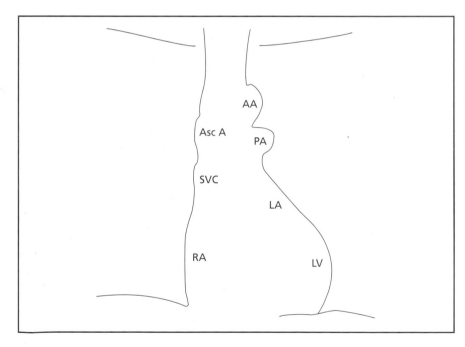

▲ **Fig. 116** Schematic diagram of cardiac silhouette on CXR. AA, arch aorta; Asc A, ascending aorta; LA, left atrial appendage; LV, left ventricle; PA, pulmonary artery; RA, right atrium; SVC, superior vena cava.

wall thickness, cavity dimensions and function.

Aortic enlargement

This is seen in hypertension, aortic aneurysm or aortic regurgitation:

- prominent aortic arch;

- ascending aorta protrudes further to the right side;

- tortuous descending aorta.

Mediastinal widening

This may indicate an aortic aneurysm and/or aortic dissection.

Enlarged pulmonary artery

This is seen in the following conditions.

- Pulmonary hypertension: chronic obstructive pulmonary disease, primary pulmonary hypertension and Eisenmenger's syndrome.

- Pulmonary stenosis: poststenotic dilatation as a result of turbulent blood flow.

- Collagen disorders such as Marfan's syndrome.

Left atrial enlargement

This is seen in mitral valve disease (both stenosis and regurgitation), left ventricular impairment and mitral valve replacement. The left atrium and its appendage are situated in a small concavity immediately below the left main bronchus on the left heart border. Loss of this concavity or a protrusion beyond the normal left heart border is indicative of left atrial enlargement. There is also associated elevation of the left main bronchus increasing the normal carinal angle of 75°. In massive enlargement, the left atrium forms part of the right heart border, giving rise to a double border right heart shadow. Left atrial enlargement may be mimicked by mediastinal or pleural neoplasm.

Left ventricular enlargement

This is often associated with:

- pressure overload (apex elevated and more rounded in shape);

- volume overload (widening of the cardiac shadow).

Right ventricular enlargement

The right ventricle does not normally form a cardiac border, but enlargement pushes the left ventricle posteriorly and to the left, causing widening of the heart shadow.

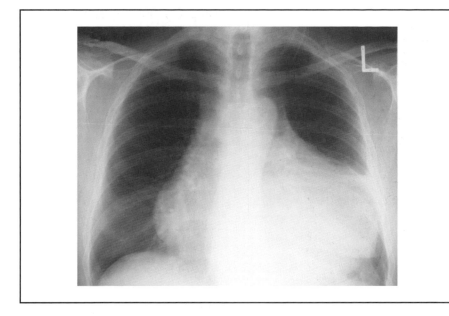

▲ **Fig. 117** Globular cardiomegaly caused by a large pericardial effusion. Note sternal wires from recent cardiac surgery.

Pericardial effusion

This may produce massive cardiomegaly, giving the cardiac contour a globular appearance, with clear lung fields (Fig. 117).

Abnormalities of pulmonary vasculature

Increased pulmonary blood flow

- Enlarged pulmonary arteries.
- Recruitment of upper lobe vessels.

Pulmonary hypertension

- Peripheral vasoconstriction (pruning).
- Further enlargement of pulmonary arteries.
- Pulmonary artery calcification.

Pulmonary venous hypertension and pulmonary oedema

In increasing order of severity:

- upper lobe blood diversion;
- interlobular septal thickening (Kerley B lines), seen as thin horizontal lines at lung bases;

- alveolar oedema, typically involving the inner two-thirds of the lung ('bat-wing' hilar shadowing);
- pleural effusions.

Pulmonary oedema is occasionally unilateral. After treatment, the radiographic appearances often lag behind clinical improvement. Prominent interstitial lines also occur in the following:

- fibrosis;
- tumour infiltration;
- interstitial pneumonia.

3.7 Cardiac biochemical markers

Principle

Heart muscle damage, usually caused by acute ischaemia, causes release of proteins that can be detected in the bloodstream.

Creatine kinase

- Creatine kinase (CK) is a cytosolic enzyme that is still measured routinely (more often, the cardiospecific myocardial-bound isoenzyme, CK-MB).
- Peak value reflects extent of heart muscle damage.
- Has a reasonable specificity, but only a moderate sensitivity.
- Rises 4–6 hours post myocardial infarction (MI) with peak at around 21–24 hours.
- Used in conjunction with the ECG to make the diagnosis of non-ST-elevation MI.
- May give equivocal results and may be uninterpretable in some circumstances, eg very high CK caused by coexisting skeletal muscle damage (note that CK-MB is also found to a small extent in skeletal muscle).

Troponin tests

These are now superseding CK-MB assays. Troponins are regulatory elements of the contractile apparatus in muscles; they exist in cardiac-specific isoforms and are highly sensitive. Rapid bedside assays for cardiac troponins T and I are available. Normally, they exist at very low levels or are undetectable in the blood and appear 4–6 hours after myocardial damage, peak at 24 hours and persist for up to 14 days (Fig. 118). Since they are cardiac specific, skeletal muscle damage does not influence their level. In addition, they are sensitive to the cardiac damage missed by CK.

- In patients presenting with acute coronary syndrome (ACS), a positive test (ie non-ST-elevation MI) is associated with a higher risk of death or MI, the higher level indicating a worse prognosis.

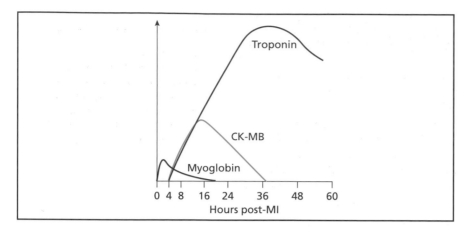

▲ **Fig. 118** Time course of cardiac markers after heart muscle damage. MI, myocardial infarction.

- They may be used to select high-risk patients with ACS likely to benefit from more aggressive treatment, eg low-molecular-weight heparin, glycoprotein IIb/IIIa receptor antagonists and early revascularisation.

- A negative test may be used in conjunction with clinical and ECG criteria to identify low-risk patients suitable for early (12-hour) discharge.

- Because of their long time window they can detect MI up to 1–2 weeks after the event.

- Whilst an elevated troponin reflects myocardial necrosis, this can occur in situations other than epicardial coronary artery occlusion, eg myocarditis, acute massive pulmonary embolus, sepsis (multiple organ failure) and severe renal failure (decreased excretion).

Myoglobin

Myoglobin is present in both skeletal and cardiac muscle, and is released about 30 minutes after heart muscle damage. Elevated values may detect infarction much sooner after the onset of chest pain than CK-MB or troponins (Fig. 118). It has a short time window and as such can miss late presentations. As a result of the poor specificity of myoglobin measurement, a positive test must be confirmed by troponin or CK-MB assay.

Brain (B-type) natriuretic peptide

This is a peptide hormone produced by the myocardium (ventricles > atria) in response to myocardial wall stress. Peripheral blood levels are elevated in patients with left ventricular dysfunction and relate to the severity of heart failure and prognosis. In terms of diagnosis it is most valuable as an exclusion test for heart failure, where a normal value virtually excludes the presence of left ventricular dysfunction. Levels can be affected by other conditions, including myocardial ischaemia (and infarction), severe airways disease and renal impairment.

FURTHER READING

Kaski JC, Holt DW, eds. *Myocardial Damage: Early Detection by Novel Biochemical Markers.* Dordrecht: Kluwer Academic Publishers, 1998.

3.8 CT and MRI

3.8.1 Multislice spiral CT

Principle

CT scanners produce multiple radiographic views of the body, which after processing are expressed in the form of digital cross-sectional images. Tissues with different densities are displayed at different grey-scale values. Current generation multislice spiral CT (MSCT) scanners are equipped with multiple, thin rows of detectors that rapidly rotate around a slowly moving patient, producing a very large number of images. To reduce motion artefacts from cardiac contraction, images are ECG gated and only data obtained during the diastolic phase of the cardiac cycle (when cardiac motion is minimal) are used for image reconstruction. These images can be reconstructed in multiple (non-axial) planes.

Indications

Pericardial disease

To detect thickening, infiltration or pericardial effusion.

Pulmonary disease

CT pulmonary angiography can image the pulmonary vasculature down to the level of the segmental branches (although ventilation–perfusion scans or invasive pulmonary angiograms are still better for smaller branches).

Thoracoabdominal vessels

To detect aortic aneurysm and/or dissection, and renal and carotid stenosis.

See Table 46 for conditions considered contraindications to CT.

TABLE 46 CONDITIONS CONSIDERED CONTRAINDICATIONS TO CT

Condition	Comment
Contrast	Known sensitivity or renal impairment (relative contraindication)
Pregnancy	Large radiation dose but depends on risk/benefit balance and uterus can be shielded (relative contraindication)
Chronic obstructive airways disease (COPD)	Patients with severe COPD may not be able to hold their breath for the 20-second duration of the scan, thereby introducing motion artefacts (relative contraindication)
Extensive coronary calcification	Calcium is high in density and results in artefacts
Irregular and fast heart rhythm	Atrial fibrillation, frequent extrasystoles and fast heart rhythm can result in significant motion artefacts

Potential applications for CT

Emerging clinical indications:

- Imaging of coronary arteries: coronary angiography is becoming increasingly possible with current MSCT machines (sensitivity and specificity of detecting luminal narrowings of >50% is around 90%). This includes imaging patency of most coronary stents (Fig. 119). Images are acquired during a single breath-hold of 20 seconds. Motion artefacts can be reduced with beta-blockade to achieve a heart rate of ≤70 bpm and reduce ventricular extrasystoles.

- Imaging of coronary bypass grafts: MSCT can be used to detect occluded venous bypass grafts (sensitivity 97–100%, specificity 98%). However, MSCT is not as accurate at diagnosing non-occlusive stenosis in venous grafts or imaging arterial grafts (Fig. 120).
- Coronary calcium score: presence of calcium in the coronary tree is a surrogate for the presence of atherosclerosis. Several prospective studies have demonstrated that a high calcium score is associated with a higher risk of future coronary events. However, current data are conflicting and results from large randomised follow-up trials are awaited.

Possible future clinical applications:

- Determination of atherosclerotic plaque composition: MSCT can potentially be used to detect lipid and fibrous composition of non-calcified atherosclerotic plaques. This information might help to identify potentially vulnerable plaques.

3.8.2 MRI

Principle

Atomic nuclei with odd (ie unpaired) numbers of protons, neutrons or both have a net charge and hence a magnetic moment. This magnetic property is exploited in MRI. Hydrogen atoms are the major constituent of the body with a magnetic moment, and are the nuclei imaged by cardiac MRI.

The principle of MRI is simple. A large superconducting magnet produces a very strong external magnetic field (eg 1.5 T, equating to a magnetic field 1500 times stronger than the earth's magnetic field). Electromagnetic energy is transmitted from coil to nuclei in the body, exciting them to a higher energy state. As nuclei return to equilibrium the excess energy is

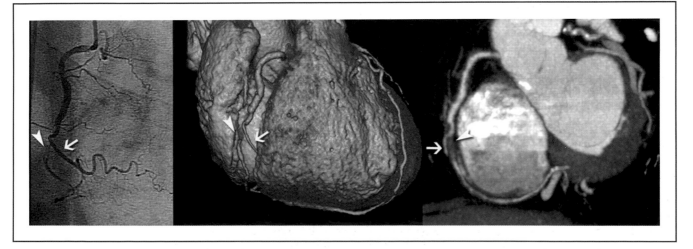

▲ **Fig. 119** Comparison between angiography (**a**) and MSCT images of the right coronary artery (expressed in two different processed image modalities, **b** and **c**). (Adapted with permission for the BMJ Publishing Group, from Mollet NR, Cademartiri F and de Feyter PJ. Non-invasive multislice CT coronary imaging. *Heart* 2005; 91: 401–7.)

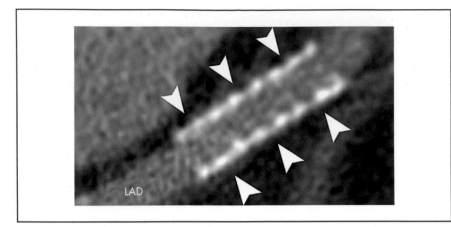

▲ **Fig. 120** Cross-sectional MSCT image of a patent coronary stent. (Adapted with permission for the BMJ Publishing Group, from Mollet NR, Cademartiri F and de Feyter PJ. Non-invasive multislice CT coronary imaging. *Heart* 2005; 91: 401–7.)

released in the form of electromagnetic waves. This energy is detected by the scanner. As different tissues return to equilibrium at different rates, complex mathematical techniques (Fourier transformation) can be used so that the structure comprising the tissues can be reconstructed. As for cardiac CT scanning, images are ECG gated (only acquired during diastole when the heart is relatively still). Irregular rhythms and tachycardia result in poorer image quality.

Indications

Anatomy

- Imaging of non-cardiac vessels: MRI can be used to acurately image thoracoabdominal and head and neck vessels including aortic aneurysms, dissection and coarctation, and stenosis of carotid and renal arteries. In aortic dissection, MRI flow studies can differentiate between the true and false lumens. Reproducibility of MRI makes it particularly attractive for the long-term follow-up of aortic coarctation and dissection repairs.

- Congenital heart disease: MRI produces a very detailed three-

dimensional anatomy used for initial diagnosis as well as follow-up.

- Cardiac mass and tumours: MRI enables the precise definition of tumour size, site of attachment and myocardial invasion. It can also be used to characterise a tumour as solid, cystic or vascular.

- Cardiomyopathies: MRI is useful in diagnosing cardiomyopathies secondary to sarcoidosis, amyloidosis and iron overload. It can also detect localised fat infiltration in the right ventricle, which gives rise to arrhythmogenic right ventricular cardiomyopathy.

- Pericardial disease.

- Coronary arteries: current MRI technology has a much lower resolution compared with multislice spiral CT, and the role of MRI is restricted to imaging of the proximal section of the coronary arteries, identification of aberrant arteries and saphenous vein bypass grafts.

Function

- Left ventricular function, volume and mass: three-dimensional cine-MRI images enable accurate

detection of left ventricular function, wall motion abnormalities as well as calculation of myocardial mass. Using contrast agents (gadolinium-enhanced), areas of myocardial scarring can also be detected.

- Myocardial perfusion.

Contraindications

The following are considered contraindications to MRI.

- Embedded ferromagnetic objects (eg intracranial clips, foreign bodies and early Starr–Edwards valves).

- Permanent pacemakers or implantable defibrillators (the magnetic field interferes with their function).

- Most current prosthetic valves and sternal wires are safe, but will cause an artefact.

- Selected coronary stents must not be imaged early after implantation (refer to manufacturer's recommendations).

FURTHER READING

Heatlie GJ and Pointon K. Cardiac magnetic resonance imaging. *Postgrad. Med. J.* 2004; 80: 19–22.

Mollet NR, Cademartiri F and de Feyter PJ. Non-invasive multislice CT coronary imaging. *Heart* 2005; 91: 401–7.

3.9 Ventilation– perfusion imaging

Principle

This investigation compares ventilation and perfusion in the lungs in order to detect areas of mismatch (ie ventilated but not perfused) that occur in acute pulmonary embolism (PE). Many other conditions (eg tumour or consolidation) cause perfusion defects, but these are generally matched by ventilation defects and associated with CXR abnormality.

Indication

A suspected PE, preferably with a normal CXR. Ventilation–perfusion scans are useful if perfusion is normal and PE therefore excluded, or if definite unmatched defects are seen and the diagnosis is confirmed; however, many scans do not produce clear-cut results and are reported as being of intermediate probability. The diagnostic yield is improved by correlation with clinical suspicion, but there are still many cases where other imaging modalities are required.

Contraindications

There are none. It is safe in pregnancy, although some centres modify the dose.

Practical details

- Inhalation of radioisotope [krypton-81m, xenon-133 or technetium-99m (^{99m}Tc)]: patient needs to be able to inhale sufficiently.

- Injection of ^{99m}Tc-labelled albumin macroaggregates or microspheres.

- Scanning after each; some centres only perform a ventilation scan if perfusion is abnormal.

- Duration of about 40 minutes.

FURTHER READING

The PIOPED Investigators. Value of the ventilation/perfusion scan in acute pulmonary embolism. *JAMA* 1990; 263: 2753–9.

3.10 Echocardiography

Principle

A piezoelectric crystal within a transducer generates ultrasonic waves in pulses that travel through tissue. Most of the sound waves are absorbed or scattered within the body but some are reflected back towards the transducer every time an ultrasound wave crosses the interface between tissues that have different densities, typically the junctions between blood, myocardium and heart valves. Frequencies of 2–5 MHz are required for routine adult cardiac work. Several modes of imaging are recognised.

M-mode

Ultrasonic pulses are transmitted and received along a single scan-line, and the interfaces are displayed as a graph of depth against time. It is especially useful for recording moving structures, timing events within the heart and measuring cardiac dimensions (Fig. 121).

Two-dimensional echocardiography

The information is displayed as a fan-shaped image. Detailed information about cardiac structures and their movement can be obtained. Standard transthoracic views include parasternal long and short axes, and two-, three- and four-chamber apical long-axis views of the heart (Fig. 122).

Doppler echocardiography

Velocity measurements can be derived, using the Doppler principle, from the frequency shift that occurs between transmitted and reflected ultrasound waves from moving red blood cells. Continuous and pulsed-wave Doppler recordings enable direct velocity measurements within the heart and across valves. Intracardiac and valvar pressure gradients are determined from the measured velocities (v) according to the modified Bernoulli equation, ie

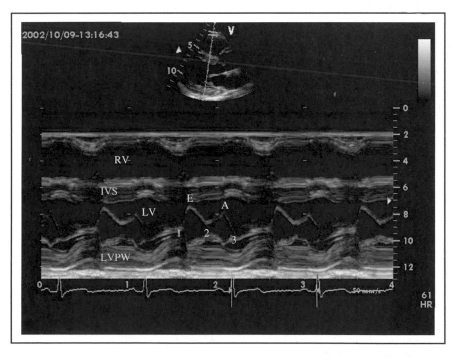

▲ **Fig. 121** Parasternal long-axis M-mode at the level of the mitral valve leaflets. 1, At the end of systole the mitral valve begins to open; E, maximum excursion of anterior mitral leaflet. 2, Initial diastolic closing wave; D, diastole; A, reopening of mitral valve caused by atrial systole. 3, Mitral valve closes at onset of ventricular systole; RV, right ventricle; LV, left ventricle; IVS, interventricular septum; LVPW, left ventricular posterior wall.

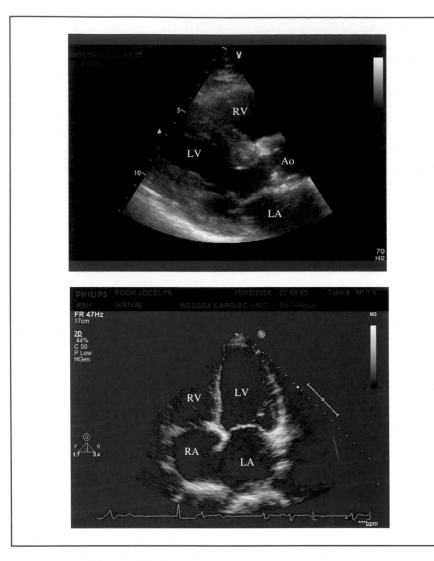

▲**Fig. 122** (**a**) Parasternal long-axis and (**b**) apical four-chamber views of the heart. LA, left atrium; LV, left ventricle; RA, right atrium; RV, right ventricle; Ao, aorta.

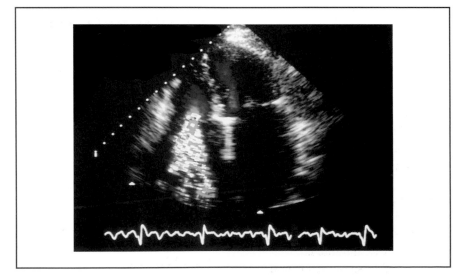

▲**Fig. 123** Tricuspid regurgitation: a broad band seen mainly as blue extends back into the right atrium. (Courtesy Dr J. Chambers.)

pressure gradient (in mmHg) $= 4v^2$. An example is shown in Fig. 123. Thus, in patients with depressed cardiac function and reduced myocardial blood velocity, valve gradients and therefore stenosis severity may be underestimated with this technique. In this situation, the valve area should be calculated. Colour-encoded Doppler velocity displayed on a two-dimensional image enables semi-quantitative assessment of valve regurgitation severity. Velocities directed towards the transducer are displayed in red and those away in blue. Increasing velocities are displayed as progressively lighter shades.

Transoesophageal echocardiography

Transoesophageal echocardiography (TOE) consists of a transducer incorporated at the tip of a gastroscope-like instrument. Because of the proximity of the oesophagus and the heart, TOE is especially useful in assessing the interatrial septum, left atrial appendage and aortic pathology. It should also be considered when poor transthoracic views are obtained and for prosthetic valve evaluation.

Stress echocardiography

This technique has comparable accuracy to myocardial perfusion imaging and MRI for diagnosis of coronary artery disease and mortality prediction in patients with ischaemic heart disease. Cardiac stress is usually achieved with dobutamine infusion but exercise, dipyridamole or pacing may be used. Worsening of left ventricular regional wall motion under stress signifies ischaemia in that territory. Other applications of stress echocardiography include:

- determination of myocardial viability in patients with poor left ventricular function and coronary artery disease;

- assessment of dynamic valve gradients in mitral and aortic stenosis;

- prediction of functional recovery in patients with severe aortic stenosis and poor left ventricular function;

- assessment of dynamic left ventricular outflow tract obstruction in hypertrophic cardiomyopathy.

New echocardiographic imaging modalities

Tissue Doppler imaging enables myocardial motion to be displayed over time, enabling the quantification of regional and global myocardial function in systole and diastole. This allows diagnosis of complex cardiomyopathies, quantification of ischaemia during dobutamine stress and detection of intracardiac dyssynchrony. Intravenous contrast agents enable improved endocardial border definition in poor echogenic patients. Three-dimensional reconstruction of the heart is now possible from a single acquisition of data obtained from three heart beats. All these new echocardiographic imaging modalities should improve future assessment of myocardial and valvar structure and function.

Indications

Echocardiography enables evaluation of regional and global ventricular systolic and diastolic function, assessment of valvar and heart muscle disease, and detection of myocardial ischaemia and viability.

Contraindications

- Stress echocardiography: unstable angina, myocardial infarction in the preceding 48 hours and ventricular arrhythmia.

- TOE: recent gastro-oesophageal bleed, known pharyngeal pouch or severe oesophageal disease. If there is unexplained dysphagia, arrange barium swallow before considering TOE.

Practical details

Transoesophageal echocardiography

- Nil by mouth for 4 hours; consider antibiotic prophylaxis if prosthetic valve.

- Obtain written consent.

- Insert intravenous cannula.

- Check for loose teeth; remove false teeth and dentures.

- Position patient on left side.

- Give sedation, eg midazolam or diazepam.

- Monitor peripheral oxygen saturation continuously.

- Insert mouthguard and perform test, ensuring that mouth secretions are cleared using suction.

- Monitor recovery; allow the patient home with an escort once they are free of sedation.

Stress echocardiography

The patient should be starved for 4 hours. Intravenous access is required. Dobutamine is administered in stepwise fashion until target rate is achieved or an ischaemic response seen.

Images are acquired at baseline, low-dose dobutamine, peak-dose dobutamine and recovery. Images are stored in digital quad screen format for offline analayis. At each stage of the test, symptoms, 12-lead ECG and BP are recorded. Following the test, the patient is monitored until disappearance of symptoms and resolution of echocardiographic and ECG changes.

Complications

Transoesophageal echocardiography

- Oesophageal trauma ranging from inflammation to rupture.

- Aspiration.

Important information for patients undergoing transoesophageal echocardiography

Explain the following:

- the benefits and risks of the procedure;
- the need for sedation, such that they may not remember the test;
- that they will be drowsy afterwards, should not drive for the rest of the day and will need to be escorted home;
- that they may have a sore throat for the next 1 or 2 days.

Stress echocardiography

- Supraventricular tachyarrhythmia.

- Ventricular tachycardia/ ventricular fibrillation: 1 in 5,000 treadmill tests.

- Death as a result of resistant ventricular fibrillation: 1 in 10,000 tests.

- Precipitation of acute coronary syndrome.

Important information for patients undergoing stress echocardiography

Stop beta-blockers for 48 hours before the test. Inform patients about the procedure and chosen stress modality. Make sure that they are aware that they may experience chest pain during the test. Explain risk of arrhythmias.

FURTHER READING

Bach DS and Armstrong WF. Dobutamine stress echocardiography. *Am. J. Cardiol.* 1992; 69: 90.

Chambers J. *Clinical Echocardiography*. London: BMJ Publishing Group, 1995.

Sengupta PP and Khandheria BK. Transoesophageal echocardiography. *Heart* 2005; 91: 541–7.

3.11 Nuclear cardiology

3.11.1 Myocardial perfusion imaging

Thallium-201 is actively taken up by myocardial cells in a manner similar to potassium. Its concentration in the myocardium depends on both perfusion and integrity of the myocardial cell membrane. A graded colour representation of perfusion is obtained, enabling comparison between regions. Absolute values of blood flow are not obtained.

A scan after exercise or pharmacological stress with dipyridamole or adenosine is followed by a resting scan at 2–4 hours. Defects seen during stress, which are not present at rest, represent ischaemia. Defects present in both scans ('fixed perfusion defect') usually indicate infarction (Fig. 124). The sensitivity for detection of significant coronary

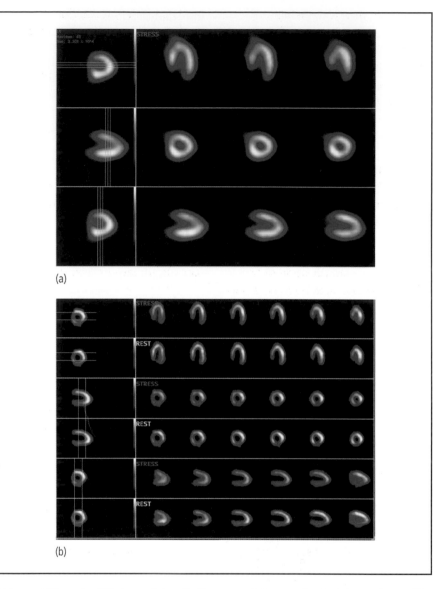

▲**Fig. 124** (**a**) Normal and (**b**) abnormal stress thallium-201 perfusion scan, showing inferior ischaemia (b). (Courtesy of Dr Jan).

artery disease is 80–85% and specificity >90%.

Indications
Nuclear techniques are expensive. In most cases, myocardial perfusion imaging should be used only when ECG morphology or patient morbidity precludes the interpretation or use of exercise ECG testing. Indications in common with exercise testing include the following:

- prognostic stratification after myocardial infarction;

- identification of ischaemia in symptomatic patients, especially atypical pain;

- risk stratification in patients with known or high risk of coronary artery disease before non-cardiac surgery.

3.11.2 Radionuclide ventriculography

Technetium-99m is used to label a patient's red blood pool and can be detected with the use of a gamma camera. The number of counts is linearly related to the blood volume and by using ECG gating to identify different parts of the cardiac cycle, the ejection fraction can be calculated. It is an accurate and reproducible technique for calculating left and right ventricular ejection fractions.

3.11.3 Positron emission tomography

This technique uses positron-emitting radionuclides to produce tomographic images of coronary flow and metabolism. The technique also enables quantification of blood flow within specified regions of the heart. Rest and pharmacological stress scans are performed in a similar manner to thallium imaging. Myocardial viability is suggested by maintained glucose metabolism in an area with a fixed perfusion defect.

FURTHER READING

Dilsizian V and Bonow RO. Current diagnostic techniques of assessing myocardial viability in patients with hibernating and stunned myocardium. *Circulation* 1993; 87: 1–20.

Kotler TS and Diamond GA. Exercise thallium-201 scintigraphy in the diagnosis and prognosis of coronary artery disease. *Ann. Intern. Med.* 1990; 113: 684–702.

3.12 Cardiac catheterisation

Principle

Catheters are introduced into the arterial and venous system, and advanced to the left and right heart, respectively, allowing the following:

- visualisation of the chambers of the heart, vessels and coronary arteries;

- pressure measurements in the cardiac chambers and major vessels;

- oxygen saturations may be sampled throughout the circulation and heart, allowing identification of shunts and calculation of cardiac output.

Indications

Left heart catheterisation

- Angina, with evidence of ischaemia at low/moderate workload.

- Prior to heart valve surgery.

Right heart catheterisation

Investigation of pulmonary hypertension and occasionally for investigation of pulmonary emboli.

Left and right heart catheterisation

- Mitral stenosis and selected cases of mitral regurgitation.

- Congenital heart disease.

- Pretransplant assessment.

- Heart failure.

- Suspected constrictive pericarditis.

Contraindications

- Severe vascular disease preventing arterial access.

- Severely deranged coagulation.

- Iodine allergy.

- Pulmonary oedema: may lead to radiographic deterioration and even death.

Renal failure may be worsened by the contrast: in vulnerable patients prescribe intravenous fluids before the procedure to prevent dehydration and stop drugs with adverse effects on renal haemodynamics (angiotensin-converting enzyme inhibitors, angiotensin receptor antagonists, NSAIDs) prior to the procedure. Inform the patient that renal function may deteriorate and, if the patient has severe pre-existing renal impairment, that dialysis is occasionally required.

Practical details

Before investigation

- FBC, urine and electrolytes and, if on warfarin, INR.

- ECG.

- Informed consent.

- Intravenous access.

The investigation

Lead shields are worn by the staff to prevent radiation exposure. Aseptic technique is used. Arterial access may be femoral, radial or brachial. Venous access can be from the femoral, central or brachial veins. Local anaesthetic is infiltrated. Using the modified Seldinger technique a sheath is placed in the artery. Preshaped catheters are passed through the sheath (on a long J-tipped guidewire in the arterial system) and guided using continuous-pressure monitoring and fluoroscopic guidance. A three-lead ECG is monitored continuously. At the end of the procedure the sheath is removed and direct pressure applied, or a closure device is used.

Examples of the images obtained from a coronary angiogram are shown in Fig. 125. Normal pressure measurements are given in Table 47. Oxygen saturations from a case of right-to-left shunting are shown in Fig. 126.

TABLE 47 NORMAL PRESSURE MEASUREMENTS

Pressure	Range (mmHg)
RA (mean)	5–6
RV (systolic)	15–30
RV (end diastolic)	1–8
PA (systolic)	15–30
PA (diastolic)	5–12
PA (mean)	9–16
Pulmonary capillary wedge (mean)	5–13
LA (mean)	2–12
LV (systolic)	90–140
LV (end diastolic)	5–12

Size of shunt

The size of a shunt can be estimated using a formula derived from the Fick equation:

$$Q_p/Q_s = (Ao - MV)/(PV - PA)$$

where Q_p is pulmonary flow, Q_s systemic flow, Ao aortic saturation, MV mixed venous saturation, PV pulmonary venous saturation and PA pulmonary artery saturation. Pulmonary venous saturation is not usually measured but is assumed to be 97%. A shunt greater than 1.5:1 is regarded as significant.

Complications

Minor

- Bruising in 50%.
- Haematoma.

Major

- Femoral artery damage requiring repair.
- Stroke, myocardial infarction, death: risk 1 in 1,000 for each.

3.12.1 Percutaneous coronary intervention

Principle

A catheter-delivered balloon with or without stent is inflated at the site of stenosis or arterial occlusion.

Indications

- Acute myocardial infarction (primary percutaneous coronary intervention).
- After failed thrombolysis for acute myocardial infarction (rescue percutaneous coronary intervention).
- Non-ST-elevation myocardial infarction.
- Flow-limiting stenosis in one or more arteries, for relief of angina.

Contraindications

- Severe peripheral vascular disease making femoral or radial catheterisation impossible.

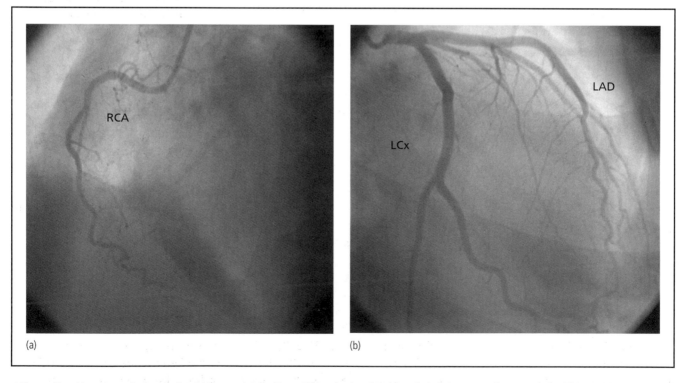

(a)   (b)

▲**Fig. 125** Normal coronary arteriogram: the right coronary artery is small (non-dominant) in (a), with the left coronary demonstrated in (b). LAD, left anterior descending artery; LCx, left circumflex artery; RCA, right coronary artery.

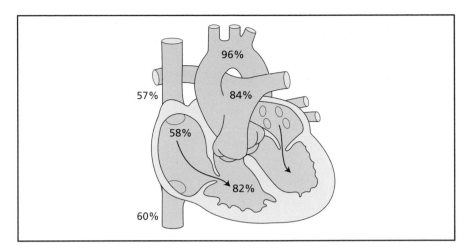

▲ **Fig. 126** Oxygen saturation measurements showing a 'step-up' in the right ventricle, indicating a ventricular septal defect with left-to-right shunt.

- Active bleeding preventing administration of antiplatelet agents.

- Thrombocytopenia.

- Allergy to iodine (contrast contains iodine).

- Inability to lie flat: intubation may be necessary if the patient has resistant pulmonary oedema.

- Patients who cannot take oral antiplatelet agents.

As for cardiac catheterisation, the contrast may worsen renal impairment.

Practical details

Before the procedure

This is the same as for cardiac catheterisation. Consent should include advice about risk of death (0.3%), emergency cardiac surgery (0.6%), myocardial infarction (0.3%), stroke (0.3%) and groin haematoma (2%).

The procedure

Access is via the radial or femoral arteries. Intravenous heparin is administered. A guidewire is introduced via the catheter into the artery and manipulated into the correct branch using screening.

The position is confirmed using radio-opaque contrast. Patients who are at high risk of thrombotic stent occlusion, such as diabetics, will then be given an intravenous bolus, followed by an infusion, of glycoprotein IIb/IIIa antagonist.

The lesion may be dilated with a balloon, usually for around 10 seconds at 1200 kPa (12 atm), and then a balloon covered with an expandable stent is placed to cover the lesion. When the balloon is inflated, the stent expands and remains in position on deflation of the balloon. Confirmation of a good angiographic result is important to ensure that there have been no complications (Fig. 127). A metal or drug-eluting stent may be used: the latter has a lower chance of restenosis.

To confirm the severity of stenosis, a pressure wire may be passed beyond the stenosis and intracoronary adenosine administered to dilate the coronary bed. A fractional flow reserve of less than 75% indicates a significant stenosis. Intravascular ultrasound is used to image complex plaques or to confirm good stent deployment (Fig. 128). Heavily calcified plaques may be difficult to crack with a balloon, so atherectomy devices (eg Rotablader) can be

deployed to reduce the burden of atheroma, allowing stent placement.

After the procedure

The femoral artery is usually sealed with a closure device. Patients are prescribed aspirin and clopidogrel for 1 year.

Complications

- Perforation of a coronary artery may lead to tamponade, in which case a covered stent can be placed over the hole, with pericardiocentesis required to remove the fluid in some cases.

- Coronary artery dissection exposes the endothelium causing thrombotic occlusion of the artery. This is controlled by stenting the site of the dissection.

- Acute stent thrombosis: occasionally a small dissection can be missed, and hours or days later these patients re-present with pain and ST elevation, requiring further stenting and administration of glycoprotein IIb/IIIa antagonists.

- Late stent thrombosis: there is a small risk of thrombotic stent occlusion months after the procedure. This may relate to hypotensive episodes, eg during surgery, or to cessation of clopidogrel. Drug-eluting stents have higher rates of stent thrombosis, hence patients remain on clopidogrel for at least 1 year.

3.12.2 Percutaneous valvuloplasty

Principle

A catheter-delivered balloon is passed through a stenosed valve and inflated, widening the valvular orifice. This technique is mainly reserved for mitral stenosis.

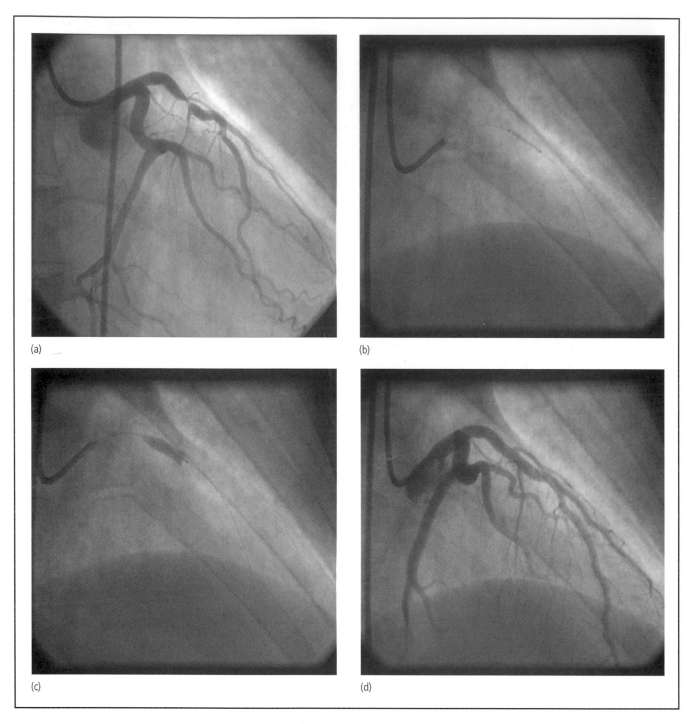

(a)

(b)

(c)

(d)

▲ **Fig. 127** Coronary artery stenting: (**a**) left coronary angiogram showing a tight stenosis in the left anterior descending artery; (**b**) positioning of stent mounted on an angioplasty balloon; (**c**) inflation of balloon to deploy stent; (**d**) final result.

Indications

Severe symptomatic mitral stenosis.

Contraindications

- Heavily calcified mitral valve leaflets.

- Severe mitral regurgitation.

- Pulmonary oedema.

- INR <2.

- Left atrial thrombus.

Practical details

Before the procedure

Transoesophageal echocardiography is performed to exclude left atrial

thrombus and assess suitability for valvuloplasty. The INR should be 2.0–2.5. During consent, the patient is alerted to the risk of stroke and pericardiocentesis for tamponade.

The procedure

Venous and arterial access are obtained. A bolus of intravenous

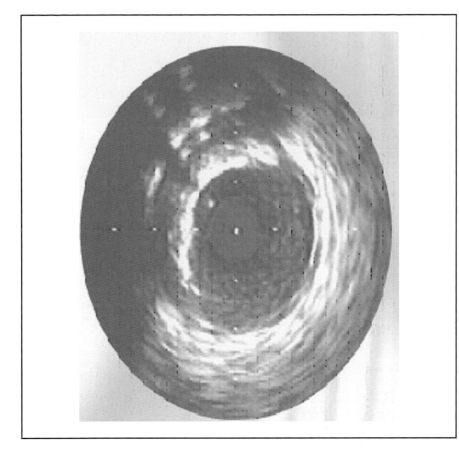

▲ **Fig. 128** Intravascular ultrasound of a coronary artery. In the centre is the catheter, around which is a heavily calcified atheromatous plaque that appears bright white.

heparin is administered and the activated clotting time is checked. A long sheath is introduced via the right femoral vein and the interatrial septum is penetrated with a needle, with pressures measured continuously. A pigtail catheter is then introduced via the femoral artery and advanced to the left ventricle, allowing simultaneous left atrial and left ventricular pressure measurements. The mean gradient is calculated. A balloon is advanced through the mitral valve and inflated to high pressure for a few seconds (Fig. 129). The mean gradient is recalculated, and the procedure is repeated if the gradient has not decreased sufficiently.

After the procedure

The sheaths are removed once the activated clotting time is less than 150 seconds. Warfarin is continued.

Complications

- Stroke.

- Tamponade requiring pericardiocentesis.

- Severe mitral regurgitation.

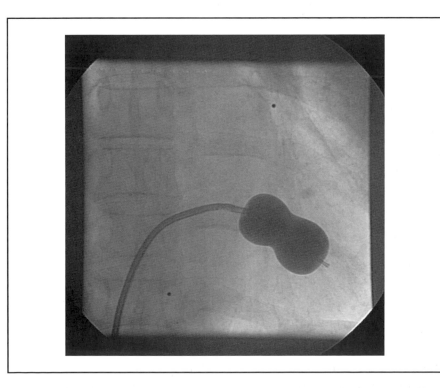

▲ **Fig. 129** Mitral valvuloplasty: a trans-septal puncture allows an Inoue balloon to be advanced into a stenotic mitral valve and inflated.

4.1 Self-assessment questions

Question 1

Clinical scenario

A 48-year woman is referred to the rapid access chest pain clinic by her GP with chest tightness. This occurs on exertion but also occasionally after meals. Her only past medical history is hypertension and permanent atrial fibrillation. Her only medication is digoxin and warfarin.

Question

Which of the following regarding exercise tests is true?

Answers

A A fall in BP with increasing exercise is a non-significant finding

B Providing that a heart rate >75% of that predicted is achieved and no ECG changes are documented, ischaemic heart disease can be confidently excluded

C Digoxin therapy makes interpretation of exercise tests difficult

D Exercise testing should not be performed in patients with a previous history of ventricular arrhythmias

E There is a higher false-positive rate in males compared with females

Question 2

Clinical scenario

A 56-year old man is admitted to the Emergency Department with chest pain and dizziness. He had an anterior myocardial infarction 2 years previously for which he received a drug-eluting stent. Figure 130 shows his ECG.

Question

Which of the following statements regarding broad-complex tachycardias is *incorrect*?

Answers

A May be caused by atrioventricular re-entry tachycardia using an accessory pathway

B The origin of ventricular tachycardia (VT) can be

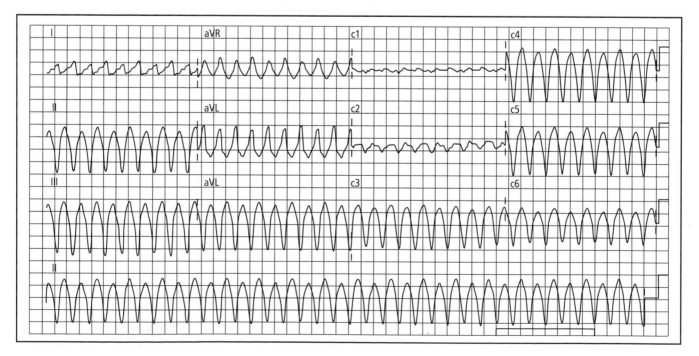

▲Fig. 130 Question 2.

identified from the 12-lead ECG

C Fusion beats are diagnostic of VT

D VT is not usually terminated by adenosine

E Amiodarone is an effective alternative treatment to implantable cardioverter defibrillators in the treatment of VT

Question 3

Clinical scenario

A 47-year old man is found to have bifascicular block on his ECG during a pre-admission assessment prior to a hernia repair. He is asymptomatic. The anaesthetist has requested an opinion as to whether he should have a temporary pacemaker for the procedure.

Question

Which of the following statements regarding pacing is correct?

Answers

A This patient should have a temporary pacemaker for his operation

B Transient complete heart block in a patient following an acute inferior myocardial infarction requires a temporary pacemaker

C Patients undergoing atrioventricular node ablation for troublesome atrial fibrillation require pacing

D Hypothermic patients with bradycardia require temporary pacing

E Patients with a 2.5-second pause after carotid sinus massage require permanent pacing

Question 4

Clinical scenario

A 24-year-old woman with a previous history of eating disorder presents with increasing shortness of breath. A CXR shows cardiomegaly and normal lung fields. A transthoracic echocardiogram shows a dilated right ventricle with mild tricuspid regurgitation and a peak pulmonary artery pressure estimated at 70 mmHg (normal pressure <30 mmHg). The left heart is normal, laboratory investigations are normal and a pregnancy test is negative.

Question

Which one of the following investigations would you consider first?

Answers

A Ventilation–perfusion scan

B Right and left heart catheterisation

C Transoesophageal echocardiography

D Cardiopulmonary exercise test

E Thrombophilia screen

Question 5

Clinical scenario

A 32-year-old woman with a history of congenital heart disease is planning to start a family. She has no other significant medical history and is currently symptomatically stable on a small dose of loop diuretic.

Question

Which one of the following conditions is associated with an unacceptably high risk in pregnancy?

Answers

A Corrected tetralogy of Fallot

B Perimembranous ventricular septal defect

C Secundum atrial septal defect

D Coarctation of the aorta

E Pulmonary hypertension of any cause

Question 6

Clinical scenario

A 67-year-old man presents with a 6-week history of malaise, low-grade pyrexia and rigors 6 months after having a prosthetic aortic valve replacement. His C-reactive protein is 150 mg/dL (normal <5 mg/dL) and his creatinine 150 µmol/L (normal <120 µmol/L). A transoesophageal echocardiogram confirms vegetation on the aortic prosthesis.

Question

Which of the following organisms is most likely to be responsible?

Answers

A *Staphylococcus aureus*

B *Streptococcus viridans*

C *Staphylococcus epidermidis*

D *Escherichia coli*

E *Candida albicans*

Question 7

Clinical scenario

A 32-year-old athlete presents with severe interscapular pain after training. He is of slim build and tall (210 cm). He has a sinus tachycardia and his BP is 180/100 mmHg with no deficit between his right and left arm. There are no murmurs and all his peripheral pulses are palpable. The rest of his physical examination is normal. A CXR shows widened mediastinum and a CT confirms an aortic dissection distal to the left subclavian artery that does not involve the aortic arch.

Question

Which of the following is the most appropriate intervention?

Answers

A Intravenous calcium antagonist

B Intravenous labetalol

C Urgent cardiothoracic surgical referral

D Transoesophageal echocardiography

E Oral angiotensin-converting enzyme inhibitor

Question 8

Clinical scenario

A 45-year-old builder with one episode of unexplained syncope has a transthoracic echocardiogram that is suggestive of hypertrophic cardiomyopathy.

Question

Which two of the following features are *not* associated with a high risk of sudden death?

Answers

A History of ventricular tachycardia (VT) or resuscitated ventricular fibrillation

B Recurrent syncope

C Strong family history of sudden death

D Breathlessness on exertion

E Extreme left ventricular hypertrophy (septal thickness >3 cm)

F Non-sustained VT on Holter monitoring

G Syncope while running

H Diagnosis in childhood

I Resting outflow tract gradient >25 mmHg

J BP drops on exercise

Question 9

Clinical scenario

A 70-year-old man, known to have ischaemic heart disease and who has had a coronary artery bypass graft in the past, presents with progressive breathlessness. He is haemodynamically stable but has clinical signs of congestion and a CXR confirms pulmonary oedema. An ECG shows sinus rhythm with anterior Q waves, QRS complex of 180 ms duration (normal <120 ms) with a left bundle-branch block pattern. Transthoracic echocardiography shows systolic left ventricular dysfunction with an ejection fraction of 25% (normal 50–60%).

Question

Which two of the following interventions would *not* be associated with an improved mortality in this patient?

Answers

A Loop diuretic

B Lisinopril

C Statin

D Implantable cardioverter defibrillator

E Eplerenone

F Biventricular pacing

G Carvedilol

H Spironolactone

I Bisoprolol

J Diltiazem

Question 10

Clinical scenario

A 32-year-old woman who is 22 weeks' pregnant is admitted to the maternity ward and found to be hypertensive with a BP of 180/100 mmHg. This is her first pregnancy and it is otherwise uncomplicated. She has no other relevant medical history and her urinalysis is normal, as is renal and liver function.

Question

Which of the following should *not* be used to control her BP?

Answers

A Hydralazine

B Methyldopa

C Labetalol

D Ramipril

E Amlodipine

Question 11

Clinical scenario

A 60-year old man is admitted with an acute inferior myocardial infarction. He is thrombolysed with streptokinase, and treated with aspirin and clopidogrel. Two hours later you are asked to see him as his BP has decreased from 110/70 mmHg to 70/40 mmHg, although he is pain-free. Examination reveals a clear chest, normal heart sounds and a raised JVP. His ECG shows complete resolution of the ST-segment elevation.

Question

What is the appropriate course of action?

Answers

A Administer intravenous diuretic

B Administer 250 mL 0.9% saline intravenously

C Administer inotropes

D Wait for 30 minutes to see if his BP picks up

E Administer hydrocortisone

Question 12

Clinical scenario

A 36-year-old man is knocked off his motorbike on his way to work. There is no head injury and he remains conscious throughout. He does, however, complain of some chest discomfort on the way to hospital in the ambulance.

Question

Which of the following statements regarding traumatic heart disease is correct?

Answers

A Motor vehicles are not the commonest cause

B Creatine kinase is a useful indicator of myocardial injury

C The ascending portion of the aorta is most commonly involved

D Glycoprotein IIb/IIIa inhibitors are the treatment of choice in a patient with an acute coronary syndrome associated with trauma

E Postpericardiotomy (Dressler's) syndrome is associated with traumatic heart disease

Question 13

Clinical scenario

A 63-year-old man is brought into the Emergency Department having collapsed and has had a series of shocks from his implantable cardioverter defibrillator (ICD). He has a history of a myocardial infarction (MI) 3 years previously and of coronary artery bypass grafting last year.

Question

Which two of the following statements regarding ICDs are *incorrect*?

Answers

A ICDs are indicated in patients who have had a previous MI and an ejection fraction <40%

B Shock therapy may be delivered for ventricular fibrillation and ventricular tachycardia

C ICDs may be indicated in patients with hypertrophic cardiomyopathy

D This patient will not be allowed to drive for at least 3 months

E Interrogation of the ICD following the collapse will identify the exact rhythm that caused the collapse

F ICDs also have the ability to pace for bradycardias

G It is important to check the electrolytes following shock therapy

H Several shocks may be delivered by the ICD to terminate an abnormal rhythm

I ICDs may be indicated in patients who have not had a previous history of MI

J It may be possible to discharge this patient from hospital later the same day

Question 14

Clinical scenario

A 45-year-old woman is brought into the resuscitation room having collapsed on her driveway at home. On arrival the paramedics found her to be in ventricular fibrillation and successfully cardioverted her to sinus rhythm with a single shock.

She is maintaining her airway but cannot be roused. Her heart rate is regular and she is maintaining a good BP. A neighbour told the paramedics that she had recently visited her doctor but was not sure why. Figure 131 shows her ECG.

Question

Which two of the following are *least* likely to have caused the appearances seen on her ECG?

Answers

A Sotalol

B Terfenadine

C Erythromycin

D Atenolol

E Amitriptyline

F Diltiazem

G Amiodarone

H Chloroquine

I Haloperidol

J Domperidone

Question 15

Clinical scenario

A 68-year-old man, previously fit and well, presents with anterior

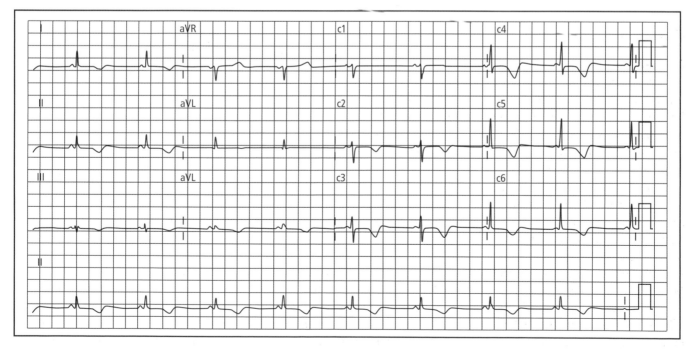

▲**Fig. 131** Question 14.

myocardial infarction (MI) for which he receives appropriate thrombolysis, antiplatelet therapy and diamorphine. Over the next 4 hours he complains of increasing dyspnoea. His pulse rate is 110 bpm (sinus), BP 160/90 mmHg and arterial saturation is 92% on 60% inspired oxygen. His CXR is shown in Fig. 90.

Question

What is the most appropriate intravenous pharmacological treatment?

Answers

A Atenolol
B Dobutamine
C Enalapril
D Furosemide
E Nitrate

Question 16

Clinical scenario

A 32-year-old woman has been referred to you by her doctor after complaining of syncope and breathlessness. Her sister died suddenly in her twenties. Clinically she has a loud second heart sound. An ECG shows changes compatible with right ventricular hypertrophy and strain.

Question

What would be the most appropriate investigation to consider next?

Answers

A CT pulmonary angiography
B Echocardiography
C Holter ambulatory monitoring
D Right and left heart catheterisation
E Ventilation–perfusion scan

Question 17

Clinical scenario

A patient with documented systolic dysfunction has permanent atrial fibrillation. His resting heart rate is 100 bpm and systolic BP 120 mmHg; there is no evidence of fluid retention. Creatinine is normal and he is already receiving appropriate doses of furosemide and an angiotensin-converting enzyme inhibitor.

Question

Which two of the following would be the most appropriate drugs to add?

Answers

A Amiodarone
B Aspirin
C Atenolol
D Bisoprolol
E Candesartan
F Digoxin
G Diltiazem
H Enoxaparin
I Sotalol
J Warfarin

Question 18

Clinical scenario

A 50-year-old man without any prior history is referred to the outpatients department for assessment of increasing exertional dyspnoea. An examination reveals no abnormalities, and his BP is 120/60 mmHg and his pulse 70 bpm in sinus rhythm. His ECG shows left bundle-branch block and echocardiography confirms moderate impairment of left ventricular function. His GP has already started him on oral furosemide and he is now virtually asymptomatic.

Question

What would be the most appropriate treatment to add next?

Answers

A Angiotensin-converting enzyme inhibitor
B Angiotensin receptor blocker
C Aspirin
D Beta-blocker
E Spironolactone

Question 19

Clinical scenario

A 59-year-old man is admitted breathless following an episode of syncope while shopping. There is no previous history of syncope. Past history includes multiple stab ligations for bilateral varicose veins 4 weeks previously, mild asthma and borderline hypertension (not on treatment). He has received 500 mL of volume expansion in the Accident and Emergency Department. On examination he is breathless at rest, apyrexial, pulse 104 bpm (regular) and BP 90/50 mmHg. His heart sounds are normal. Chest examination reveals a few scattered wheezes. ECG shows sinus tachycardia with inverted T waves in leads V1–V3. CXR is normal. Oxygen saturation is 92% on 40% oxygen. Peak expiratory flow rate is 300 L/min.

Question

What investigation would be most helpful in directing his immediate treatment?

Answers

A CT pulmonary angiogram
B D-dimer
C Transoesophageal echocardiography
D Troponin
E Ultrasound of leg veins (bilateral)

Question 20

Clinical scenario

Five days after total hip replacement a 70-year-old man with known chronic obstructive airways disease (COPD) becomes short of breath with a cough. He has left-sided pleuritic chest pain and a low-grade temperature. His CXR is consistent with long-standing COPD, but no other abnormalities are seen. His arterial blood gases on air demonstrate pH 7.34, P_{CO_2} 4.0 kPa and P_{O_2} 10.2 kPa. After 2 hours of oxygen therapy (F_{IO_2} 30%) his P_{O_2} has risen to 11.0 kPa, but the other parameters are unchanged. By this stage his FBC results show haemoglobin 14 g/dL, white cell count 4×10^9/L and platelets 600×10^9/L. Biochemistry shows sodium 131 mmol/L, potassium 5.2 mmol/L, urea 14 mmol/L and creatinine 170 μmol/L.

Question

What is the most likely cause for his clinical picture?

Answers

A Infective exacerbation of COPD
B Left-sided pneumonia
C Acute pulmonary embolus
D Small pneumothorax
E Panic attack

Question 21

Clinical scenario

A 50-year-old man is being investigated for carcinoma of the colon. He presents to hospital with a 1-week history of becoming progressively unwell. He reports intermittent sweats and a loss of appetite. On examination he appears pale, has low-grade pyrexia and is tachycardic. He has a non-tender rash on his feet. His heart sounds are normal, but there is an aortic systolic murmur and a faint aortic diastolic murmur. His lung fields are clear. His abdomen is mildly tender but there is no evidence of peritonism. There is no hepatomegaly, but the tip of his spleen is palpable.

Question

Which one of the following investigations will be most helpful in providing a diagnosis for his subacute deterioration?

Answers

A CXR
B Abdominal ultrasound

C Biopsy of the skin lesion
D Colonoscopy
E Multiple blood cultures

Question 22

Clinical scenario

A 30-year-old woman is referred for assessment of her hypertension. Multiple readings have demonstrated a BP of over 160/98 mmHg. She has been intermittently depressed since the death of her sister 1 year ago. During this period she has gained 15 kg in weight. She also reports menstrual irregularity, tiredness and weakness, which have all been attributed to her depression. On examination she has generalised obesity. There are multiple stretch marks on her abdomen. Her ankles are moderately swollen and she has bruises on her legs.

Question

Which one of the following conditions best describes the aetiology for her high BP?

Answers

A Severe depression
B Polycystic ovarian syndrome
C Diabetes mellitus
D Essential hypertension
E Cushing's syndrome

Question 23

Clinical scenario

A 45-year-old man is referred to the medical outpatient clinic as he is found to have an abnormal ECG at a routine medical screening. The ECG shows left ventricular hypertrophy (LVH). He is otherwise well but has had occasional BP measurements above normal.

Question

Which one of the following statements is true with regard to LVH?

Answers

A Aortic regurgitation typically gives rise to concentric LVH
B Eccentric LVH is the hallmark of hypertrophic cardiomyopathy
C Hypertensive LVH is not altered by drug treatment
D LVH is an independent risk factor for cardiovascular death
E Assessment of the apex beat cannot distinguish pressure overload from volume overload

Question 24

Clinical scenario

A 56-year-old woman with a murmur is about to have a cystoscopy. The urology team asks you to assess her with regard to the need for antibiotic prophylaxis prior to the operation.

Question

Which one of the following cardiac conditions and which one of the following procedures require antibiotic prophylaxis?

Answers

A Patent foramen ovale
B Ventricular septal defect (VSD)
C Eisenmenger's syndrome secondary to VSD
D Surgically ligated patent ductus arteriosus
E Atrial fibrillation
F Cystoscopy
G Dobutamine stress echocardiography
H Cardiac catheterisation
I Transoesophageal echocardiography
J Myocardial perfusion imaging

Question 25

Clinical scenario

A transthoracic echocardiogram is performed to investigate an 18-year-old man who collapsed whilst playing football. The parasternal long-axis view is shown in Fig.132.

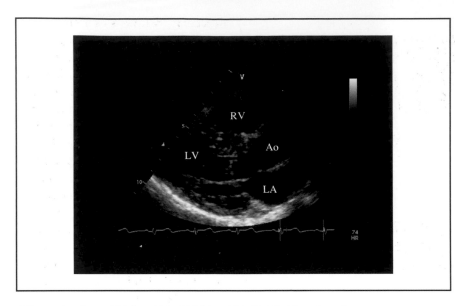

▲ **Fig. 132** Question 25: LV, left ventricle; RV, right ventricle; LA, left atrium; Ao, aorta.

Question

Which two of the following are correct concerning his diagnosis?

Answers

A The second heart sound will be soft

B A loud systolic murmur is likely

C A thrusting displaced apex beat is likely

D The ECG is likely to be normal

E Exercise testing is contraindicated

F Cardiac catheterisation is required to confirm the diagnosis

G An implantable defibrillator may be indicated

H Antibiotic prophylaxis is not required

I Sotalol improves the prognosis

J Angiotensin-converting enzyme inhibitors improve the prognosis

Question 26

Clinical scenario

An 84-year-old woman is admitted with a left hemiplegia and expressive dysphasia. Her family tells you that she has a previous cardiac history but they are unsure what this is. Transthoracic echocardiography is normal and so it is recommended that you request transoesophageal echocardiography.

Question

Transoesophageal echocardiography is superior to transthoracic echocardiography for the diagnosis of which of the following?

Answers

A Left ventricular apical thrombus

B Left atrial appendage thrombus

C Left ventricular non-compaction

D Hypertrophic cardiomyopathy

E Ventricular septal defect

Question 27

Clinical scenario

A 57-year-old lawyer is admitted as an emergency with profound breathlessness. He has been fit and well previously but is awaiting endoscopy for indigestion. On admission he is found to be hypotensive with a gallop rhythm and bilateral inspiratory crackles. His CXR confirms an increased cardiothoracic ratio and pulmonary oedema.

Question

Which of the following is true of heart failure?

Answers

A The detection of bilateral crackles on auscultation of the lung bases is unreliable as an indicator of pulmonary oedema

B The history and physical examination will be sufficient for diagnosis in most cases

C Verapamil is useful even if the patient is in sinus rhythm

D Beta-blockers must be avoided

E Oral drug treatment can improve symptoms but cannot improve the ejection fraction

Question 28

Clinical scenario

A 32-year-old woman is 32 weeks into her first pregnancy. She is complaining of profound lethargy, palpitations and dizziness. The obstetricians are otherwise happy with her progress, but have asked for a medical review.

Question

Which of the following is normal in pregnancy?

Answers

A Anaemia

B Atrial fibrillation

C A fourth heart sound

D A diastolic murmur at the lower left sternal edge

E Hypotension

Question 29

Clinical scenario

A 54-year-old woman is admitted with acute dyspnoea and hypoxia on arterial blood gas analysis. Her ECG is abnormal. Echocardiography demonstrates a dilated right ventricle.

Question

Which of the following would you *not* expect to see on her ECG?

Answers

A Sinus tachycardia

B Right-axis shift

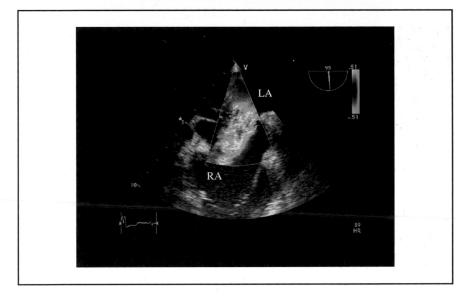

▲**Fig. 133** Question 30.

C Changes that disappear in a few days

D Right bundle-branch block

E Prolonged QT interval

Question 30

Clinical scenario

A 36-year-old woman presents with 12 months of increasing breathlessness. She has otherwise been well. She smokes 15 cigarettes a day. Transoesophageal echocardiography is performed as part of her investigations. Figure 133 is an image from this investigation.

Question

Which of the following statements is true concerning her diagnosis?

Answers

A The second heart sound has paradoxical splitting

B A loud murmur is likely

C The ECG is likely to show left bundle-branch block

D Surgery is the only treatment option

E Antibiotic prophylaxis is mandatory

4.2 Self-assessment answers

Answer to Question 1

C

A reduction in haemodynamic performance with exercise may represent significant coronary artery disease and should be investigated further. Generally, a heart rate >85% of that predicted is accepted as a target to achieve. The ST-segment changes associated with digoxin use make the exercise ECG very difficult to interpret, a matter further complicated by this patient's atrial fibrillation.

Answer to Question 2

E

In Wolff–Parkinson–White syndrome, delta waves are secondary to antegrade conduction down the accessory pathway and cause a broad-complex tachycardia. Atrioventricular re-entry tachycardia (AVRT) secondary to concealed accessory pathways exhibits antegrade conduction through the atrioventricular (AV) node and retrograde conduction through the accessory pathway and so does not show delta waves. Ventricular tachycardia (VT) with right bundle-branch block morphology will most probably originate from the left ventricle, and vice versa with left bundle-branch morphology. Fusion beats are an intermediate morphology of the QRS complex between the broad complex of VT and the narrow complex of sinus rhythm. Fusion beats are found in about 5% of VTs.

Adenosine exerts its action on the AV node. Since the majority of VTs do not include the AV node in the re-entry mechanism, adenosine will not terminate the rhythm. However, in atrioventricular nodal re-entry tachycardia/AVRT with aberrant conduction (and hence broad complex), adenosine is highly effective. Most of the large prospective studies comparing amiodarone with implantable cardioverter defibrillators (e.g. SCDHeFT) have shown a clear superiority of implantable cardioverter defibrillators in preventing death in patients with VT. The major studies suggest that amiodarone may be no better than placebo in preventing death.

Answer to Question 3

C

Temporary pacing for a bifascicular (and possibly trifascicular) block should only be considered in patients who give a history of presyncope or syncope. Complete heart block, even if transient, should lead to insertion of a temporary pacing lead in the context of an acute anterior myocardial infarction.

In inferior myocardial infarction, complete heart block is often transient, does not confer a bad prognosis and does not require temporary pacing. Of course, ablation of the atrioventricular node will leave the patient in either complete heart block or ventricular standstill. At all costs, try to avoid placing a temporary pacing lead in patients who are bradycardic as a result of hypothermia. The ventricles are often 'irritable' and ventricular fibrillation is easily induced. The mainstay of treatment is slow rewarming. A 3.0-second pause is usually taken as the criterion for pacing in carotid sinus hypersensitivity.

Answer to Question 4

A

Although this woman may have primary pulmonary hypertension, which has associations with the use of appetite suppressants, it is important to first exclude pulmonary thromboembolic disease. Subsequent investigations may then focus on excluding other secondary causes of pulmonary hypertension.

Answer to Question 5

E

Pulmonary hypertension of any cause is associated with a 50% maternal mortality. Other high-risk cardiac conditions are severe mitral, pulmonary or aortic stenosis and Marfan's syndrome with a dilated aortic root. Intracardiac shunts without pulmonary hypertension are relatively safe but require closer follow-up. Operated tetralogy of Fallot without residual pulmonary stenosis is lower risk; coarctation is associated with dissection and is intermediate risk.

Answer to Question 6

C

Although streptococci are the most common cause of native valve endocarditis, postoperatively staphylococci are most likely and the history is suggestive of *Staphylococcus epidermidis*. *Staphylococcus aureus* is more likely to present in the early postoperative period and follows a more fulminant course.

Answer to Question 7

B

This man has a type B dissection and so the main treatment is to control the BP. A beta-blocker would be the first-choice agent as this reduces the shear wall stress of the aorta. Cardiothoracic referral is indicated in type A dissection, and in type B dissection if there is evidence of ongoing dissection with organ or limb ischaemia.

Answer to Question 8

D and I

Dyspnoea with exertion and resting outflow tract gradient are not associated with an increased risk of sudden death.

Answer to Question 9

A and J

Loop diuretics may improve symptoms, but there is no evidence that they improve mortality. Dihydropyridine calcium antagonists are contraindicated in heart failure. Spironolactone and eplerenone are aldosterone antagonists and have been shown to improve mortality in patients with significant systolic left ventricular dysfunction who present with decompensated heart failure and in those with heart failure post myocardial infarction, respectively. Angiotensin-converting enzyme inhibitors and beta-blockers improve mortality in systolic heart failure. Defibrillators reduce mortality from sudden death in post-myocardial infarction patients with low ejection fraction (<30%). Biventricular pacemakers also improve prognosis in patients with ejection fraction <30% and left bundle-branch block. Statins in the presence of proven coronary artery disease have been shown to improve outcome.

Answer to Question 10

D

Angiotensin-converting enzyme inhibitors are contraindicated in pregnancy. The others have all been used safely in pregnancy.

Answer to Question 11

B

This is likely to be a right ventricular infarct. Fluid should be administered, and an echocardiogram organised.

Answer to Question 12

E

Vehicular accidents are by far the most common cause. Creatine kinase will inevitably be raised with skeletal muscle injury; troponin would be a better marker in this situation. The ligamentum arteriosum is the most common site for aortic trauma as this is where the aorta is tethered to other mediastinal structures. It is also the site of greatest shearing forces. Glycoprotein IIb/IIIa inhibitors are contraindicated due to the increased bleeding risk; percutaneous coronary intervention may be an option, although the risk of bleeding remains with antiplatelet agents. Dressler's syndrome is a well-documented sequel of traumatic heart disease and may result in pericardial effusion with or without tamponade.

Answer to Question 13

A and D

A previous history of myocardial infarction (MI) and impaired left ventricular function is an indication for an implantable cardioverter defibrillator (ICD); the cut-off point for ejection fraction is 30–35%. ICDs can deliver pacing to terminate ventricular tachycardia (VT) in some circumstances but will have the ability to shock in either ventricular fibrillation (VF) or VT where pacing is unsuccessful. ICDs may be indicated in cases of hypertrophic cardiomyopathy and in patients with other conditions that may put them at risk of ventricular arrhythmias, irrespective of whether they have had a previous MI. Interrogation of the device will identify the exact rhythm and, if electrolytes are normal, then the patient may be discharged the same day with adjustments to the ICD programming or alteration of antiarrhythmic medication. Following shock therapy for VT or VF, patients may not drive for a minimum of 6 months.

Answer to Question 14

D and F

Her ECG demonstrates a very prolonged QT interval. This is a risk factor for developing torsade de pointes and cardiac arrest. A prolonged QT can be part of the inherited long QT syndrome but can be acquired. All the drugs, apart from atenolol (which can be used to treat a long QT) and

diltiazem, are associated with torsade de pointes.

Answer to Question 15

E

This man has developed acute pulmonary oedema secondary to acute myocardial infarction. He has an elevated BP and as such the optimal initial therapy is intravenous vasodilator. Intravenous nitrate is the most attractive option listed, to be followed by an oral angiotensin-converting enzyme (ACE) inhibitor (studies of early intravenous ACE inhibition have not demonstrated early benefit). Subsequent small aliquots of loop diuretic may be required.

Answer to Question 16

B

Given the history, lack of signs (except accentuated P2) and family history of sudden death, the most likely diagnosis is pulmonary hypertension. Echocardiography is the key initial investigation to evaluate cardiac structure and provide a non-invasive estimate of right heart pressures. If confirmed, other investigations directed towards establishing aetiology will be warranted.

Answer to Question 17

D and J

Beta-blockers have prognostic and symptomatic benefit in heart failure. In the UK bisoprolol, carvedilol and nebivolol are licensed for this use. Digoxin can improve symptoms in cases of severe heart failure, but should not be used at the expense of a beta-blocker. This patient has permanent atrial fibrillation (AF) and as such there is no benefit in trying to restore sinus rhythm, either

chemically or electrically. Impaired left ventricular function and AF carries a significant risk of thromboembolic complications and hence anticoagulation with warfarin should be recommended unless contraindicated.

Answer to Question 18

A

Although this man is now asymptomatic, he has been rendered such by diuretic therapy. Prognostically he will benefit from using both a long-term angiotensin-converting enzyme inhibitor (ACEI) and a beta-blocker. Most guidelines recommend the addition and then increased titration of an ACEI as first-line therapy, followed by a beta-blocker. A recent trial, CBIS III, supports this approach. In practice many would commence treatment with an ACEI, and at some stage increase its titration and add a low-dose beta-blocker.

Answer to Question 19

A

This clinical presentation is highly suggestive of life-threatening pulmonary embolism. He remains hypotensive (he normally tends to be hypertensive) and tachycardic. The next step must be to confirm the presence of proximal pulmonary embolism and to consider thrombolysis (surgery 4 weeks previously for varicose vein stab ligation is not a contraindication). CT pulmonary angiography would be the most desirable investigation. Whilst transthoracic echocardiography would be of value in demonstrating a dilated right heart, this is not specific for pulmonary embolic disease and can be seen in other instances, for example severe pneumonia.

Transoesophageal echocardiography would carry substantial risk in this haemodynamically compromised man. An elevated troponin (right ventricular ischaemia) in the context of pulmonary embolism indicates a worse prognosis and many would suggest that this would add weight to thrombolytic therapy.

Answer to Question 20

C

This patient has hypoxaemia with low normal P_{CO_2}. The two main differentials are pulmonary embolus and chest infection. However, there is nothing in his results to suggest a chest infection. The CXR does not demonstrate cosolidation and/or other changes of a chest infection, and furthermore there is no increase in the white blood cell count.

Answer to Question 21

E

The most likely diagnosis in this man is infective endocarditis. He demonstrates multiple non-specific features of insidious-onset infective endocarditis (low-grade pyrexia, sweats, heart murmur of aortic insufficiency, mild splenomegaly and rash). Colonic malignancy is a recognised risk for endocarditis.

Answer to Question 22

E

High BP, depression, fatigue, weakness, weight gain, menstrual irregularity and bruising can all be the result of Cushing's syndrome. Polycystic ovarian syndrome can result in insulin resistance, weight gain and menstrual irregularity but does not cause hypertension. Patients with severe depression often lose weight.

Answer to Question 23

D

Aortic regurgitation leads to volume overload and therefore to eccentric hypertrophy. Hypertrophic cardiomyopathy typically produces asymmetrical (or focal) left ventricular hypertrophy. Regression of hypertrophy in treated hypertension is well recognised. Recent studies also show that prognosis can be improved by treatments that result in regression of hypertrophy. In pressure overload, the apex beat is prominent but not displaced and is referred to as concentric hypertrophy. Displacement of the apex beat occurs as a result of ventricular dilatation in volume overload and is called eccentric hypertrophy.

Answer to Question 24

B and F

All valve lesions, prosthetic valves and cardiac lesions with high-pressure jets require antibiotic prophylaxis. In Eisenmenger's syndrome the pressures have equalised and a surgically ligated patent ductus arteriosus will have no residual flow. Any procedures that induce transient bacteraemia require antibiotic prophylaxis.

Answer to Question 25

B and G

The echocardiogram demonstrates asymmetrical hypertrophy of the septum with systolic anterior motion of the mitral valve leaflet causing left ventricular outflow tract obstruction. These features are highly suggestive of hypertrophic cardiomyopathy (HCM). Clinical features of HCM include jerky pulse, double apex beat, third and fourth heart sound and harsh ejection systolic murmur if obstruction is present. Cases with mild hypertrophy and no obstruction often have a normal cardiac examination. The ECG is often abnormal, even when the echocardiogram is normal. The diagnosis is usually made from a combination of clinical features, ECG and echocardiogram. Cardiac catheterisation is inferior to echocardiography for the diagnosis, but may provide useful information on coronary anatomy in cases suitable for percutaneous alcohol ablation treatment. Once a diagnosis is made, all patients should have exercise testing and 48-hour ambulatory ECG. The presence of non-sustained ventricular tachycardia and a drop in BP during exercise testing are markers of poor prognosis. Other poor prognostic features are a history of syncope, family history of sudden death, left ventricular wall thickness >3 cm and severe resting outflow tract obstruction. High-risk patients should have an implantable defibrillator. Medical therapy does not improve prognosis.

Answer to Question 26

B

For transoesophageal echocardiography (TOE) the transducer is positioned against the left atrium, and hence this technique is superior for visualisation of the left atrium, interatrial septum, pulmonary veins and the aortic arch. The low signal-to-noise ratio also makes TOE superior for prosthetic valve assessment. The left ventricular apex lies in the far field and is foreshortened with TOE. Transthoracic echocardiography is therefore superior for left ventricular apical disease, especially if used in conjunction with intravenous contrast agents.

Answer to Question 27

A

The positive predictive value of basal crackles is very poor, and a CXR is needed to confirm the presence of pulmonary oedema. The clinical diagnosis of congestive cardiac failure turns out to be correct in only one-third of cases. Verapamil is negatively inotropic and not indicated in this situation. Digoxin can improve symptoms in some individuals, even if they are in sinus rhythm. Beta-blockers are an important part of the treatment of heart failure, but should be introduced only when heart failure is stabilised on diuretics and an angiotensin-converting enzyme inhibitor (ACEI). Improved ejection fraction is well documented after treatment with an ACEI and beta-blockers.

Answer to Question 28

A

The increase in blood volume causes anaemia (dilution), systolic flow murmurs and a third heart sound. It also contributes to the increase in cardiac output, which counteracts the decrease in systemic vascular resistance, leaving BP largely unchanged. Most palpitations in pregnancy are caused by ectopics, although supraventricular tachycardias also occur.

Answer to Question 29

E

The clinical picture is of significant pulmonary embolism. All the listed factors, apart from prolongation of the QT interval, are relatively common in this context. The classical S1Q3T3 is seen sometimes but not commonly.

Answer to Question 30

E

The echocardiogram demonstrates bidirectional flow between the left atrium and right atrium, diagnostic of an atrial septal defect (ASD). Clinical features of ASD include atrial fibrillation and wide fixed split second heart sound. A soft systolic and diastolic flow murmur may be heard. Large defects, as in this example, will have bidirectional flow and the murmur is often inaudible. Advanced cases will have signs of pulmonary hypertension and right heart failure. The ECG typically demonstrates right bundle-branch block and right-axis deviation in the case of secundum defects and left-axis deviation with primum defects. If there is a suitable rim around the ASD, percutaneous closure is an acceptable alternative to surgery.

RESPIRATORY MEDICINE

Authors:

P Bhatia, SJ Fowler, S Kaul, DKC Lee and A Pawlowicz

Editor:

SJ Fowler

Editor-in-Chief:

JD Firth

1.1 History-taking

1.1.1 New breathlessness

Letter of referral to respiratory outpatient clinic

Dear Doctor,

Re: Mr Norman Boothroyd, aged 52 years

This man presents with a 2-month history of increasing breathlessness. His appetite is variable, but he suspects he may be losing weight as his clothes are becoming loose since returning from holiday abroad in the Far East about 6 months ago. He works as an automobile mechanic in a family-run business and is very worried because his father died of a respiratory complaint. My colleague prescribed some inhalers but these have not helped his breathing. I would be grateful for your expert opinion with regards to further investigation and management of his breathlessness.

Yours sincerely,

Introduction

Breathlessness or dyspnoea is defined as difficult, laboured or uncomfortable awareness of breathing. It is a feature of many cardiac and respiratory conditions. The physician must seek to make a clinical diagnosis before attempting a definitive test. The main diagnostic categories are shown in Table 1. An important concern is to identify any malignant diseases as early as possible.

History of the presenting problem

When and how?
A careful description of the dyspnoea is required. Let the patient tell his story in his own words, but clarify the following points if they do not emerge spontaneously.

- Is the dyspnoea really new or is this a progression of previously mild symptoms? Airways disease in particular often becomes a 'new' problem when the patient is unable to perform a particular task.

- When is it worse? Exertional dyspnoea is a non-specific symptom, but the specific complaint of orthopnoea suggests heart failure (or rarely bilateral diaphragm paralysis), although any patient with very severe breathlessness will not want (or be able) to lie down.

- If the symptoms are worse lying on one side, then this may suggest unilateral lung disease, eg a patient with right lung collapse may report a preference for sleeping on the right side.

- Nocturnal dyspnoea usually makes the clinician think of heart failure, but asthma is also worse at night.

Is the patient a smoker?
Does the patient smoke, currently or previously? Does the patient have cancer? These points needs to be clarified early. In a smoker, lung cancer requires positive exclusion if there are ominous associated symptoms (particularly weight loss, as seems to have occurred in this case, or haemoptysis). New breathlessness may also indicate a new perception of

TABLE 1 **CAUSES OF SLOW-ONSET NEW BREATHLESSNESS**	
Ferquency	**Cause**
Common	Airways disease
	Cardiac disease
	Pleural effusion/disease
	Lobar/lung collapse (caused by obstructing tumour)
Must consider	Thromboembolic disease
	Anaemia
Other conditions	Pulmonary arterial hypertension
	Interstitial lung disease
	Neuromuscular disease
	Chest wall disease

previously unrecognised airflow obstruction.

What is the patient's job?

The incidence of mesothelioma is set to peak in 2015. These symptoms could fit, especially if associated with unilateral pain and if the patient's employment history indicates asbestos exposure. Some periods of such employment may have been temporary; hence, when relevant, it is necessary to reconstruct the patient's full work CV (see Section 2.6).

> It is extremely important to obtain a full occupational history in any patient presenting with a respiratory problem. Go through things carefully: 'What was the first job you had after leaving school . . . and then . . . and then.'

Does the patient have any pets or unusual hobbies?

Although the answer is usually no, this question is quick to ask and may be relevant.

Features suggesting infection

Infection would not be a common cause of a dyspnoea of 2 months' duration. The exceptions to this are tuberculosis or a lung abscess, so you should therefore ask about fever, shivering attacks and sputum production. Is the patient at high risk of tuberculosis (eg an immigrant from an endemic area or living on the streets)?

Other relevant history

Previous pulmonary disease

A previous history of asthma, wheeziness or colds 'going to my chest' clearly raises the likelihood of airflow obstruction being the diagnosis. Remember that the patient may have had undiagnosed asthma at school (and therefore been unable to play sport or have disliked the playground in the winter) and grown out of it, only to have it relapse.

Cardiac disease

Although breathlessness with weight loss suggests a respiratory cause, it will be important to probe the patient's history thoroughly for any previous cardiac problems, chest pain or discomfort that might be due to coronary ischaemia, and also for ankle swelling that might be a sign of congestive cardiac failure.

Features to suggest pulmonary embolism

This would not be a common cause of this presentation but needs to be considered, so ask particularly about any previous known thromboembolism, unilateral leg swelling or discomfort/pain, pleuritic chest pain or haemoptysis (although malignancy would be the immediate concern if this patient had coughed up blood).

Plan for investigation and management

Chest radiograph

The CXR is almost an extension of the physical examination, and indeed most new patients attending the chest clinic have a CXR before seeing the doctor. Frequently this will show an abnormality that initiates a standard diagnostic pathway, eg pleural effusion, a solitary lung mass or apical alveolar shadowing. It is important to check for cardiac enlargement, and if the CXR appears to be normal then carefully review the apices, mediastinum and bony structures.

Blood tests

These are of limited value in the assessment of slow-onset new dyspnoea. The haemoglobin will exclude anaemia (and polycythaemia if there has been long-standing hypoxia). Blood tests may be diagnostic where the history and/or examination suggests a specific diagnosis, eg extrinsic allergic alveolitis, and clinical clues of malignancy should be pursued (eg measurement of liver function tests). Sarcoid is notoriously variable in its presentation: measurement of serum angiotensin-converting enzyme and calcium are indicated where this diagnosis is entertained.

Lung function tests

Lung function measurements are the next investigation for the breathless patient in whom the CXR is non-contributory. Look for evidence of airflow obstruction or a restrictive lung defect. Lung volumes and gas transfer measurements are required where the diagnosis is genuinely uncertain.

Additional investigations

Further investigations are guided by the clinical features and results of the CXR and lung function tests. They might include:

- CT thorax (including high-resolution images);

- ECG and echocardiogram (possibly with contrast);

- bronchoscopy;

- thoracoscopy;

- lung biopsy;

- respiratory muscle function tests.

Further discussion

- Patients with an inhaled foreign body often have to be prompted to enable this diagnosis, which is suggested by lobar collapse or a persistent cough.

- A patient with dyspnoea and pain may have a pneumothorax. This is usually of sudden onset, but not always, and may be forgotten by the patient. A CXR taken in expiration may demonstrate the condition, as shown in Fig. 1.

- Consider respiratory muscle weakness if there is a restrictive defect with a normal or supernormal gas transfer in the presence of a normal CXR. A good screening test is to compare the erect and supine vital capacity, when a drop of >20% suggests bilateral diaphragm paralysis.

1.1.2 Solitary pulmonary nodule

Letter of referral to respiratory outpatient clinic

Dear Doctor,

Re: Mr Stephen Norman, aged 56 years

I would be grateful for your opinion on this marketing manager who had a CXR as part of his company's health screening programme. The report indicates that there is a 'pulmonary nodule' in the left upper lobe. He denies any history of haemoptysis. His appetite and weight remain unchanged. He lives with his wife who is fit and well. Examination of his respiratory system remains unremarkable. Please advise on his further management.

Yours sincerely,

Introduction

There are many causes of a solitary pulmonary nodule (Table 2). The most important cause is lung

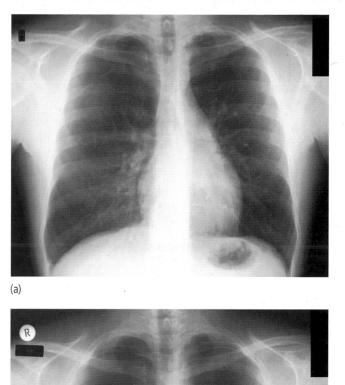
(a)

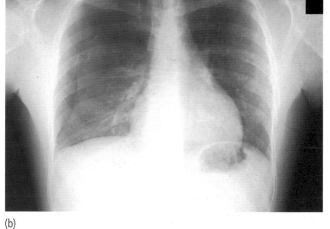
(b)

▲**Fig. 1** A pair of radiographs taken in a patient with a right-sided pneumothorax. On the inspiratory film (a) the pneumothorax is around 20%, which increases to around 60% on the expiratory film (b).

	TABLE 2 CAUSES OF A SOLITARY NODULE	
Instance	**Cause**	
Common	Primary lung cancer Old tuberculous nodule Secondary metastasis	
Rare	Infection (abscess) Benign tumour (adenoma or hamartoma) Arteriovenous malformation Active granulomatous disease (tuberculosis, sarcoid, Wegener's granulomatosis, rheumatoid nodule)	

cancer. Other likely causes include an old tuberculous nodule, a lung secondary and a benign adenoma. It is important to look for any external clues that will point towards a diagnosis. Old CXRs are extremely helpful in this situation. Ask the patient if he has ever had an X-ray, perhaps in another hospital and sometimes prior to elective surgery.

History of the presenting problem

Lung cancer

With respect to lung cancer it is important to ascertain the following.

- Smoking history: current, ex or never? If the patient is a current smoker or ex-smoker, then calculate pack-years [(number of cigarettes smoked per day/20) × number of years the patient has been a smoker].

- Occupational history: the patient may not have always been in a managerial post (see Section 2.6).

- Any history of cough and/or haemoptysis?

- Any chest wall pain, brachial plexus symptoms (numbness, tingling or weakness in hand muscles)? These are symptoms associated with a superior sulcus tumour.

- Any history of shortness of breath?

- Any change in the character of the patient's voice? Hoarseness may indicate recurrent laryngeal nerve palsy.

- Any history of night sweats?

- Any history of weight loss or anorexia?

- Any symptoms that might arise from systemic manifestations of cancer and paraneoplastic syndromes? These include

loss of balance, dizziness (paraneoplastic cerebellar), bone pain from hypercalcaemia or metastases, and weakness from Eaton–Lambert syndrome (proximal more than distal weakness).

Tuberculosis

With respect to tuberculosis (TB) consider the following.

- Past history of TB: details of treatment (if possible) and whether any course of treatment was completed.

- Has the patient taken steroids or any immunosuppressants, which would increase the risk?

- Does the patient have any history of alcohol abuse, which is associated with TB?

- Is there any history of liver disease (this may alter therapeutic regimen)?

- Family history: clearly an important element in this case. Is there any family history of TB? If so, which relatives were involved? Details of treatment (if possible) and whether courses of treatment were completed.

Other considerations

- Benign tumour: haemoptysis unlikely.

- Lung secondary: any history of other tumours the patient may have had (breast and ovarian in women, testicular in men).

Other relevant history

- General health: malaise, fatigue, lethargy. These non-specific signs could be associated with either TB or neoplastic disease.

- Past medical history: rheumatoid arthritis (including current and past treatments).

- Inhaled foreign body or severe respiratory illness: associated with lung abscess.

- History of unexplained anaemia or anaemia known to be associated with bleeding from the gastrointestinal tract: arteriovenous malformation.

- History of sinusitis, red eyes, hearing loss or renal problems: consider Wegener's granulomatosis.

Plan for investigation and management

After explaining to the patient that under normal clinical circumstances you would examine him to confirm that there are no abnormalities, as stated in the letter from the GP, you would plan as follows.

Chest radiograph

Repeat the CXR today for immediate comparison with the one obtained at the health screening.

> Always make strenuous efforts to review old CXRs: the nodule that was present 5 years ago and has not changed is unlikely to be sinister.

Sputum

If this is not obtainable, then sputum induction with the help of a physiotherapist may be required: request microscopy, culture and sensitivity, including acid-fast bacilli (specifically) and cytology.

Computed tomography

Conduct CT scans of thorax, liver and adrenals (Fig. 2).

Bronchoscopy

Conducted after a CT scan, ideally within 1 week of it. Bronchial biopsies should be sent in formalin

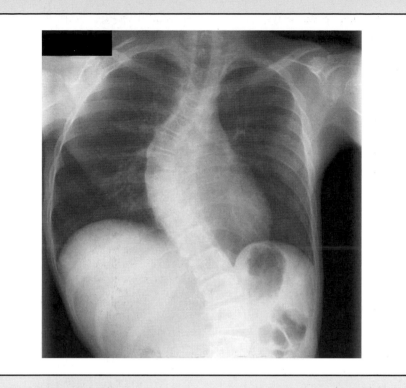

▲**Fig. 2** CT scan showing a solitary pulmonary nodule in the posterior aspect of the right lower lobe, which was difficult to see on the plain CXR (lymphoma was eventually diagnosed).

for histology, and in saline for microscopy and culture if TB is suspected.

Mantoux/Heaf test
Perform if you suspect TB.

Blood tests

- FBC.

- Coagulation screen.

- C-reactive protein/erythrocyte sedimentation rate.

- Urea/creatinine.

- Electrolytes.

- Liver function tests.

- Bone function tests: hypercalcaemia is associated with non-small-cell lung cancer, whereas syndrome of inappropriate antidiuretic hormone (hyponatraemia) and ectopic adrenocorticotropic hormone production (hypokalaemia, hyperglycaemia

and alkalosis) are associated with small-cell carcinoma.

- Serum angiotensin-converting enzyme (marker for sarcoid).

Arrange to review the patient in clinic when the results of these tests are available.

Further discussion

Benign tumours
About 2–5% of primary lung tumours are benign. These are a heterogeneous group of neoplastic lesions originating from pulmonary structures, including bronchial adenomas, hamartomas and a group of even more uncommon neoplasms (eg chondromas, fibromas, lipomas, leiomyomas, hemangiomas, teratomas, pseudolymphomas and endometriosis). Resection is normally recommended to avoid complications of bronchial obstruction, haemoptysis and

mitotic transformation (present in 2% of adenomas). The rate of growth of the tumour and the patient's general condition enter the risk–benefit equation.

Pulmonary arteriovenous malformations
Only treat if these are symptomatic. They can be locally embolised under radiological guidance and lung resection is rarely necessary.

1.1.3 Exertional dyspnoea with daily sputum

Letter of referral to respiratory outpatient clinic

Dear Doctor,

Re: Mr Kevin Power, aged 24 years

Could you please advise on the further management of this man? Six months ago he took his first job as a hospital physiotherapist and since then he has presented with exertional dyspnoea and has been coughing up a cupful of sputum daily. There is no history of wheeze. He also complains of intermittent abdominal pain which he has had for the last 8 months, and which initially was attributed to the stress of taking his final exams and starting his job. The only other history of relevance is that he has smoked over 40 cigarettes daily since the age of 15 years. Physical examination is entirely normal, as is his spirometry. Do you think that he might be developing chronic bronchitis/chronic obstructive pulmonary disease (COPD)?

Yours sincerely,

Introduction

This young man presents with pulmonary and abdominal symptoms, which may or may not be part of the same underlying condition. When considering the differential diagnoses take into account the patient's age. Always rule out ongoing infection first, as this requires prompt investigation and treatment, as well as contagious disorders, so that appropriate steps are taken to protect others.

The causes of a productive cough to be considered in a young patient are:

- COPD (chronic bronchitis), perhaps associated with α_1-antitrypsin deficiency (see Section 2.3);

- bronchiectasis/cystic fibrosis (see Sections 2.4 and 2.5);

- lung abscess (see *Infectious Diseases*, Section 1.1.1);

- pulmonary tuberculosis (TB) (see *Infectious Diseases*, Section 2.6.1);

- asthma/allergic bronchopulmonary aspergillosis (see Section 2.2.3);

- hypogammaglobulinaemia (see *Rheumatology and Clinical Immunology*, Sections 1.1.1 and 2.1.1).

History of the presenting problem

You must make sure there is no ambiguity regarding the patient's history.

- Was he really perfectly well prior to his recent episode? Could he play games at school and keep up with his friends when he played football?

- Does he remember frequent visits to his GP for the treatment of coughs/colds?

- Did he have measles, pertussis (whooping cough) or pneumonia as a child? This may suggest bronchiectasis.

- What is the colour of his sputum? Does the colour and quantity of his sputum change? Has he every noticed any blood in his sputum? Bronchiectasis and lung abscess can produce purulent sputum, which may be offensive and blood-tinged. Mucoid or mucopurulent sputum is characteristic of chronic bronchitis.

- Intermittent abdominal pain could be caused by a variety of problems (see *Gastroenterology and Hepatology*, Section 1.1.6).

Other relevant history

- General health: is there anything to suggest pulmonary TB (eg weight loss or night sweats)? Has he had any recent contact with a person diagnosed with TB?

- Is there any history of nasal/sinus problems? If so, it may suggest hypogammaglobulinaemia or cystic fibrosis (CF) in this case.

- Has he got any symptoms that might suggest diabetes (polydipsia, polyuria or weight loss), which would also suggest CF?

- Is there a family history of similar symptoms? Does he have any brothers/sisters/cousins, and do they (or could they) have CF?

- Is there a family history of COPD/emphysema/cirrhosis of the liver? This might indicate emphysema secondary to α_1-antitrypsin deficiency.

> **Do not forget to take a family history: CF or hypogammaglobulinaemia become the most likely diagnoses in this case if other family members are similarly affected.**

Plan for investigation and management

In a patient presenting with exertional dyspnoea and daily sputum production the following should be considered.

Chest radiograph

Perform to help exclude pulmonary TB, lung abscess and heart failure. It may reveal features suggestive of COPD/bronchiectasis/CF and give further clues as to the likely cause of bronchiectasis, for example if dextrocardia is found. Basal emphysematous changes would strongly suggest α_1-antitrypsin deficiency.

Sputum microbiology

Use routine culture and sensitivity, and direct staining and culture to check for acid-fast bacilli.

Lung function tests

These will determine if there is any airway obstruction, which may be found in COPD, asthma, bronchiectasis and CF.

Blood tests

A raised white cell count with neutrophilia or raised C-reactive protein suggests an underlying infection. A low serum α_1-antitrypsin level may suggest hereditary emphysema. Raised fasting glucose may point towards CF-related diabetes. Liver function tests can assess hepatic involvement in both CF and α_1-antitrypsin deficiency. Check serum immunoglobulins.

Arterial blood gases

Indicated if Sao_2 is <94% in order to check for any evidence of respiratory failure.

ECG

Perform this to look for any evidence of cor pulmonale.

Sweat sodium concentration

A value greater than 60 mmol/L is indicative of CF, but a normal test may be observed in approximately 1% of patients with CF who have unusual genotypes.

High-resolution CT scanning of the chest

This has become the best imaging modality for the detection of bronchial wall thickening and dilatation characteristic of bronchiectasis, with a sensitivity of 97%. It may reveal emphysema and suggest allergic bronchopulmonary aspergillosis if proximal bronchiectasis is seen.

Ultrasound examination of the hepatobiliary system

Conduct to look for any evidence of cirrhosis/gallstones.

Abdominal radiograph

This may show underlying gallstones or a partial intestinal obstruction (meconium ileus equivalent in CF).

Plan to review the patient in clinic when the results of tests are available.

Further discussion

In this scenario the presence of pulmonary and abdominal symptoms in a young man may suggest a late presentation of CF. Up to 7% of patients with CF are diagnosed at ≥18 years of age, when they are more likely than children to present with gastrointestinal symptoms and diabetes mellitus. Intermittent abdominal pain in CF can be caused by intermittent partial obstruction, low-grade appendicitis, duodenal irritation as a result of failure to buffer gastric acid or cholelithiasis. A further clue may be culture of *Staphylococcus aureus* from the sputum. The most appropriate initial

tests should therefore be directed towards the presumed diagnosis of CF in this case.

Hypogammaglobulinaemia is certainly another possibility, especially since by profession the patient is at increased risk of exposure to bacterial and viral infection.

Pulmonary TB and lung abscess are rather unlikely because of the time-scale involved and lack of other systemic symptoms, but should be excluded by a CXR.

The patient is too young to have COPD or even emphysema secondary to α_1-antitrypsin deficiency, because most patients with α_1-antitrypsin deficiency present between 32 and 41 years and rarely before 25 years of age. He does not meet the criteria for chronic bronchitis either, which is a diagnosis of exclusion. This is defined as the presence of chronic cough with sputum production that occurs most days of the week, at least 3 months a year, for more than two consecutive years and in the absence of other specific causes.

1.1.4 Dyspnoea and fine inspiratory crackles

Letter of referral to respiratory outpatient clinic

Dear Doctor,

Re: Justin Banks, aged 56 years

Thank you for seeing this man who has been complaining of dyspnoea on exertion for the last 8 months. He denies any wheeze or chest pain but also gives a history of having a dry cough for over a year. He has never smoked and works as a clerk in the local council. His past medical history includes appendicectomy and he was diagnosed with rheumatoid arthritis 3 years ago. Apart from regular NSAIDs, he is not on any treatment. Examination reveals fine bibasal crackles only. Please advise about diagnosis and management.

Yours sincerely,

Introduction

Dyspnoea on exertion with fine inspiratory crackles is a very common symptom and can be due to both cardiac and respiratory causes (Table 3).

History of the presenting problem

Because dyspnoea on exertion with fine inspiratory crackles can be due to congestive cardiac failure or respiratory problems it is important to pursue both possibilities in your history-taking.

Related to the cause of breathlessness

- Chest pain, especially retrosternal tightness related to exertion, would strongly suggest a cardiac cause. Orthopnoea, paroxysmal nocturnal dyspnoea, ankle swelling and weight gain, all of which point towards fluid retention, would also support the diagnosis of congestive cardiac failure (see *Cardiology*, Section 2.3).

- Expectoration of copious amounts of sputum would suggest bronchiectasis.

- A history of smoking with wheeze, mucoid phlegm and cough strongly suggests COPD (see Section 2.3). Much less commonly wheeze may be seen in eosinophilic pneumonia, as many patients with this condition also have asthma.

TABLE 3 CAUSES OF BREATHLESSNESS WITH FINE INSPIRATORY CRACKLES

Cardiac	Congestive cardiac failure
Respiratory	Chronic obstructive pulmonary disease (COPD)
	Bronchiectasis
	Diffuse parenchymal lung disease (DPLD)
	• Idiopathic: usual interstitial pneumonia (UIP), sarcoidosis, cryptogenic organising pneumonia
	• Fibrosing alveolitis associated with autoimmune rheumatic disorder: rheumatoid arthritis, scleroderma, systemic lupus erythematosus (SLE), ankylosing spondylitis, mixed connective tissue disorder, polymyositis–dermatomyositis
	• Associated with occupational and environmental exposure: silicosis, asbestosis, berylliosis, aluminium oxide fibrosis, farmer's lung, malt worker's lung, mushroom worker's lungs, bird fancier's lung, stannosis
	• Autoimmune: primary biliary cirrhosis, Wegener's granulomatosis, inflammatory bowel disease
	• Drug induced: amiodarone, penicillamine, busulfan, bleomycin, crack cocaine inhalation
	• Other causes: radiotherapy, amyloidosis, Langerhans' cell histiocytosis, post infections (eg tuberculosis), pulmonary alveolar proteinosis, lymphangioleiomyomatosis, eosinophilic pneumonia, acute respiratory distress syndrome, lymphangitic carcinomatosis

• Patients with DPLD usually present with shortness of breath, but a cough may be prominent in patients with lymphangitis carcinomatosis, sarcoidosis, UIP and eosinophilic pneumonias.

• Pleurisy may occur in up to 50% of patients with SLE and 25% of patients with rheumatoid arthritis, but it is rare in UIP.

• Pneumothorax, unlikely to be relevant in this case, may be the presenting reason for the onset or worsening of breathlessness in patients with a range of respiratory conditions, including rarities such as lymphangioleiomyomatosis and Langerhans' cell histiocytosis. This diagnosis should be suspected whenever a patient reports a sudden change in their breathing.

In addition, always ask about symptoms like haemoptysis and weight loss that may suggest the occurrence of adenocarcinoma in patients with underlying DPLD.

Related to the severity of breathlessness

It is also important to assess how disabling the symptoms are by asking how far the patient can walk. A useful objective way of assessing dyspnoea is by using the Medical Research Council (MRC) Dyspnoea Scale.

The MRC Dyspnoea Scale

1 Not troubled by breathlessness except on strenuous exercise.
2 Is short of breath when hurrying or walking up a slight hill.
3 Walks slower than contemporaries on the level because of breathlessness, or has to stop for breath when walking at own pace.
4 Stops for breath after about 100 metres or after a few minutes on the level.
5 Is too breathless to leave the house, or breathless when dressing or undressing.

Other relevant history

• Relevant past history: childhood respiratory infections, and perhaps also childhood history of measles or pertussis, would suggest

bronchiectasis (see Section 2.4). Ask specifically about tuberculosis (TB).

• Joint pains: suggestive of connective tissue disorders and sarcoidosis; sacroiliac joints are affected in ankylosing spondylitis (usually upper-zone fibrosis).

• Eyes: hazy vision or decreased acuity, eye pain and photophobia with red eyes all suggest possible uveitis due to sarcoidosis or autoimmune disease.

• Skin problems: a photosensitive rash would suggest SLE.

• Drug history: drugs can cause pulmonary fibrosis. In routine practice check any drug in the *British National Formulary*, but note especially those detailed in Table 3. It is also worth asking specifically about amiodarone: 'Have you been given any drugs to control or steady the heart rate?'

• Occupational history: this man now works as a council clerk, but he may not always have done so.

• Hobbies: breeding pigeons can lead to extrinsic allergic alveolitis and eventually cause pulmonary fibrosis. In routine clinical practice patients may not mention this because they do not know that it is relevant or because they fear that it is; in PACES, the surrogate's briefing notes are more than likely to say 'Don't mention hobbies unless you are asked directly'.

Plan for investigation and management

Having taken a history and examined the patient, the next step is to arrange investigations to confirm the diagnosis and find a cause for the underlying condition.

Chest radiograph

This is very likely to reveal a diffuse reticulonodular pattern with 'small lungs'. Bilateral hilar lymphadenopathy may be seen in sarcoidosis. In cases of asbestos exposure pleural plaques may be visible. Look for cardiomegaly and Kerley B lines suggesting congestive cardiac failure. In old healed TB and ankylosing spondylitis, apical fibrosis will be seen.

Blood tests

- FBC to check for polycythaemia (due to hypoxia).

- Autoimmune screen, including rheumatoid factor, antinuclear antibodies and circulating antineutrophil cytoplasmic antibody (Wegener's granulomatosis).

- Serum angiotensin-converting enzyme levels (raised in sarcoidosis).

- Relevant precipitins (when extrinsic allergic alveolitis is suspected, eg bird fancier's disease).

- Clotting screen (in anticipation of the need for lung biopsy).

ECG

Look for features of pulmonary hypertension: right-axis deviation, P pulmonale in lead II and dominant R in V1 may be seen in pulmonary diseases causing hypoxia. Cardiac sarcoidosis may present with heart block.

Pulmonary function tests

These will almost certainly show a restrictive disorder with reduced forced expiratory volume in 1 second (FEV_1) and forced vital capacity (FVC), but a normal FEV_1/FVC ratio, reduced carbon monoxide transfer factor and reduced total lung capacity as well as residual volume.

Arterial blood gases

If S_p0_2 <92% to decide if there is need for oxygen theapy.

High-resolution CT scanning

This is the investigation of choice (see Section xxx) and can detect DPLD not visible on the CXR (sensitivity is 94% versus 80%). Areas of ground-glass opacity can be targeted when planning biopsy, thus increasing the diagnostic yield.

Bronchoscopy and bronchoalveolar lavage

Bronchoalveolar lavage is used to sample cells from the lower respiratory tract. An increase in granulocytes, particularly neutrophils and eosinophils, is typically seen in cases of fibrosing alveolitis occurring alone or with connective tissue disorders and asbestosis. Increased numbers of lymphocytes are seen in drug-induced lung disorders and granulomatous lung disorders.

Lung biopsy

A histological diagnosis can be made by lung biopsy.

- Transbronchial lung biopsy: sampling error is common and samples are often too small to make a diagnosis. It is useful in granulomatous disorders, metastatic disorders, eosinophilic pneumonia, alveolar proteinosis and infections. It is a safe procedure and can be performed as a day case, although pneumothorax occurs in about 1–2% of cases (higher in some series).

- Open lung biopsy: provides good-quality specimens and can be performed from the diseased area.

- Video-assisted thoracoscopic lung biopsy: performed under general anaesthesia and can yield good-size samples.

- Percutaneous (CT-guided) biopsy.

Management

Specific management will depend on the underlying cause. General measures include the following.

- Withdraw any drugs responsible.

- Treat any airflow obstruction with bronchodilators.

- Stop smoking.

- Oxygen therapy as per blood gas results.

- Pulmonary rehabilitation to improve overall fitness.

- Pneumonia vaccination and yearly influenza vaccination.

Specific treatment Idiopathic forms of DPLD and those associated with autoimmune rheumatic disorder are often treated with corticosteroids or other immunosuppressive drugs. In general the evidence of efficacy is not strong, but see Section 2.7 for further discussion. Single lung transplantation may be offered to selected patients.

1.1.5 Nocturnal cough

Letter of referral to respiratory outpatient clinic

Dear Doctor,

Re: Mrs Nicola Cook, aged 36 years

Thank you for seeing this teacher who has a 5-month history of dry nocturnal cough. She has never smoked, is otherwise well and her physical examination is normal. She has tried various over-the-counter cough medications with no relief. I am at a loss as to the diagnosis: can you help?

Yours sincerely,

Introduction

Chronic cough is defined as cough persisting for over 8 weeks. It is the single most common complaint of adult patients to their GPs. It can be a very distressing symptom and may result in matrimonial disharmony, affect job prospects, and can generally undermine the patient's confidence. There are many causes (see Table 4): a systematic approach can help reach a diagnosis and hopefully cure this annoying symptom.

In studies of patients referred to tertiary care practices, the first three conditions listed in Table 4 are found to be the cause of chronic cough in 65–95% of patients, and in many cases combinations of these are present. Proper history-taking, examination and basic investigations can help in diagnosing most cases, but the remainder will need detailed investigations.

History of the presenting problem

An appropriate history will help narrow down the causes.

- How long has the cough been present? A very long history militates against a sinister cause.

- Did it start after an upper respiratory tract infection? This clearly suggests post-infective bronchial hyperresponsiveness.

- Is the cough worse with exertion? In cough variant asthma, the cough is worse during or after exertion and at night.

- Is there any wheeze? This would indicate asthma or CCF. In cough variant asthma, there is normally no wheeze or dyspnoea.

- Is there any heartburn, sour belches, indigestion or hoarseness of the voice in the morning? These signs would suggest GORD or oesophageal dysmotility.

- Has the patient had any headaches/tenderness over the sinuses, a blocked or running nose, sneezing bouts or a dripping sensation at the back of the throat? These symptoms would indicate upper airway cough syndrome.

- Is the patient a smoker and is there haemoptysis? Always consider bronchogenic carcinoma in such a case.

- Is the cough accompanied by expectoration of copious phlegm that would be suggestive of bronchiectasis?

- The combination of haemoptysis with weight loss, night fever and chest pain would point towards tuberculosis.

- Are the symptoms worse at work? If so, this would clearly indicate that occupational exposure is an important factor.

- Does the patient have any painful rashes on the legs, with joint pains and itching of the eyes (iritis)? Remember sarcoidosis in such cases.

- Is there dysphagia and recurrent lower respiratory infections? If so, consider oesophageal dysmotility and Zenker's diverticulum.

Other relevant history

Is there any other medical history that could suggest a diagnosis?

- Has the patient been a smoker?

- Does she have a past history of asthma?

- Does she have a past history of rhinitis, sinusitis, nasal polyps or nasal blockage?

- Are the symptoms seasonal? If yes, could this be allergic rhinitis?

TABLE 4 CAUSES OF CHRONIC COUGH	
Frequency	**Causes**
Common	Asthma syndromes: cough variant asthma; post-infective bronchial hyperresponsiveness; and eosinophilic bronchitis (see Section 2.8.5)
	Upper airway cough syndrome (UACS), also known as post nasal drip syndrome
	Gastro-oesophageal reflux disease (GORD)
	Smoking and chronic obstructive pulmonary disease
Less common	Lung cancer
	Drug induced [angiotensin converting enzyme inhibitors (ACEI) and β-blockers]
	Bronchiectasis
	Tuberculosis (TB)
	Foreign body inhalation
	Occupational exposure
	Sarcoidosis
	Cryptogenic fibrosing alveolitis
	Congestive cardiac failure (CCF)
	Pertussis
Rare	Oesophageal dysmotility syndromes
	Zenker's diverticulum
	Tracheobronchomalacia
Controversial	Psychogenic

- Has the patient or any close contacts had tuberculosis in the past?

- Has the patient had any oesophageal disorder such as Barrett's oesophagus? This can predispose to reflux oesophagitis and cough.

- What is the patient's drug history: enquire about angiotensin-converting enzyme inhibitors and beta-blockers in particular.

- Does she suffer from any autoimmune rheumatic disorder?

- Up to 4% of patients with rheumatoid arthritis may have bronchiectasis presenting as cough.

- Is there any history of ankle swelling, orthopnoea, paroxysmal nocturnal dyspnoea and ischaemic heart disease? If so, think of CCF.

Plan for investigation and management

After explaining to the patient that under normal clinical circumstances you would examine her to confirm that there are no abnormalities as stated in the letter from her GP, you would plan as follows.

Chest radiograph

All patients with a chronic cough should have a CXR to look for evidence of malignancy, diffuse parenchymal lung disease (DPLD), infection or CCF. At times a fluid level behind the cardiac shadow will point towards a hiatus hernia with a cough due to associated GORD.

Peak expiratory flow monitoring

A peak expiratory flow (PEF) recording showing diurnal variation is helpful in establishing the diagnosis of asthma as a cause of the chronic cough. If such variation is seen, then a therapeutic trial of

bronchodilator is warranted before proceeding with further investigation.

Pulmonary function tests

These are essential both for diagnosing COPD and assessing its severity. In DPLD, lung function will show a restrictive disorder.

Sputum examination

Sputum, if present, should be collected for microscopy and bacterial, mycobacterial and fungal culture, and for a differential cell count (eosinophilia in asthma).

Other investigations

Depending on the clinical findings and the results of the above investigations, then the following may also be appropriate.

Ears/nose/throat opinion, nasendoscopy and imaging (radiography and/or CT scan of sinuses) Look for nasal polyps, rhinitis and sinusitis.

Twenty-four hour ambulatory oesophageal pH monitoring A probe is inserted into the oesophagus to enable monitoring of pH for 24 hours. Patients wear a device called a digitrapper, through which they record incidents of cough, heartburn, chest pain or other symptoms. When the monitoring period is over, analysis seeks to determine how fluctuations in acidity relate to the patient's symptoms.

Oesophageal manometry Sometimes referred to as an oesophageal function or oesophageal motility study, this test is used to check how well the muscles of the oesophagus are working. It also measures the strength of the lower oesophageal sphincter or 'valve' that prevents the backward flow of food from the stomach into the

oesophagus. It is helpful in assessing patients with a cough due to oesophageal dysmotility syndrome.

High-resolution CT scan of the lungs This can identify patients with pulmonary fibrosis and may be diagnostic.

Bronchial challenge test Using direct bronchoconstrictors such as methacholine or histamine, asthmatics demonstrate both airway hypersensitivity (reacting at a lower dose) and hyperreactivity (greater bronchoconstriction per unit given) than non-asthmatic patients. A bronchial challenge test is indicated when asthma is a possibility but when other tests such as diurnal PEF measurement or bronchodilator reversibility are not diagnostic.

Bronchoscopy/CT staging scan If there is a lung mass, bronchoscopy is essential for obtaining a tissue diagnosis. If a diagnosis of bronchogenic carcinoma is made (exceedingly unlikely in this young non-smoking woman), a staging CT scan of the lungs will establish whether the disease is operable. It will also help monitor disease response in patients treated with chemotherapy or radiotherapy.

ECG Patients with CCF causing a nocturnal cough may have clues to the cause evident on the ECG, such as old infarcts or left ventricular hypertrophy (due to hypertension).

Echocardiogram Patients suspected of having CCF should undergo echocardiography to assess left ventricular function.

Further discussion

Most causes of nocturnal cough can be diagnosed by a proper history and basic investigations, but some patients may need referral to an ears/nose/throat specialist or a gastroenterologist.

Once a diagnosis is reached, patients with GORD may also need advice about lifestyle modifications such as:

- stopping smoking;

- eating smaller meals;

- avoiding tea, coffee and alcohol;

- elevating the head end of the bed by 15 cm.

- avoidance of recumbency for 3 hours postprandially;

- weight reduction;

- decreasing fat intake.

1.1.6 Daytime sleepiness and morning headache

Letter of referral to respiratory outpatient clinic

Dear Doctor,

Re: Mrs Jennifer Barclay, aged 44 years

Thank you for seeing this woman who has been complaining of daytime sleepiness and morning headaches for the last 8 months. She has smoked 25 cigarettes per day for the last 20 years. Though she weighs 96 kg, she is otherwise well and physical examination is normal. I wonder if she has a respiratory reason for this and would welcome your opinion.

Yours sincerely,

Introduction

Excessive daytime sleepiness is due to abnormal nocturnal sleep, which may be insufficient or inefficient (poor-quality sleep). The causes of excessive daytime sleepiness are

TABLE 5 CAUSES OF EXCESSIVE DAYTIME SLEEPINESS

Prevalence	Cause
Common	Insufficient sleep
	Chronobiologic disorder (1)
	Sleep-disordered breathing disorders (2)
	Restless leg syndrome/periodic limb movement disorder
Rare	Narcolepsy
	Idiopathic hypersomnia
	Post-traumatic hypersomnia

Notes
(1) Jet-lag syndrome, shift work, etc.
(2) Obstructive, central sleep apnoea and upper airway resistance syndrome: patients may sleep for the required seven to eight hours every night but there may be frequent arousals preventing slow wave sleep [stage three and four non-rapid eye movement (REM) and REM sleep] resulting in daytime somnolence.

shown in Table 5. When combined with a morning headache, a sign of CO_2 retention, the causes can be narrowed down to disorders causing chronic respiratory failure (ventilatory failure).

Causes of chronic respiratory failure resulting in high CO_2 that produces morning headaches are shown in Table 6.

> Morning headaches and sleepiness during the day: always consider CO_2 retention.

History of the presenting problem

It is clearly important to take an appropriate sleep history.

- Obtain details of waking time, sleeping time, any daytime naps, appropriateness of bedroom for sleeping (no distractions) and times of drinking any caffeine-based drink.

- Is there any reason for insufficient sleep, such as shift work, poor sleep hygiene (daytime naps), uncomfortable sensations in the leg with an urge to move the limb resulting in sleep fragmentation?

TABLE 6 CAUSES OF CHRONIC RESPIRATORY FAILURE CAUSING CO_2 RETENTION

Prevalence	Cause
Common	Chronic obstructive pulmonary disease (COPD)
	Sleep-disordered breathing disorders
Less common	Other causes of chronic lung disease
	Thoracic cage deformities (kyphosis, scoliosis and thoracotomy)
	Central alveolar hypoventilation syndrome (Pickwickian syndrome)
Rare	Motor neuron disease and motor neuropathies: amyotrophic lateral sclerosis, poliomyelitis, Guillain–Barré syndrome, syringomyelia, phrenic nerve palsies and hereditary sensorimotor neuropathies
	Muscle diseases: congenital myopathies, Duchenne's muscular dystrophy, myotonic dystrophy, polymyositis, acid maltase deficiency and limb girdle dystrophy
	Neuromuscular junction disorders: myasthenia gravis

- Do the headaches improve as the day goes by? If not, then this throws doubt on the suggestion that they are caused by CO_2 retention.

- How long have the sleepiness and headaches been present? A very long history would suggest a slowly progressive condition such as thoracic deformity.

- Is there a history of snoring, apnoeic spells and choking sounds at night? All these are suggestive of OSA. Ask directly 'Has anyone ever told you that you snore a lot or make odd sounds with your breathing at night or seem to stop breathing when you're asleep?' Did the onset of the patient's symptoms coincide with any recent weight gain? This is a risk factor for the development of OSA.

> When probing for a history of OSA, always try to get a history from the patient's sleeping partner.

- Is the patient on any sedatives and how much alcohol does she consume? These are exacerbating factors for OSA because they reduce pharyngeal tone.

- History suggestive of narcolepsy: cataplexy, sleep paralysis, hypnagogic and hypnopompic hallucinations (frightening hallucinations occurring at sleep onset and end of sleep, respectively) or disturbed nocturnal sleep.

- How bad is the daytime sleepiness? The Epworth sleepiness score is useful for assessing subjective daytime somnolence (see Section 2.1).

Other relevant history

- As the patient is a smoker, enquire about a history of wheeze, cough with phlegm or dyspnoea, which are suggestive of COPD. COPD is a well-known cause of chronic respiratory failure presenting as morning headache, and disturbed sleep in such patients can also lead to daytime somnolence.

- Is there any history suggestive of congestive cardiac failure? Up to 50% of patients with severe congestive cardiac failure (left ventricular ejection fraction <45%) have central sleep apnoea, and the nocturnal apnoeas can cause fragmented sleep with daytime somnolence.

- Is there a family history of neuromuscular disorders?

- Does the patient have a past history of polio? The post-polio syndrome can develop decades after the initial illness and presents with functional deterioration of the muscles.

Plan for investigation and management

After explaining to the patient that under normal circumstances you would examine her to confirm that there are no abnormalities, as stated in the GP's letter, you would plan as follows.

Chest radiograph

Perform to exclude lung disease or cardiomegaly, and to confirm thoracic cage deformity.

Arterial blood gases

During the day these may show hypercapnia, which may be associated with normal pH and raised bicarbonate (compensated respiratory failure) or acidic pH and normal bicarbonate (not yet compensated). Hypoxia may also be present. Arterial blood gases measured at 7 a.m. are a good reflection of nocturnal blood gases and can help decide whether the patient needs nocturnal oxygen therapy or non-invasive positive-pressure ventilation (NIPPV).

Pulmonary function tests

These may confirm the presence of COPD in a smoker, which may require treatment. In cases of diaphragmatic palsy due to phrenic nerve lesions, the vital capacity should be measured in the upright and supine positions. Normally, vital capacity in recumbence decreases by 10%. In unilateral paralysis, the upright vital capacity shows a decrease to 70–80% of the predicted level, usually with a slightly more significant decrement in the supine position. In contrast, patients with bilateral diaphragmatic paralysis show a 50% decrease in vital capacity when they are supine because of cephalad displacement of their abdominal contents.

Overnight pulse oximetry

This can be done at home. It records Sao_2 continuously overnight and has been used both as a screening test for OSA and to assess nocturnal hypoxia in patients with COPD or disorders of ventilation.

Transcutaneous Pco_2 monitoring

This enables monitoring of CO_2 levels during sleep. In patients with disorders causing hypoventilation, CO_2 levels are high during the night. This is due to both an altered ventilation/perfusion ratio and a decrease in central respiratory drive, particularly in REM sleep.

Polysomnography

If sleep-disordered breathing is suspected, the gold standard is polysomnography with electroencephalography, electromyelography, electrooculography, Sao_2, and thoracic and abdominal movement sensors. This can be

Station 2: History Taking　　**203**

combined with ECG and BP monitoring.

Blood tests

- FBC looking for polycythaemia, which may occur due to nocturnal hypoxia.

- Thyroid function test: hypothyroidism may present with weight gain and tiredness, and may contribute to either OSA or obesity hypoventilation syndrome.

Cardiac tests

- ECG: may show right heart strain or left ventricular hypertrophy (patient may have undiagnosed hypertension).

- Echocardiogram: in patients with features of congestive cardiac failure an echocardiogram should be arranged; if left ventricular function is impaired, it should be treated with angiotensin-converting enzyme inhibitors and diuretics.

Further discussion

The diagnosis of most disorders causing ventilatory failure is quite easy. However, once the diagnosis is made treatment is likely to require referral to a specialist in sleep medicine. In cases of obesity, weight reduction is an important measure along with domiciliary non-invasive ventilation.

In cases of motor neuron disease and genetic muscle disorders, a decision to start NIPPV should be made following discussion with the patient and the family. At the same time, a plan for future level of care should be made: for example, would all parties consider treatment on a high-dependency unit acceptable, but not intubation and ventilation?

Once a patient is started on NIPPV, regular follow-up is required:

check for compliance, equipment replacement due to wear and tear (mask and tubes), servicing of the machine and if the pressures selected are adequate.

1.1.7 Lung cancer with asbestos exposure

> ### Letter of referral to respiratory outpatient clinic
>
> Dear Doctor,
>
> **Re: Mr Anthony Edwards, aged 56 years**
>
> I would be grateful for your opinion on this taxi driver who came to see me last week with a 4-month history of right-sided nagging chest ache. A CXR was requested and the report indicated that he has right-sided pleural thickening associated with a moderate pleural effusion. He has previously worked in numerous labouring jobs, including as a lagger. He is an ex-smoker of 6 years. His appetite is poor of late and he has lost a stone in weight in the last 3 months. I fear the worst, but please advise on his further investigation and management.
>
> Yours sincerely,

Introduction

Your main concern is that this patient has asbestos-related lung disease and that this could be mesothelioma, although asbestos also causes other pathology:

- pleural plaques;

- benign asbestos-related pleural thickening;

- asbestos-related interstitial fibrosis (asbestosis);

- lung cancer.

It is clearly vitally important to take a detailed occupational history in this case.

> **How to take an occupational history**
>
> - The easiest way of recording employment is by asking the patient what he did immediately after leaving school and then recording positions chronologically; people tend to remember their jobs most easily this way.
> - Do not forget holiday jobs from school or casual employment (Steve McQueen, the American actor, worked with asbestos for 6 months before he became famous, and he died of asbestos-related lung disease).
> - Did anyone in the patient's family work in an asbestos factory and bring the dust home on their clothes?
> - On a more short-term basis, particularly if you are worried about the patient's current employment (say in relation to occupational asthma), do the symptoms worsen during the working week and improve at the weekend and during holidays?

History of the presenting problem

It will clearly be appropriate to take a full history of respiratory symptoms and functional status, as described in previous history scenarios in this module, but the crucial element in this case will be to focus on taking the occupational history.

Occupational history

- If the patient remembers working with asbestos, how long was this for? How close was the contact and for what length of the working day? For example, was the patient working in the holds of ships unloading bags of asbestos? Were the patient's clothes covered in asbestos dust?

- Did the patient wear protective clothing or masks? Were these provided by the employers?

- Record the names of the companies worked for (they may be helpful for later reference).

Smoking history

This is essential because if there is both asbestos and tobacco exposure, then it is necessary to quantify both for legal purposes.

> **Take an accurate smoking history and record in the notes when and if the patient has stopped smoking. If the patient claims compensation at a later date, this information will be required.**

Symptoms

- Has the patient had any chest pain? If so, how long does it last? Does it keep him awake at night?

- Has the patient been short of breath at rest or during exercise?

- Has it been more difficult of late for the patient to lie down without feeling breathless?

- Has the patient experienced any loss of weight or had a history of anorexia?

- Persistent pain or rapid progression of symptoms are poor predictive features.

Other relevant history

It is important to ascertain whether there have been any previous episodes of chest problems. Did the patient suffer from chest problems as a child? Many chest pathologies can result in pleural thickening (Fig. 3):

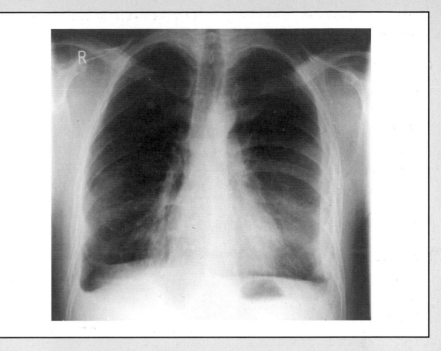

▲ **Fig. 3** CXR showing obvious left-sided pleural thickening caused by asbestos exposure. (Courtesy of Dr R. Rudd.)

- asbestos exposure;

- trauma;

- previous chest infection/empyema;

- previous haemothorax;

- old tuberculosis.

Plan for investigation and management

Chest radiograph

In this case, the patient presented with a chest film. In routine clinical practice look carefully for any pleural thickening: it is easy to miss. Is there any calcification, particularly over the diaphragm? Do not forget to look for areas of fibrosis.

CT scan of chest

This is invaluable when assessing the extent of disease and checking whether there is pleural thickening, fibrosis (requires high-resolution scanning) or malignancy (Fig. 4). If appropriate, a CT scan may be followed by CT-guided biopsy. In cases of bronchogenic cancer and asbestos exposure the presence of fibrosis supports the argument that the patient was exposed to significant quantities of asbestos.

Pleural biopsy and aspiration

> ⚠ **A 'blind' pleural biopsy with an Abrams' needle can only be carried out in the presence of a moderate to large pleural effusion, otherwise you may puncture the lung and give the patient a pneumothorax. A CT-guided biopsy is preferred when there is localised pleural thickening.**

> **Make sure that you send pleural biopsy samples to microbiology for microscopy and culture (including TB, in saline rather than formalin), as well as to histology. The diagnosis may not be malignancy, or there may be dual pathology.**

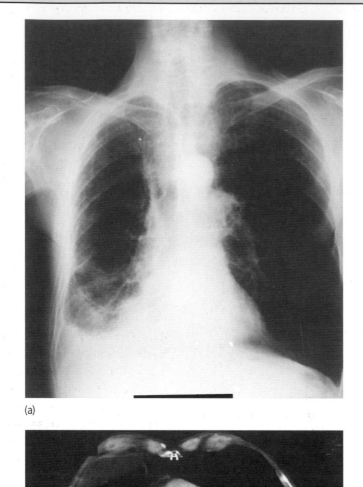

(a)

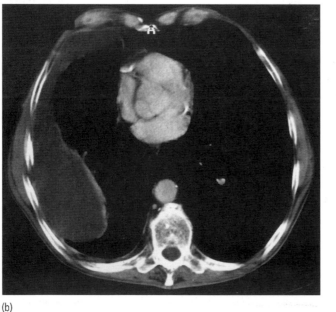

(b)

▲**Fig. 4** **(a)** CXR and **(b)** CT scan of patient with mesothelioma causing right-sided pleural thickening, volume loss and mediastinal shift, with invasion into the right hemithorax.

Thoracoscopy

This is generally only available in specialist centres, where it can be performed by chest physicians and/or cardiothoracic surgeons. It has a far higher diagnostic success rate than blind biopsy (95% in combination with aspiration versus 70% for Abrams' biopsy plus aspiration), and pleurodesis can also be performed at the same time if malignancy is confirmed.

Other tests

It will clearly be appropriate to check the patient's FBC (might reveal anaemia) and clotting screen (in expectation of biopsy); electrolytes and renal, liver and bone function tests (for evidence of metastatic disease); and lung function tests (to establish baseline).

Management

Specific management will depend on the precise diagnosis, but given the high likelihood of malignant disease with a poor prognosis, this patient may require referral to palliative care services in the not-too-distant future.

1.1.8 Breathlessness with a normal chest radiograph

Letter of referral to respiratory outpatient clinic

Dear Doctor,

Re: Mr Colin MacDonald, aged 44 years

I would be grateful for your advice regarding this man who has presented with a 6-month history of breathlessness. He has smoked 20 cigarettes a day since the age of 16, but has recently cut down to five per day. A trial of inhaled steroids and diuretics was unhelpful. At present his only medication is a steroid nasal spray for his rhinitis. His younger daughter suffers from asthma.

I could not find anything abnormal on physical examination. His CXR is reported as being within normal limits. His spirometry shows forced expiratory volume in 1 second (FEV_1) of 2.6 L (83% predicted), forced vital capacity (FVC) 3.1 L (79% predicted) and an FEV_1/FVC ratio of 83%. Oxygen saturation (on air) is 93%. I wonder whether he suffers from primary hyperventilation?

Yours sincerely,

Introduction

The most likely causes of chronic breathlessness with a normal CXR are shown in Table 7.

Normal spirometry makes COPD unlikely. Asthma as a sole diagnosis would also be improbable given that significantly reduced oxygen saturation is associated with normal spirometry. Low oxygenation rules out the possibilities of primary hyperventilation or anaemia as the primary cause of dyspnoea.

In DPLD, lung function usually shows a restrictive pattern. However, remember that some patients have preserved lung volumes or airflow obstruction, and hence it is inappropriate to use restrictive lung function as a criterion to exclude the diagnosis.

Although the most common presentation of PE is pleuritic chest pain with or without haemoptysis, isolated dyspnoea may be the only symptom and the possibility of chronic PE must be considered in this case. Exertional dyspnoea is also the most common presentation of early pulmonary hypertension, a rare condition that is frequently underdiagnosed. In view of a history of rhinitis and a family history of asthma, Churg–Strauss syndrome should be also excluded in this case.

History of the presenting problem

A complete history is important to narrow the differential diagnosis. Ask specifically about the following.

Initial presentation

Was it insidious or did it follow any environmental/dust exposure?

Mode of presentation

Was it chronic or episodic? Episodic presentation narrows the diagnostic field to extrinsic allergic alveolitis (EAA), eosinophilic pneumonia, vasculitis and cryptogenic organising pneumonia. However, there is considerable variation in the time frame of presentation of many DPLDs. For example, eosinophilic

pneumonia, cryptogenic organising pneumonia and Churg–Strauss syndrome may present acutely, episodically or chronically. Others, such as drug-induced DPLDs may be acute or chronic.

Other chest symptoms

Patients with DPLDs may have an unproductive cough. A productive cough makes DPLD rather unlikely. Other chest symptoms are uncommon in DPLDs, but if present are of importance as they may further narrow the differential diagnosis. Pleuritic chest pain may occur in DPLDs associated with systemic lupus erythematosus (50% of cases), rheumatoid arthritis (25% of cases) and mixed connective tissue disease. Some patients with chronic PE may recall pleuritic chest pain at the time of initial presentation. Substernal discomfort or pain is common in sarcoidosis. Wheezing may occur in chronic eosinophilic pneumonia and Churg–Strauss syndrome. Haemoptysis may be present in chronic PE and vasculitis. Symptoms of recurrent flu-like illness are often a feature of EAA or vasculitis (see Sections 2.7 and 2.8 and *Cardiology*, Section 2.18.1).

Risk factors of PE

Assess the clinical probability of PE (see *Cardiology*, Sections 1.4.6 and 2.18.1) by asking about previous episodes of thromboembolism, risk factors (immobility, etc.) and family history.

Drug history

Take a detailed history of all previous and current medication, both prescribed and non-prescribed. Many classes of drugs cause DPLD, so in routine clinical practice always consult the drug datasheet or *British National Formulary*. The variable timing of onset of symptoms from

---

TABLE 7 CONDITIONS PRESENTING CHRONICALLY WITH BREATHLESSNESS AND A NORMAL CXR

Prevalence	Cause
Common	Chronic obstructive pulmonary disease (COPD) Asthma Anaemia
Less common	Pulmonary vascular disorders: pulmonary embolism (PE), pulmonary hypertension Diffuse parenchymal lung disease (DPLD) Primary hyperventilation
Rare	Pulmonary vasculitis, eg Churg–Strauss syndrome

---

drug-related DPLD is well known, and some drugs such as cyclophosphamide and amiodarone may have been taken for up to several years before drug-induced alveolitis develops. Do not forget to enquire directly about appetite suppressants, a known cause of pulmonary hypertension (see *Cardiology*, Section 2.12).

Lifetime occupations
Review in chronological order, including specific duties and known exposures to dust, gases and chemicals. Record details of occupational processes, the exposure level and type of respiratory protection provided.

Recreational interests
Enquire specifically about exposure to birds.

Family history
Sarcoidosis, cryptogenic fibrosing alveolitis (now known as usual interstitial pneumonia), pulmonary hypertension and chronic PE may rarely be familial.

Travel history
Travelling predisposes to infection with parasites, which may cause pulmonary eosinophilia and is also a risk factor for PE.

Other relevant history
Enquire about other systemic disorders associated with lung diseases and their symptoms (arthralgia or arthritis, rash, dry or red or painful eyes, dry mouth and Raynaud's phenomenon) (see *Rheumatology and Clinical Immunology*, Section 1.1.9).

A cardiac history is also crucial in this case. This patient had a clear chest, but those with basal crackles due to DPLD are frequently prescribed diuretics for

an erroneous diagnosis of heart failure. A lack of response to diuretics is usual in chronic DPLD, but does not exclude cardiac failure, which can complicate chronic PE and pulmonary hypertension.

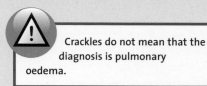

Crackles do not mean that the diagnosis is pulmonary oedema.

A past or current history of asthma and rhinitis may suggest Churg–Strauss syndrome.

A past history of cancer and radiotherapy may explain drug-induced/radiation pneumonia.

Plan for investigation and management
The priority as always is to decide on the basis of history (and in routine practice the clinical examination) which of the differential diagnoses are most likely in the individual scenario and direct the investigations accordingly.

After explaining to the patient that under normal clinical circumstances you would examine him to confirm his GP's findings, you would consider the following.

Chest radiograph
This should be repeated, particularly if performed more than 3 months ago, to assess whether there is any new change. Remember that the CXR is normal in as many as 10% of patients with some forms of DPLD, particularly those with hypersensitivity pneumonia.

Laboratory lung function tests
Check for any change in spirometry and for early signs of a restrictive defect, such as reduced total lung capacity, residual volume and carbon monoxide transfer factor.

Arterial blood gases
To confirm hypoxaemia as suggested by oximetry.

High-resolution CT
A combination of clinical information and high-resolution CT enables a correct diagnosis in up to 80% of patients with DPLD.

CT pulmonary angiography or ventilation/perfusion lung scanning
Perform if there is high clinical probability of chronic PE.

Blood tests
- FBC: to check for anaemia and eosinophil count.

- Urea, creatinine and electrolytes.

- Liver and bone function tests: calcium may be elevated in sarcoidosis.

- Antinuclear antibodies and rheumatoid factor: any signs of autoimmune rheumatic disease.

- Precipitins (including avian and *Micropolyspora faeni*) if EAA (eg bird-fancier's lung or farmer's lung) is suspected.

- D-dimer if there is low or moderate clinical probability of PE. If there is a high probability of PE, go directly to imaging tests.

- Antineutrophil cytoplasmic and glomerular basement membrane antibodies if vasculitis is suspected.

If there is high clinical suspicion of PE, do not measure D-dimer levels but proceed directly to appropriate imaging tests, ie CT pulmonary angiography or ventilation/perfusion lung scanning.

Urine dipstick

To exclude haematuria and proteinuria that might indicate vasculitis or autoimmune rheumatic disease.

ECG

This may show the right heart strain seen in PE or primary pulmonary hypertension.

Echocardiography

Perform if pulmonary hypertension is suspected. Echocardiography can also detect some occult cardiac causes of pulmonary hypertension (shunts and valvular and left ventricular abnormalities).

Further discussion

If DPLD is confirmed by high-resolution CT scan, lung biopsy may not be required in the appropriate clinical setting if the appearances are characteristic. For patients in whom lung biopsy is required, high-resolution CT images can help to decide whether transbronchial biopsy or open lung biopsy would be the best option and determine the most appropriate areas from which the biopsy samples should be taken.

If chronic PE is confirmed, a search for an occult malignancy must be considered: women should have a thorough clinical breast examination, all patients should have a pelvic examination and there should be a low threshold for investigation of gastrointestinal or other symptoms.

If the echocardiogram suggests pulmonary hypertension, further investigations are needed to exclude its known causes, as is right heart catheterisation to determine prognosis and optimise treatment.

1.2 Clinical examination

1.2.1 Coarse crackles: bronchiectasis

Instruction

This man complains of breathlessness and daily cough with sputum production. Please examine his respiratory system.

General features

- Look in the sputum pot: note the quantity and character of the patient's sputum.

- Is the patient cachexic, of short stature, clubbed, cyanosed or oedematous (hypoproteinaemic/cor pulmonale)? If this is the case in a young patient (<40 years old), consider cystic fibrosis (CF).

- Is there an indwelling venous line or Portacath? These are commonly found in patients requiring frequent courses of intravenous antibiotics.

Respiratory examination

The auscultatory findings are only part of the picture.

Trachea

This is not likely to be deviated, but is there a scar from previous tracheostomy?

Percussion

Areas of dullness likely to indicate underlying consolidation.

Auscultation

Is expiration prolonged, thereby indicating chronic obstructive pulmonary disease (COPD)? Bronchial breathing indicates underlying consolidation.

Crackles (typically coarse) over a particular area suggests bronchiectasis. Reduced breath sounds over an area is consistent with pleural effusion (lung base) or lung abscess (relatively uncommon).

In routine clinical practice you would clearly perform a full physical examination. This is not possible in the PACES station, but note if the abdomen is swollen (may indicate cirrhosis/ascites) and if there is a gastrostomy feeding tube (percutaneous endoscopic gastrostomy tubes are often used to support the nutrition of patients with CF).

Further discussion

Diagnosis

In any patient presenting with chronic exertional dyspnoea and sputum production, consider:

- COPD (take a history of smoking, listen for wheeze and check spirometry);

- bronchiectasis (and any condition associated with bronchiectasis);

- bronchial asthma (check history of wheeze, and ask if it is episodic);

- lung abscess and pneumonia (usually of acute onset and accompanied by fever).

In a young patient with chronic exertional dyspnoea and sputum production, consider:

- bronchiectasis (may be caused by CF);

- α_1-antitrypsin deficiency;

- hypogammaglobulinaemia (may be suggested by recurrent pneumonia or sinusitis).

In any patient with breathlessness and clubbing, consider:

- bronchiectasis;
- diffuse parenchymal lung disease, ie usual interstitial pneumonia/ cryptogenic fibrosing alveolitis;
- lung abscess (less likely in PACES);
- carcinoma of the lung (less likely in PACES).

Investigations

Chest radiograph A CXR is helpful for excluding an acute infection. It may also reveal features of COPD, bronchiectasis, interstitial fibrosis, lung abscess or cardiomegaly in congestive cardiac failure. Dextrocardia may be present.

Sputum examination Send for microscopy, culture and sensitivity, including acid-fast bacilli.

Lung function tests These will determine if there is airway obstruction, and in cases of COPD will help evaluate treatment. It is important to request full lung function tests comprising static lung volumes, spirometry and transfer factor.

High-resolution CT Can diagnose bronchiectasis, interstitial lung diseases, emphysema or presence of bullae.

Arterial blood gases Indicated if fingertip Sao_2 is below 94% in order to check whether there is respiratory failure (type I or II).

Other investigations

- Blood tests: a raised white cell count with neutrophilia suggests underlying bacterial infection. Secondary polycythaemia suggests chronic hypoxia. Serum α_1-antitrypsin level may be low,

suggesting its deficiency and underlying emphysema. Liver function tests can exclude hepatic involvement in both CF and α_1-antitrypsin deficiency.

- ECG: is there cor pulmonale?

- Sweat sodium concentration: in CF the sweat sodium concentration is usually high (>60 mmol/L).

- Ultrasound examination of the hepatobiliary system: check for cirrhosis and/or gallstones.

Management

- CF: see Section 2.5.

- Bronchiectasis: see Section 2.4.

- COPD: see Section 2.3.

- Pulmonary infections (lung abscess/ pneumonia): see *Infectious Diseases*, Sections 1.1.1. and 1.3.4.

- Hypogammaglobulinaemia: see *Rheumatology and Clinical Immunology*, Section 1.1.1 and 2.1.1.

1.2.2 Fine crackles: interstitial lung disease

Instruction

This man has had increasing exertional breathlessness and a dry cough for 6 months. Please examine his respiratory system.

General features

- Look for cachexia, clubbing and cyanosis.

- Signs of systemic disease.

  - Skin: rash (including erythema nodosum) and scleroderma/ calcinosis/Raynaud's phenomenon.

  - Arthropathy.

- Eyes: scleritis/uveitis.

- Lymphadenopathy.

- Look also for signs of treatment of a disease, such as the side effects of steroids.

Respiratory examination

Trachea

This may be pulled towards the side if there is severe and asymmetric fibrosis.

Palpation

There will be reduced expansion on affected side(s)/zone(s).

Percussion

This is normal in interstitial lung disease.

Auscultation

Typical crackles suggestive of pulmonary fibrosis are described as fine end-inspiratory 'popping' or a 'shower', and are likened to the sound of Velcro being prised apart or of drawing pins falling onto a tiled floor. They will not clear with coughing. The distribution of crackles has some relation to the underlying condition (Table 8).

Further discussion

The terms 'interstitial lung disease' or 'diffuse parenchymal lung disease' are used to describe pathological processes involving the lung parenchyma. If the parenchyma becomes stiff because of fibrosis or infiltration, then the small airways it surrounds may snap open during inspiration, the origin of the typical fine end-inspiratory crackles. Many different classification systems have been applied to these diseases, with the result being much confusion. It is easiest to start by classifying them by aetiology, as shown in Table 9, but note that it may be difficult clinically and radiographically to

TABLE 8 DISTRIBUTION OF CRACKLES AS A GUIDE TO UNDERLYING DISEASE

Distribution	Disease
Upper zones	Inhalational diseases (eg extrinsic allergic alveolitis, pneumoconioses) Ankylosing spondylitis
Lower zones	Usual interstitial pneumonia (previously known as cryptogenic fibrosing alveolitis) Pulmonary oedema
Anywhere	Sarcoid

predominantly the lung bases that do not ordinarily respond to immunosuppressive treatment.

> ⚠ Do not become anxious about the classification of the various forms of interstitial lung disease. If asked what the cause of the fine crackles might be, simply say: 'There are a range of conditions that can cause pneumonia and lung fibrosis: primary, which used to be called cryptogenic fibrosing alveolitis but is now classified into different subtypes; and secondary, with autoimmune rheumatic disorders, sarcoid and drugs being the commonest types.'

differentiate between these conditions and pulmonary oedema, and this should always be considered as an alternative diagnosis.

More confusion surrounds the classification of idiopathic interstitial pneumonia. Previously known as cryptogenic fibrosing alveolitis or idiopathic pulmonary fibrosis, these are now classified (more-or-less) universally as shown in Table 9. By far the commonest entity is usual interstitial pneumonia, which is analogous to cryptogenic fibrosing alveolitis and characterised by a progressive fibrosing process involving

Investigations

Chest radiograph In interstitial lung disease this typically shows reticular and nodular shadowing, perhaps with honeycombing, volume loss and traction bronchiectasis in the worst affected areas. The heart border and diaphragm may have a 'moth-eaten' appearance. In sarcoid there may be hilar lymphadenopathy.

Lung function tests These typically reveal a restrictive picture with a proportionate decrease in both spirometric (forced expiratory volume in 1 second and forced vital capacity) and static lung volumes (eg total lung capacity). The carbon monoxide transfer factor is also often reduced. It is important to establish a baseline.

Pulse oximetry All patients should have pulse oximetry performed at rest, and on exertion if symptoms are marked.

High-resolution CT The diagnostic test of choice in patients with suspected interstitial lung disease.

Lung biopsy The need for tissue sampling in the diagnosis of interstitial lung disease should be addressed in a specialist clinic.

TABLE 9 CLASSIFICATION OF DIFFUSE PARENCHYMAL LUNG DISEASE

Class of disease	Examples
Idiopathic	See below
Drugs (1)	Methotrexate Amiodarone Bleomycin Cabergoline
Autoimmune rheumatic disease	Rheumatoid arthritis Systemic sclerosis Ankylosing spondylitis
Pulmonary eosinophilic	Acute eosinophilic pneumonia Churg–Strauss syndrome
Inhalational injury	Extrinsic allergic alveolitis Crack cocaine/heroin/cigarettes Inorganic dusts: asbestosis, silicosis and coal worker's pneumoconiosis
Infection	*Pneumocystis carinii*
Malignancy	Lymphangitis carcinomatosa Bronchoalveolar cell carcinoma
Miscellaneous	Sarcoidosis Langerhans' cell histiocytosis/histiocytosis X Radiation fibrosis

Note
(1) This is only a 'top four', many other drugs have also been implicated. For further details see www.pneumotox.com

In short, where the combination of clinical and radiographic features are diagnostic (eg in usual interstitial pneumonia), then a biopsy is not required. If this is not the case, then the choice of biopsy technique (transbronchial biopsy versus open lung/video-assisted biopsy) depends again on the likely diagnosis. For example, in sarcoidosis and cryptogenic organising pneumonia the former is usually diagnostic, whereas larger structurally intact (ie surgical) biopsies are required to diagnose conditions such as Langerhans' cell histiocytosis or non-specific interstitial pneumonia.

Other investigations

It is worth considering the following.

- FBC and clotting screen (in anticipation of biopsy).

- Inflammatory markers (C-reactive protein, erythrocyte sedimentation rate).

- Creatinine, electrolytes, and liver and bone function tests (to check for any evidence of multisystem disorder and hypercalcaemia in sarcoid).

- Autoimmune and vasculitis screen (rheumatoid factor, antinuclear antibodies, extractable nuclear antigen and antineutrophil cytoplasmic antibodies).

- Serum angiotensin-converting enzyme (sarcoid).

- Precipitins (including avian and *Micropolyspora faeni*) if extrinsic allergic alveolitis (eg bird-fancier's lung or farmer's lung) is suspected.

- Also check urine dipstick for blood and protein (autoimmune rheumatic or vasculitic disorder).

Management

- Treatment, as ever, depends on the underlying condition.

- Where inhalational or systemic exposure is implicated, removal of the toxin if possible, or the patient from that environment if not, is necessary.

- In usual interstitial pneumonia the use of immune suppression (with prednisolone as first-line therapy) needs to be instigated with care, especially as only a minority of patients will respond. Serial objective measures (eg radiographic and lung volumes) must be taken so that improvements (or sometimes only a slowing of decline) can be appreciated.

- Usual interstitial pneumonia has a poor prognosis (50% of sufferers die within 5 years of diagnosis) and palliative care services should be involved, preferably before the rapid terminal decline that typically occurs.

- Oxygen therapy may be required (either long-term oxygen therapy or short-burst therapy to improve symptoms and/or exercise tolerance).

1.2.3 Stridor

Instruction

This man has had increasing difficulty in breathing. Please examine his respiratory system.

General features

- From the bedside, note if there is a high-pitched sound with each inspiration.

- Look for respiratory distress and cyanosis.

- Look for clues to the underlying aetiology, eg tracheostomy scar,

goitre and hypothyroidism (see *Endocrinology*, Sections 2.3.1 and 2.3.3).

Although unlikely in PACES, in routine clinical practice look for evidence of malignancy (neck lymph nodes, clubbing, cachexia, tar staining of fingers and superior vena cava obstruction) and in an acute presentation look for signs that suggest anaphylaxis (facial/tongue oedema, erythema and wheeze).

> In a case of stridor, look very carefully at the neck for a tracheostomy scar.

Respiratory examination

- Confirm the patient has stridor (as opposed to wheeze).

- Is the trachea deviated?

- There will be no abnormal signs in the chest if the problem is confined to the upper airway.

Further discussion

Stridor and wheeze are both caused by turbulent airflow through the airways. Wheeze is predominantly an expiratory sound and results from intrathoracic airflow obstruction. Stridor is heard during inspiration and indicates extrathoracic airflow obstruction, which may be fixed or variable (see Section 3.6.2).

Consider the causes of stridor (Table 10).

Investigations

To determine the presence and cause of chronic extrathoracic airway obstruction, check the following:

- flow–volume loops (fixed obstruction or variable extrathoracic obstruction);

TABLE 10 DIFFERENTIAL DIAGNOSIS OF STRIDOR

Acute (see Section 1.4.6)	Angio-oedema • Allergic • C1 esterase deficiency Inhaled foreign body
Subacute/chronic due to progressive obstruction (may also present acutely when stenosis becomes critical)	Extrinsic compression in the neck or upper mediastinum: • Goitre • Lymph node mass • Mediastinal fibrosis • (Obstructive sleep apnoea – see Section 1.1.6) Intrinsic • Tracheal/laryngeal tumour • Vocal cord dysfunction • Gastro-oesophageal reflux • Infection: epiglottitis, abscess (retropharyngeal or peritonsillar) • Stenosis post endotracheal intubation or tracheostomy Neurogenic • Myasthenia gravis • Stroke

• laryngoscopy with or without bronchoscopy;

• contrast-enhanced CT of the neck and upper mediastinum.

Management

Whilst a case of acute stridor is extremely unlikely to appear in any postgraduate examination, prompt recognition and appropriate management are life-saving in clinical practice (see Section 1.4.6).

After emergency treatment to ensure the airway is secure and ventilation adequate, further treatment depends on the underlying cause. Specific treatment of the stenosis (for example in malignancy or post-intubation stenosis) includes laser therapy or bypass (ie tracheostomy).

1.2.4 Pleural effusion

Instruction

This man has had increasing difficulty in breathing for the last 2 months. Please examine his respiratory system.

General features

The primary things to check for are respiratory distress, tachypnoea and cyanosis. Look for clues to the underlying aetiology, as detailed below.

Malignancy

There are several signs that would suggest this:

• sputum pot;

• cachexia;

• hoarse voice;

• clubbing;

• tar staining of fingers;

• jaundice (hepatic metastasis);

• Horner's syndrome (ptosis, miosis, anhydrosis and enophthalmos);

• neck lymphadenopathy;

• superior vena cava obstruction;

• scar (from previous thoracic/breast surgery, CT-guided lung biopsy or pleural biopsy);

• breast abnormalities (nipple retraction, deviation and mass).

Tuberculosis

• Sputum pot.

• Lymphadenopathy.

Systemic lupus erythematosus

• Rash.

Rheumatoid arthritis

• Joint deformity.

• Nodules.

Respiratory examination

General inspection

Look for:

• thoracotomy scar;

• chest wall deformity (thoracoplasty);

• asymmetric chest wall movement (reduced on side of effusion).

Trachea

If deviation is present, this will be away from the side of a massive pleural effusion, or towards that side if there is coexisting ipsilateral collapse.

Palpation

• Examine the supraclavicular and cervical nodes as above.

• Expansion is decreased on the side of the pleural effusion.

Percussion

Check for dull sound on percussion on the side of the pleural effusion (it will be 'stony dull' if the effusion is large enough).

Auscultation

• Reduced or absent breath sounds (same area as above).

• Reduced vocal resonance/tactile vocal fremitus (same area as above).

TABLE 11 LIGHT'S CRITERIA FOR DISTINGUISHING EXUDATIVE AND TRANSUDATIVE PLEURAL EFFUSIONS

Discriminator	Exudate	Transudate
Protein concentration in effusion	>30 g/L	<30 g/L
Ratio of pleural fluid protein to serum fluid protein >0.5	Yes	No
Pleural fluid LDH more than two-thirds higher than the normal upper limit for serum LDH	Yes	No
Ratio of pleural fluid LDH to serum fluid LDH >0.6	Yes	No

LDH, lactate dehydrogenase.

TABLE 12 CAUSES OF A PLEURAL EFFUSION

Type	Prevalence	Cause
Transudate	Common	Congestive cardiac failure
	Uncommon	Cirrhosis
		Nephrotic syndrome
	Rare	Myxoedema
		Peritoneal dialysis
Exudate	Common	Malignancy
		Bacterial infection (parapneumonic, empyema, TB)
	Uncommon	Pulmonary emboli
		Haemothorax
		Autoimmune rheumatic disorder
	Rare	Drug induced (amiodarone, methotrexate or nitrofurantoin)
		Gastrointestinal disease (pancreatitis or subphrenic abscess)
		Yellow nail syndrome
		Chylothorax

TB, tuberculosis.

probably the single most useful test, with empyema strongly suggested by a pH <7.2, which is an indication for insertion of an intercostal drain.

If there is no associated pneumonia, is the fluid a transudate or an exudate? Measure the fluid and serum protein and the LDH (Table 11). In addition organise the following as standard tests:

- microscopy and culture (both anaerobic and aerobic, and for TB);

- cytology (Table 13);

- pH.

And in cases where diagnostic uncertainty remains, check the following.

- Glucose: a value <1.6 mmol/L typically occurs in an effusion associated with TB or rheumatoid arthritis.

- Rheumatoid factor: suggests rheumatoid arthritis is the cause of the effusion.

- Amylase: suggests pancreatitis.

Further discussion

Pleural effusions are divided into exudates and transudates on the basis of Light's criteria (Table 11).

The PACES examiner is likely to ask what diagnoses you would consider in a patient with a pleural effusion who presents on the general medical take (Table 12).

Investigations

Chest radiograph Perform to confirm the presence of an effusion (Fig. 5).

Pleural fluid If there is associated pneumonia, is the fluid parapneumonic or is it an empyema? If it is opaque/turbid and with a foul smell, then it is clearly an empyema. In cases that are less clear-cut the pleural fluid pH is

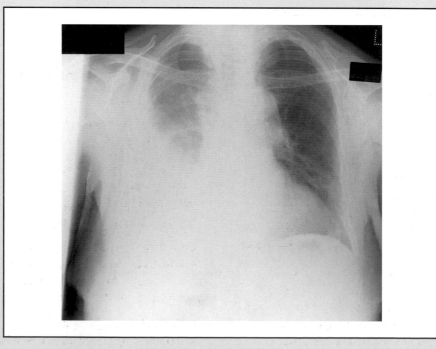

▲**Fig. 5** CXR showing a large right pleural effusion.

TABLE 13 CYTOLOGY OF PLEURAL EFFUSIONS

Cytological finding	Possible diagnoses or inference
Red cells >100 × 10^9/L	Trauma, malignancy and pulmonary embolism
White blood cells: neutrophilia (>50%)	Pyogenic infection
White blood cells: lymphocytosis (>90%)	TB, lymphoma and malignancy
White blood cells: eosinophilia (>10%)	Non-diagnostic: benign
Mesothelial cells	Absent in TB
Malignant cells	Diagnostic of malignancy if present

TB, tuberculosis.

- Adenosine deaminase: this is high in cases of TB.

Pleural (Abrams') biopsy Pleural biopsy may be indicated if initial pleural fluid analysis does not yield a diagnosis, and is of particular value in those with an exudative pleural effusion in order to exclude TB or an underlying malignancy. It is standard practice to perform this with an Abrams' needle, which is a large blunt-tipped needle with a hook to catch a sample of parietal pleura. The diagnostic yield in pleural TB is increased by 20–40%, but it is much less (around 10–20%) in malignant disease. It is important to remember that because this is a blind (unguided) procedure a negative result does not exclude any diagnosis.

Thoracoscopy Medical thoracoscopy is primarily a diagnostic procedure, but it can be used for therapeutic purposes. The most common indications are evaluation of the unknown exudative effusion, staging of diffuse malignant mesothelioma or lung cancer, and treatment by talc pleurodesis of malignant or other recurrent effusions or empyema. Local treatment of spontaneous pneumothorax is also an indication.

Indications for pleurodesis
The indications for pleurodesis are symptomatic recurrent pleural effusion or spontaneous pneumothorax. Many substances have been injected intrapleurally in an attempt to obliterate the pleural space, the mechanism for most being simply to create an inflammatory reaction that leads to fusion of the visceral and parietal pleura. Commonly used agents include talc, doxycycline, silver nitrate and povidone iodine.

1.2.5 Wheeze and crackles: chronic obstructive pulmonary disease

Instruction

This man complains of progressive exertional shortness of breath. Please examine his respiratory system.

General features
Examine for signs of the following.

- Central cyanosis.

- Bounding pulse and warm palms (signs of CO_2 retention).

- Tar-stained fingers: if there is finger clubbing, then consider concomitant lung cancer.

- Tremor: fine finger tremor secondary to β-agonist therapy; flapping tremor (indistinguishable from that associated with hepatic failure) due to CO_2 retention.

- Raised JVP during inspiration (Kussmaul's sign) may be observed in the absence of heart failure as a result of the compressive effect of lung inflation on cardiac filling.

- Signs of right heart failure (see *Cardiology*, Section 1.2.2).

- Cachexia: 20% of patients with moderate/severe chronic obstructive pulmonary disease (COPD) lose weight due to increased muscle protein breakdown as a systemic effect of COPD, but weight loss may also be a sign of concomitant lung cancer.

Examine the immediate vicinity of the patient for additional clues that indicate respiratory problems, eg inhalers, nebuliser and oxygen.

Respiratory examination

General inspection

- Obvious breathlessness at rest.

- Tachypnoea.

- Signs of hyperinflation:

  (a) Chest held near full inspiratory position at end of normal expiration.

  (b) Increased anteroposterior diameter of the chest (barrel-shaped chest).

  (c) Reduced distance between cricoid cartilage and suprasternal notch (less than the breadth of three fingers).

- 'Pump handle' (up and down) movement of the ribs, instead of normal 'bucket handle' (upwards and outwards) movement.

- Use of the accessory respiratory muscles of the neck and shoulder girdle.

- Generalised indrawing of the intercostal muscles and/or supraclavicular spaces on inspiration (Hoover's sign) due to hyperinflation.

- Pursed-lip breathing: expiration through pursed lips maintains a higher airway pressure, thus keeping the distal airways open longer during expiration and decreasing the work of breathing.

Palpation

- Poor bilateral chest movement: expansion <5 cm suggests significant airflow obstruction.

Percussion

- Hyperresonant percussion note (but be aware that this is not a robust physical sign).

- Obliteration of cardiac and hepatic dullness.

- Low position of diaphragm with limited caudal motion.

Auscultation

- Reduced breath sounds.

- Prolonged expiratory phase of respiration: an excessively prolonged forced expiratory time (>4 seconds, when measured with the stethoscope placed over the trachea) suggests a significant degree of airflow limitation.

- Wheezes: these may be initially heard on forced expiration only and may disappear if there is severe airflow limitation because of low rate of airflow.

- Coarse crackles (during early inspiration and often in expiration): these may clear or alter as the secretions are shifted on coughing or deep breathing.

- Heart sounds may become distant with displacement of the point of maximal intensity to the subxiphoid region.

Further discussion

In early COPD a physical examination may be normal or may show prolonged expiration and/or wheezes on forced expiration only. As the disease progresses, abnormal signs will become apparent and in advanced stages many are almost pathognomonic.

At the time of presentation consider asthma as a differential diagnosis (Table 14) and α_1-antitrypsin deficiency in a patient presenting between the ages of 30 and 45.

Expect to be asked how you would confirm the diagnosis of COPD with lung function tests and how you would treat a patient presenting chronically with the condition or with an acute exacerbation (see Sections 2.2.2 and 2.3).

1.2.6 Cor pulmonale

Instruction

This woman complains of breathlessness on exertion. Please examine her chest.

General features

The key features to establish the diagnosis of cor pulmonale will be cyanosis and a grossly raised JVP. If these are present, then look carefully for the following.

- Evidence of chronic obstructive pulmonary disease (COPD), such as the presence of features typical of a 'blue bloater'.

- Features of an autoimmune rheumatic disorder, which would suggest the presence of a secondary interstitial lung disease.

- Obesity, which may indicate obstructive sleep apnoea or alveolar hypoventilation disorder.

- Severe chest wall deformity such as kyphoscoliosis.

- Evidence of a neurological disease, such as wasting of the muscles or the presence of muscle fasciculation.

- Clubbing, which would point towards a diagnosis of interstitial lung disease or bronchiectasis.

Respiratory examination

The findings in the chest will be determined by the underlying pathology, but particularly look for:

- hyperinflation and wheezing, which may indicate COPD;

- bibasilar fine inspiratory crackles, which are suggestive of interstitial lung disease;

TABLE 14 CLINICAL FEATURES DIFFERENTIATING COPD AND ASTHMA		
	COPD	**Asthma**
Smoker or ex-smoker	Nearly all	Possible
Symptoms under age 35	Rare	Common
Chronic productive cough	Common	Uncommon
Breathlessness	Persistent and progressive	Variable
Night-time waking with breathlessness and/or wheeze	Uncommon	Common
Significant diurnal or day-to-day variability of symptoms	Uncommon	Common

- coarse inspiratory crackles, which are suggestive of bronchiectasis.

In routine clinical practice you would clearly perform a full physical examination. This is not possible in the PACES station, but you should still look at the ankles for oedema and, if asked, say that you would particularly like to examine the abdomen to check for the pulsatile hepatomegaly caused by tricuspid incompetence.

Further discussion

The major causes of cor pulmonale are shown in Table 15.

Investigations

An appropriate strategy to investigate a patient with suspected cor pulmonale would involve the following.

Respiratory Perform CXR and lung function tests, proceeding to high-resolution CT scan of the lungs to define pulmonary pathology (use CT pulmonary angiography if you suspect thromboembolic disease or other disorder of pulmonary circulation).

Cardiac Perform ECG and echocardiography, looking in particular for evidence of right atrial/ventricular dilatation or hypertrophy. Right and left heart catheterisation in some cases.

Treatment

This will depend on the underlying diagnosis, but be aware of the issues surrounding diuretic treatment. A difficult balance needs to be struck between denying diuretics to the patient with massive uncomfortable peripheral oedema (and perhaps ascites) and rendering the patient exhausted, hypotensive and with advancing renal impairment as a result of over-diuresis. In the presence of cor pulmonale, a high right-sided filling pressure is required to generate cardiac output.

⚠️ Be aware of the difficulties of managing cor pulmonale with diuretics.

1.2.7 Pneumonectomy/ lobectomy

Instruction

This man has long-standing exertional dyspnoea. Please examine his chest.

General features

Look for signs related to chronic hypoxic lung disease:

- cyanosis (central and peripheral), bounding pulse or coarse flap (CO_2 retention);

- signs of right heart failure.

Also, check for signs related to possible underlying malignancy.

- Muscle wasting or signs of weight loss.

- Tar-stained fingers/moustache.

- Clubbing: this also occurs in chronic suppurative lung disease, another possible reason for pneumonectomy or lobectomy.

- Lymphadenopathy: supraclavicular (especially behind the medial end of the clavicle) and neck nodes.

- Superior vena cava obstruction, indicated by facial and/or upper limb oedema, and fixed raised JVP.

- Horner's syndrome: suggested by unilateral partial ptosis, miosis with or without anhydrosis.

Also take note of oxygen, sputum pot, and nebulisers/inhalers.

Respiratory examination

General inspection
Observe for:

- respiratory distress and tachypnoea;

- asymmetric chest wall movement;

TABLE 15 CAUSES OF COR PULMONALE

General cause	Prevalence[1]	Example
Lung disease	Common	COPD Cystic fibrosis Interstitial lung disease
Disorder of ventilatory control	Common Uncommon	Obstructive sleep apnoea Primary central hypoventilation
Thoracic cage deformity	Common	Kyphoscoliosis
Neuromuscular disorder	Uncommon Rare	Amyotrophic lateral sclerosis Bilateral diaphragmatic paralysis Poliomyelitis/post-polio syndrome Guillain–Barré syndrome Muscular dystrophy Myasthenia gravis
Disorder of the pulmonary circulation	Uncommon Rare	Chronic recurrent pulmonary thromboembolism Primary pulmonary hypertension Pulmonary veno-occlusive disease Schistosomiasis Sickle cell anaemia

1. Prevalence of cor pulmonale in developed countries.

TABLE 16 REASONS FOR LUNG RESECTION	
Frequency	**Cause**
Common	Lung cancer
Less common	Massive pulmonary haemorrhage
	Tuberculosis (also thoracoplasty)
	Aspergilloma
	Bronchiectasis
	Lung abscess/necrotising pneumonia
	Trauma

- thoracotomy scar;

- chest wall deformity (thoracoplasty).

Trachea
Check carefully for deviation.

Palpation
Examine supraclavicular and neck nodes as above. Expansion is decreased on the side of pneumonectomy, as detailed below.

- Upper lobectomy: decreased in upper zone anteriorly.

- Lower lobectomy: decreased at base.

- Middle lobectomy: may not be clinically detectable, as it is of relatively small volume (surface anatomy: axilla and lower anterior chest wall).

Percussion

- Dull to percussion: the same areas as for expansion.

Auscultation

- Breath sounds will be reduced in the affected area. Bronchial breathing, and increased vocal resonance (or tactile vocal fremitus), can sometimes be heard.

Further discussion
Consider possible reasons for pneumonectomy or lobectomy (Table 16).

Thoracoplasty, removal of the chest wall with consequent collapse of the underlying lung (usually the upper lobe), was a common procedure for pulmonary tuberculosis. The signs are as for upper lobectomy apart from the obvious deformity.

The first investigation that you would request would obviously be a CXR.

1.2.8 Apical signs: old tuberculosis

Instruction

This patient had tuberculosis (TB) in the past. Please examine his respiratory system.

General features

- If there is bronchiectasis (known to occur with TB), the patient may be bringing up copious sputum with haemoptysis. Look for a sputum pot.

- Scars: before the antibiotic era, various surgical procedures were tried as treatment for TB, including phrenic nerve crush, thoracotomy, thoracoplasty and/or plombage (this involved collapse of the affected portion of the lung, usually the upper lobe, and filling the space with 5–18 polystyrene spheres).

Respiratory examination

Inspection

- There may be a deformity of the upper chest (thoracoplasty).

- Look for reduced movement of the upper chest wall on respiration.

Trachea
Is the trachea deviated? In fibrosis it is pulled towards the affected side.

Palpation
Confirm reduced expansion of the upper chest wall.

Percussion
The percussion note may be dull at the apex/apices.

Auscultation
Bronchial breath sounds may be heard, with or without crackles, at the apex/apices.

Further discussion
Old healed TB usually presents as pulmonary nodules in the hilar area or upper lobes, with or without fibrotic scars and volume loss. Bronchiectasis and pleural scarring may be present, with signs localised to the upper chest wall.

Differentiating active TB from inactive TB can be very difficult. It must be remembered that a CXR cannot rule out disease activity accurately. All cases should have sputum examination, but there are some features that help discriminate between active and inactive disease.

Signs suggestive of active TB

- Infiltrate or consolidation: opacification of airspaces within the lung parenchyma. Consolidation or infiltrate can be dense or patchy and might have irregular, ill-defined or hazy borders.

- Any cavitary lesion, ie lucency (darkened area) within the lung parenchyma, with or without the irregular margins that might indicate an area of surrounding airspace consolidation or infiltrates, or surrounding nodular or fibrotic (reticular) densities, or both. Calcification can exist around a cavity.

- Nodule with poorly defined margins: round density within the lung parenchyma, also called a tuberculoma. Nodules included in this category are those with margins that are indistinct or poorly defined. The surrounding haziness can be either subtle or readily apparent, and suggests coexisting airspace consolidation.

- Pleural effusion: this finding must be distinguished from blunting of the costophrenic angle, which may or may not represent a small amount of fluid within the pleural space (except in children, when even minor blunting must be considered a finding that can suggest active TB).

- Hilar or mediastinal lymphadenopathy: enlargement of lymph nodes in one or both hila or within the mediastinum, with or without the associated atelectasis or consolidation.

- Linear interstitial disease (in children only): prominence of linear interstitial (septal) markings.

- Other miliary TB: nodules of 1–2 mm distributed throughout the parenchyma.

Signs suggestive of inactive TB

- Discrete fibrotic scar or linear opacity: discrete linear or reticular densities within the lung. Calcification can be present within the lesion and then the lesion is called a 'fibrocalcific' scar.

- Discrete nodule(s) without calcification: one or more nodular densities with distinct borders and without any surrounding airspace opacification. Nodules are generally round or have rounded edges. These features enable them to be distinguished from infiltrates or airspace opacities.

- Discrete fibrotic scar with volume loss or retraction: discrete linear densities with reduction in the space occupied by the upper lobe. Associated signs include upward deviation of the fissure or hilum on the corresponding side, along with asymmetry of the volumes of the two thoracic cavities.

- Discrete nodule(s) with volume loss or retraction: one or more nodular densities with distinct borders and no surrounding airspace opacification, as well as a reduction in the space occupied by the upper lobe.

- Other: any other finding suggestive of prior TB, such as upper lobe bronchiectasis.

Expect to be asked about the management of a case of pulmonary TB. See *Infectious Diseases*, Section 2.6.1 for discussion of chemotherapy and contact tracing.

1.2.9 Cystic fibrosis

Instruction

This (20-year-old) man has been complaining of increasing shortness of breath. Please examine his respiratory system.

General features

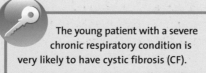

The young patient with a severe chronic respiratory condition is very likely to have cystic fibrosis (CF).

Around the bed check for:

- non-invasive ventilation (machine, circuit and mask);

- oxygen tubing;

- nebulisers/inhalers;

- sputum pot (with thick purulent secretions).

When examining the patient, look for the following.

- Does he look young for his age? Any chronic debilitating condition retards growth.

- Cyanosis.

- Cachexia.

- Current long-term intravenous access (eg Portacath) or signs of repeated attempts at intravenous access.

- Clubbing.

- Bruising (insulin injection sites).

- Rash (vasculitis or drug-induced).

- Proximal myopathy (long-term steroid therapy).

- Abdominal scars.

- Gastrostomy tube/nasogastric tube.

Respiratory examination

Findings depend on the relative contribution of bronchiectasis, airflow obstruction, air trapping and cor pulmonale in any given patient.

General inspection

- Respiratory distress and tachypnoea.

- Scar (from previous pneumothorax and from previous venous access devices).

- Raised JVP: prominent *v* waves (tricuspid regurgitation).

Station 1: Respiratory Examination

- Abdominal swelling (ascites).

- Ankle swelling.

- Nasal polyps.

Trachea

Deviation may be due to lobar collapse.

Palpation

- Expansion is generally reduced in the presence of hyperexpanded lung fields.

- Right ventricular heave.

Percussion

- May be hyperresonant throughout.

- Dullness may be present in case of lobar collapse/consolidation.

Auscultation

- Reduced breath sounds and vocal resonance/tactile vocal fremitus generally.

- Coarse crackles.

- Wheeze.

In routine clinical practice you would clearly perform a full physical examination. This is not possible in the PACES examination, but look at the ankles for oedema and, if asked, say that you would particularly like to examine for signs of cor pulmonale attributable to CF lung disease, ie raised JVP, pulsatile liver (if tricuspid regurgitation) and ankle oedema. Also check for evidence of other complications of CF: cirrhosis/portal hypertension and diabetic complications (retinopathy, absent pulses/vascular bruits, peripheral neuropathy and proteinuria).

Further discussion

See Section 2.5 for discussion of the diagnosis, complications and treatment of CF.

1.3 Communication skills and ethics

1.3.1 Lifestyle modification

Scenario

Role: you are a junior doctor in a general medical outpatient clinic.

A 52-year old builder who has smoked 10–20 cigarettes per day for many years is admitted on a general medical take with 4 month's history of exertional shortness of breath, which has got significantly worse during the last few days. He has no significant past medical history except for mild hypertension (150/95 mmHg), for which he is reluctant to accept medication, and obesity (108 kg, BMI 36.5). He has improved after treatment with oxygen, nebulised bronchodilators and antibiotics. Spirometry on discharge confirms a moderate chronic obstructive pulmonary disease (COPD).

Your task: explain to this reluctant patient that he should stop smoking and lose weight.

Key issue to explore

- Why is the patient reluctant to give up smoking?

- Has he ever made an attempt to give up smoking? If he has, then how difficult was it? For how long did he manage to refrain from smoking, and why did his attempt to quit fail?

- Has he tried to lose weight? If so, what lifestyle changes did he make in this respect and did he manage to lose any weight (and

why does he think that he was unsuccessful)?

Key points to establish

Introduce yourself appropriately.

Related to smoking

- Explain the patient's spirometry result and the cause of his breathing difficulty.

- Highlight why inhalers alone are not an effective way of treating his shortness of breath in the long term.

- Explain the benefits of quitting smoking, its effect on spirometry and the price he will have to pay if he continues to smoke (eg he is likely to have gradually decreasing exercise capacity and need repeated hospital admissions). Focus on how smoking affects his health personally (COPD and hypertension) rather than in a general way.

- Balance negative information about harm and risks with positive information about the benefits of smoking cessation.

- Demonstrate active listening skills. Encourage open and non-threatening discussion on how he sees his smoking. Make sure he does not feel pressured and avoid being judgemental. Back off if he appears annoyed. Stay positive and friendly.

- Show understanding of his fears about quitting. Keep avenues open for any changes in his mind.

- Praise him for his past achievements, however small they may seem.

- Explore options available to him to support him in his decision to quit (nicotine replacement therapy, bupropion and smoking cessation clinics).

Related to obesity

- Explain the BMI value, its implication and how obesity contributes to his breathing problem.

- Show understanding regarding the difficulty that he might have experienced while trying to lose weight.

- Suggest various strategies that may help him to lose weight (dietary change, physical activities, and drugs such as orlistat and sibutramine).

Appropriate responses to likely questions

> If something is difficult, like giving up smoking or losing weight, do not pretend to the patient that it is or should be easy.

Patient: I'm not convinced that my breathing difficulty is caused by the cigarettes. I have smoked for 36 years, so why did I become short of breath only 4 months ago?

Doctor: changes related to smoking happen gradually over many years, and may not cause any breathing problems until significant damage is done. Spirometry, the breathing test which you have had done, is the best way of detecting changes in the lungs caused by cigarettes. One of the things measured – the amount that you can blow out in 1 second, called forced expiratory volume in 1 second (FEV_1) – tells us how narrow the airways are. If this reading, the FEV_1, goes down to less than 80% of what it should be for your age and height, then this indicates chronic obstructive pulmonary disease. This is irreversible damage to the lung through smoking, and I'm afraid that that is what you've

got. It is not at all uncommon for smokers to first develop breathing difficulties in the way that you have.

Patient: if, as you said, my breathing problem is caused by smoking, why was I not short of breath earlier, all the way along, when my breathing function was getting worse?

Doctor: lots of things affect whether or not you feel breathlessness, such as your general level of fitness, weight, muscle strength, heart function and tolerance of pain and breathlessness. With the same level of problems in their airways, one patient with COPD may complain of extreme breathlessness whereas another gets mild or even no symptoms.

Patient: well, I've got to die of something and besides, it looks as if it is too late for me to give up smoking, anyway. As you said, the damage through smoking has been already done, so what's the point of quitting at this stage?

Doctor: it is true that damage due to smoking is irreversible, so if you give up you won't regain lost function. In fact your lung function will still continue to decline the same as everyone else's, but it will get worse at about the same rate as would be expected in someone who didn't smoke at all. However, if you keep on smoking it will get worse much faster. So, it is never too late to give up smoking.

Patient: I did try once to give up smoking, but gained over a stone in weight, which I have been unable to lose since then. How am I going to give up smoking and lose weight at the same time?

Doctor: I agree that it may not be easy, but I am sure that you can do it. You have at least two reasons to lose weight. Your excessive weight will certainly make your shortness

of breath worse, and it may well be the cause of your raised blood pressure. As your body mass index is well over 30, you are also at high risk of developing other serious medical conditions, particularly diabetes and heart disease. A dietitian could help you to choose a diet that is best for you and you could also consider joining a weight-loss class where you could get advice on both diet and exercise, and work along with other people with the same problems to improve things.

1.3.2 Possible cancer

Scenario

Role: you are a junior doctor in a respiratory clinic.

This 48-year-old executive has had a CXR as part of his company's health screening programme (he has never had a CXR before). It shows a pulmonary nodule in the right upper lobe. He has been informed that he has a shadow in his lung.

Your task: discuss with him the implications of his undiagnosed abnormality and address his fears that this may be lung cancer. You are not expected to examine the patient.

Key issues to explore

- What is the patient's main worry?

- Is there any particular reason why the patient is worried? In routine clinical practice patients will often not mention key reasons for their concern, and in PACES the briefing notes for the surrogate will commonly say 'Do not mention this unless specifically asked'.

- What further investigations are required?

Key points to establish

Introduce yourself to the patient and say why you have been asked to see him. Explain the proposed outline of your interview by telling him that you wish to go through the history briefly to confirm the information that you have been given, that you would then like to discuss the implications of the findings and finally address any fears or concerns that he may have.

- Ask if the patient would like anyone else to be present during this discussion.

- Admit uncertainty: this might be something sinister, but it might not be.

- Emphasise that 'something can always be done', even if the diagnosis is serious.

- Always adopt a non-judgemental attitude, eg if the patient says he will continue to smoke 40 cigarettes a day despite being informed that there is a shadow in the lung.

> Explain the medical benefits of changing behaviour but do not be judgemental, even if the patient's behaviour seems to have caused the illness.

Appropriate responses to likely questions

Patient: this was only discovered at a routine check and I feel fine, so surely it can't be serious?

Doctor: it's obviously a good thing that you feel well, and I agree that the chances of something serious would be much higher if you felt ill. But, I'm afraid I can't guarantee that the shadow on the lung isn't serious.

Patient: what could the shadow be caused by?

Doctor: there are a range of possibilities: sometimes shadows on the lung can be caused by an infection, either recent or a long time ago, sometimes they can be due to conditions that cause inflammation in the lungs, and sometimes they are due to growths of various sorts.

Patient: what are the chances that this is cancer?

Doctor: I can't tell you at the moment. I'm not hiding anything, I simply don't know. It could be due to infection or to a benign growth of some sort, but yes, I'm afraid that cancer is a possibility, and we need to find out if that is the case as soon as possible.

Patient: how are we going to find out what it is?

Doctor: we need to do some more tests. In particular we need to organise a CT scan of your lungs and probably a bronchoscopy, which means looking into the lungs with a special telescope, as well. With one or other of these tests, depending exactly on where the shadow is, we may need to perform a biopsy so that we can look at the tissue under a microscope to see what the shadow is. We will also plan to do some more blood tests to check for evidence of infection or inflammation.

Patient: what will you do when you find out what it is?

Doctor: that very much depends on what we find. If it's an infection, then antibiotics may be needed . . .

Patient: but if it's cancer, will you be able to cure it?

Doctor: I honestly don't know. There are several different sorts of lung cancer, and if it is one of those it will also depend on how far it has spread. I don't think we can really go into too much detail at the moment – because we don't know exactly what we're dealing with here – but some cases of lung cancer can be cured.

1.3.3 Potentially life-threatening illness

Scenario

Role: you are the on-call medical junior doctor

Mrs Angela Warren is a 36-year-old single mother of two who has been brought to the Emergency Department by ambulance. She developed sudden-onset pleuritic chest pain and breathlessness at rest this evening. On examination her pulse rate is 120 bpm regular and her respiratory rate is 24/minute, but otherwise there are no abnormal findings. Of her initial investigations the ECG shows sinus tachycardia, the CXR is clear and blood tests are normal except for a raised D-dimer. Arterial blood gases show a normal pH (7.44), normal P_{O_2} (11.0 kPa) and reduced P_{CO_2} (3.0 kPa). The pain is easing, she reports feeling less short of breath and she wants to go home.

Your task: to explain to Mrs Warren that pulmonary embolism is a significant possibility and that she should start treatment and be investigated as an inpatient.

Key issues to explore

- Explain the possibility of a potentially life-threatening problem.

- Find out why she is so keen to get home. In routine clinical practice patients will often not mention their reasons for wanting to leave hospital unless specifically asked, and in PACES the briefing notes for the surrogate will commonly indicate that they should do the same.

Key points to establish

Main ethical issue

- The competent patient does have the right to refuse investigation and/or treatment. It is your responsibility to put her into such a position that she is able to make decisions about her management from a well-informed standpoint.

- Is she competent? Does she understand the possible diagnosis and its potential implications? She needs to know that she is at significant risk of deterioration, and even death, from her (presumed) pulmonary embolism.

> The competent patient has a right to accept or refuse treatment.

Practical issue

Are there childcare issues (for example)? If there are, then offer to make an effort to help in sorting them out. It is unfortunately not uncommon for some doctors to 'wash their hands' of patients seen to be 'refusing treatment', but usually a compromise position can be reached with good negotiation and the examiners will be looking for your ability to make a workable plan in this scenario.

Willingness to negotiate a reasonable compromise

Negotiation may result in a treatment plan that is not necessarily ideal, but better than nothing. For example, it may be agreed that the patient is given a dose of low-molecular-weight heparin immediately, and that she returns in the morning for a ventilation–perfusion scan and review.

Appropriate answers to likely questions

Patient: I'm feeling a bit better, so there can't be anything seriously wrong.

Doctor: I'm obviously pleased that you're feeling a bit better, but I'm afraid that I can't guarantee that there isn't a serious problem here. One of the blood tests, the D-dimer, and one of the tests on the blood from an artery indicate that there may be something serious going on.

Patient: so what do you think the diagnosis is?

Doctor: it is possible that you have had a pulmonary embolus, which is a blood clot in the blood supply to the lung.

Patient: how will you find out if that is what happened?

Doctor: we'll need to perform a scan that enables us to see the blood supply and check if there are any blockages.

Patient: is having a pulmonary embolus dangerous?

Doctor: if this is a clot, then usually the body slowly absorbs it over the next week or so. But the main worry is that either this clot may extend and get bigger, or that more clots may spread to the lung. If this happens then it can be very serious indeed: it can mean that you can't

get enough oxygen into your blood, that the heart is sometimes put under too much strain and cannot pump properly, and in severe cases it may even stop completely.

Patient: what treatment do I need?

Doctor: to help prevent this clot getting worse, or more clots from forming, we need to put you on some blood-thinning medicine. Whilst we are getting the scan to confirm the diagnosis this will be in the form of an injection under the skin. If the scan confirms a clot, you will then be put on blood-thinning tablets for the next 6 months.

Patient: can I go home now?

Doctor: is there some special reason that you want to go home? Is there a problem with looking after the children or something like that, something that we might be able to arrange help for?

Patient: no, I just don't like being in hospital. I want to go home.

Doctor: I'm afraid that I don't think that's a good idea. I think that there's a high chance that you've got clots of blood in the lungs, and from the tests we've done these seem to be affecting your heart and your breathing. I think we should give you the treatment to thin the blood and get the scan done in the morning.

Patient: I hear what you say, but I'm going home. Can't I have the injection and come back for the scan in the morning?

Doctor: OK, as long as you understand that this condition can sometimes be very serious, or even life-threatening, and that is the reason I would strongly advise you to stay in hospital for now. But if you really insist on going home, then I can arrange for you to have an injection of the blood-thinning treatment now before you go. If you do get worse at home, please call an ambulance and come straight back to hospital. I'll make a note in your medical records to say that this is what I've advised.

1.3.4 Sudden unexplained death

Scenario

Role: you are the medical junior doctor working on a general medical ward.

A 56-year-old woman admitted with an exacerbation of chronic obstructive pulmonary disease (COPD) 5 days ago has died suddenly. When seen on the ward round in the morning she seemed to have been gradually improving, and certainly better than she was on admission. She had been on a prophylactic dose of low-molecular-weight heparin, but the most likely cause of death was probably massive pulmonary embolism. Her husband has been called into the hospital by the senior sister on the ward. He knows that his wife has died, but does not know the circumstances.

Your task: explain to the husband that his wife died suddenly, probably from a massive pulmonary embolism, and that you will have to discuss the case with the coroner.

Key issues to explore

- The original reason for the patient's admission and its management.

- What is the husband's understanding of the cause or causes of his wife's death?

- Explain to the husband that his wife was on proper treatment for COPD and that her death was too sudden to be due to that condition, so it is most likely that she died due to an underlying pulmonary embolism.

- Explain that there is an increased risk of thromboembolism in acutely ill medical patients, and that a prophylactic dose of low-molecular-weight heparin can reduce this risk but not eliminate it altogether.

Key points to establish

- The uncertainty regarding the cause of death, and that a definite cause of death can only be established by a post-mortem.

- That you will not be able to issue a death certificate without discussion with the coroner or the coroner's officer, who may insist on a post-mortem examination.

Appropriate responses to likely questions

Patient's husband: *it has come as a big shock. I never knew that she was so unwell.*

Doctor: I would first of all like to say how sorry we all are here, especially as her death was so sudden and unexpected. It was a shock to us all. As you know, she was admitted with exacerbation of her chronic bronchitis and emphysema. She was on treatment for this, and when we saw her on the ward round this morning she seemed to be improving.

Patient's husband: *what happened then?*

Doctor: we don't know for sure, but we think that she suffered from a massive clot on the lung. This is the most likely thing to explain her sudden collapse and death.

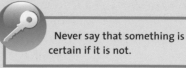

> **Never say that something is certain if it is not.**

Patient's husband: *if she had a clot, could it have been prevented?*

Doctor: pulmonary embolism or clots in the lung are known to occur in people who are confined to bed, and your wife had been in bed for much of the last week or so. These clots can be prevented by injections of blood-thinning agents, and we had been giving your wife these injections since her admission.

Patient's husband: *so why did she have a clot if you were giving her injections to stop them?*

Doctor: I'm afraid that the injections aren't 100% effective. Like all treatments they don't always work: they cut down the chances of having clots, but they don't guarantee that you won't.

Patient's husband: *but you said that you are not absolutely sure that she has had a clot in the lungs.*

Doctor: yes, that's true. We think that a massive clot in the lungs is the most likely thing, but we can't prove it and it is possible that she had something else, like a sudden heart attack.

Patient's husband: *so what happens now?*

Doctor: because we are not absolutely sure why your wife died, I cannot issue a death certificate. For this reason, and also because she died unexpectedly, I must speak to the coroner's office. It may be that they will decide that a post-mortem examination needs to be done.

Patient's husband: *can't you just sign a death certificate?*

Doctor: I'm afraid that I can't. I can only sign a death certificate if I know the cause of death and, as we've discussed, I'm not absolutely sure here. This is why I must speak to the coroner's office.

Patient's husband: I'm not keen on her having a post-mortem.

Doctor: I understand what you're saying, but I am not able to issue a death certificate because I do not know the cause of death. I have to refer the matter to the coroner.

Patient's husband: what will the coroner do?

Doctor: I can't say for certain. I will explain what happened: that your wife came into hospital because her chest was bad, that she was on treatment and seemed to be getting better, and then that she died suddenly and we think from a clot of blood on the lungs. If the coroner is willing to accept that, then I will put it on the death certificate. However, if the coroner says that he wants a post-mortem to try and find out exactly what happened, then that's his decision and we have to accept it.

1.3.5 Intubation for ventilation

Scenario

Role: you are the medical junior doctor working on a general medical ward.

Mr Ian Jones, a 74-year-old man with chronic obstructive pulmonary disease, is admitted with an acute hypercapnic exacerbation precipitated by a chest infection. He has previously been confined to his home because of exertional dyspnoea, despite the use of domiciliary oxygen and nebulised bronchodilators. Conventional medical therapy is being administered and adjuvant non-invasive ventilation is being set up for him. He still appears mentally alert.

The question of whether it would be appropriate to intubate him for ventilation is discussed on the ward round. The view of the medical team is that there would be no guarantee of success, and the process may be unpleasant for the patient. Moreover, even if intubation and ventilation were to be successful and the patient to survive this episode, he is likely to be left with even greater respiratory disability than he had prior to this illness. There is no doubt that whatever is done his medium- to long-term outlook is very poor indeed.

Your task: to approach him with the issue of whether or not he would want to be intubated for ventilation in case the current therapeutic measures are unsuccessful in resolving his ventilatory failure.

Key issues to explore

- What is the patient's understanding of his medical condition and prognosis?

- What is the patient's attitude to invasive procedures such as intubation and ventilation?

- What are the likely attitudes of his family members and carers?

Key points to establish

- Is the patient competent to make an informed decision about endotracheal intubation and ventilation? Does the patient have a realistic understanding of the advantages and disadvantages of this treatment? Can he give you an account of them?

- Has the patient discussed these issues with anyone else or written a 'living will'?

> 'Prioritising autonomy' means enabling the patient to decide what treatment he or she wants, the doctor's duty being to outline available effective treatments.

Appropriate responses to likely questions

Patient: hello Doctor.

Doctor: hello Mr Jones, I just thought I'd come and have a chat while the mask and equipment to help you with your breathing is being set up.

Patient: by all means.

Doctor: how much do you know about the sort of treatment you are receiving?

Patient: not a lot, really.

Doctor: well, we are going to ask you to breathe through a mask that is connected to a machine that will help you with your breathing. If you breathe normally then the flow of air coming from the machine will help.

Patient: OK doctor, I'll do my best.

Doctor: good, but can we talk a bit further? As you know, your breathing is pretty bad just now, and while we are hopeful that things will improve with this treatment we're just starting, it may be that they won't. If that turns out to be the case, we have to consider carefully what we should do. Is that something you've ever thought about or talked with anyone about?

Patient: what do you mean?

Doctor: some people with serious medical problems, such as your chest, have thought about exactly what treatments they would want or not want if things got really bad. Some people have talked with their family or friends about it, or have written a 'living will'. Is this something you've done?

Patient: no, what are the treatments you are talking about?

Doctor: if things get worse, we need to think about whether it would be the right thing to take you to the intensive care unit. There they could put you to sleep, place a tube into your throat and connect you up to a breathing machine, called a ventilator, that will do all the breathing for you. How do you feel about that?

Patient: well, Doctor, I'm not really sure. What are the pros and cons?

Doctor: the idea would be to help you with your breathing while we try to overcome the infection in your chest, but the treatment has its own set of risks. This includes chest infections that can be very difficult to treat, and there is a strong possibility that you may not be able to come off the breathing machine easily. In that case – if you were going to need the breathing machine for a long time – we would have to make a hole in your neck [show visually], pop a tube down into your wind-pipe and use this to connect you to the breathing machine.

Patient: if I did go onto the breathing machine, would I get better?

Doctor: I'm afraid that this can't be guaranteed. Your chest is very bad and whatever we do it isn't going to get completely better. I'm afraid that it's likely that every episode of infection such as this is going to

make things a bit worse, even if you do get over it.

Patient: what's the right thing to do?

Doctor: this isn't the sort of situation where there's a 'right' and a 'wrong' thing to do. Some people will decide that they want to try the ventilator if things get really bad, but they have to recognise that this can be very difficult for them and might not work out. Other people decide that they want to be kept comfortable if they get into that sort of situation. Whatever decision is made, we will look after you as well as we can.

1.3.6 Patient refusing ventilation

Scenario

Role: you are the medical junior doctor on call and you are asked by the nurses to speak to the daughter of a patient who was admitted on acute medical take a few nights ago.

Mrs Natalie Cooper, aged 74 years, has presented with type II respiratory failure secondary to an exacerbation of severe chronic obstructive pulmonary disease that normally limits her exercise tolerance to approximately 50 metres at best. She is well known to the respiratory team because of her recurrent hospital admissions, but on this occasion she has failed to respond to maximal medical treatment that has included a trial of non-invasive ventilation.

During previous admissions the question of escalation of treatment has been discussed with her, and she has

consistently said that she would not want to be intubated and ventilated in the event of deterioration. The respiratory team think that this is a reasonable decision for her to have made, that she is competent to make it and this has been recorded in her notes.

Your task: explain to the daughter that her mother does not want mechanical ventilation and that her views must be respected.

Key issue to explore

- What is the daughter's understanding of her mother's condition? Explain the details: a life-threatening flare-up, a poor response to medical therapy including a trial of non-invasive ventilation, and the progressive character of her underlying lung disease and its complications.

- What is the daughter's understanding of her mother's wishes?

- The impossibility of predicting the outcome of this situation accurately.

Key points to establish

- Demonstrate an understanding of the daughter's wishes, in particular if she wants to do everything to keep her mother alive.

- Ensure that the daughter understands that her mother's decision against mechanical ventilation in the future was her own, and was made on the basis of a full understanding of her condition and the probable consequences of not proceeding to mechanical ventilation.

- Explain that patients have a legal right to decline specific treatment, including treatment that is life-prolonging.

- Demonstrate sympathy with the daughter's difficulty in accepting her mother's decision.

- Reassure her that every effort will be made to keep her mother comfortable in the event that she deteriorates and is dying.

Appropriate responses to likely questions

Daughter: *as you said, my mother is very poorly and I feel that she is too ill to make such important decisions as those concerning life-and-death issues.*

Doctor: you are right, your mother is probably too ill now to make any valid judgements. However, she has discussed this with the chest team before when she was well. At that time she was fully competent to make decisions on what treatment she would wish to receive in the future, and this has been recorded in her notes.

Daughter: *exactly what has been discussed with her in the past?*

Doctor: your mother was aware that she has a chronic lung condition, which is progressing, and that her lung reserves are low. She knew that at some point she might end up in a 'do-or-die' situation, because of a flare-up or deterioration, and the possible ways of treating this, with their advantages and disadvantages, were discussed. She made a conscious decision that if such circumstances arose she did not wish to be put on a life-support machine. She, along with any other patient who can understand the implications of their decisions, has the legal right to decide what kind of medical treatment to choose or refuse.

Daughter: *I still feel that I have the right to overturn my mother's decision, while she is so poorly as not to be able to decide what is best for her.*

Doctor: I fully understand what you say, as you obviously would like your mother to receive all available treatment so that she can live for as long as possible. But your mother took the decision not to be put on a mechanical breathing machine (a ventilator), and this has been recorded in her notes. She has not changed her decision since she's been on the ward so we therefore have to respect her wishes. I am afraid that no one has a legal right to accept or decline treatment on her behalf and that includes the closest family, however distressing this may be. I fully understand that it's very difficult for you.

Daughter: *if she doesn't go onto a breathing machine, then is it definite that she will die?*

Doctor: no, it's not absolutely definite. At the moment she is very ill and we fear that she is going to die, but it's not 100% certain. Patients do sometimes come back from situations as bad as this, but we don't think that's likely, although I'd be delighted to be wrong.

Daughter: *if she did go onto a breathing machine, then would she live?*

Doctor: again, I'm afraid that's not certain. The machine would help the breathing in the short term, but there can be problems. It can sometimes be very difficult indeed to get someone off the machine and this can lead to a variety of complications. So no, it's not certain she'd live if she went onto the breathing machine.

Daughter: *I find it very difficult to accept my mother's decision. She has never told us that she would not want to be put on a life-support machine.*

Doctor: I suspect that your mother was concerned that she might become incapacitated and unable to make decisions on her own behalf. She has been on maximal medication for her chronic lung condition for some time now, and I think that she felt tired of fighting for breath and, more importantly, that the prospect of losing her independence was unacceptable to her. She must have felt that enough was enough. It was very brave of her to make up-front planning: making a decision not to pursue life-prolonging treatment is obviously not an easy one and she probably wanted to protect her loved ones from the responsibility of being involved. Our duty is to respect her values and wishes.

> Patients commonly do not talk to their relatives about end-of-life decisions because they want to protect them. Relatives often find this difficult to accept or understand.

Daughter: *it is easy for you to say this – she is not your mother.*

Doctor: I honestly think that even if your mother could be pulled through this flare-up, she might have a significantly worse quality of life. There is also a significant chance that she might end up on a ventilator permanently in order to go on living, and she probably would not wish to face this. This is not only my opinion, but also the view of other doctors who look after her. I have to say that I support your mother's decision and would also feel the same if it were my own mother. At the same time I fully understand how difficult it is for you to accept this, and I can assure you that the doctors and nurses will work together to ensure that your

Station 4: Communication Skills and Ethics   **227**

mother does not suffer, and that she continues to receive all the treatments needed to relieve her symptoms.

1.4 Acute scenarios

1.4.1 Pleuritic chest pain

Scenario

A 54-year-old previously fit woman is admitted with left-sided pleuritic chest pain that began suddenly 8 hours ago. On examination, she is tachypnoeic at rest with a respiratory rate of 28/minute.

Introduction

The visceral and parietal pleurae consist of single layers of cells separated by the pleural space. Pleuritic pain is characteristically triggered by deep inhalation, a cough or movement of the thorax. It is usually unilateral, sharp and can be referred to the shoulder, neck or abdominal wall. The diagnoses listed in Table 17 should be considered. In most cases, including this, the first priority is to exclude pulmonary embolism (PE).

History of the presenting problem

Pain

Is the pain really pleuritic? Did it develop suddenly? Sudden pleuritic chest pain is most likely to be due to PE with pulmonary infarction or a pneumothorax. A sudden onset of unilateral chest pain/discomfort and breathlessness should make you think immediately of pneumothorax, particularly in a tall thin 'marfanoid' man.

What was the patient doing in the hours before and at the moment when the pain came on? A precise history is very important: unaccustomed or vigorous activity, eg painting a ceiling, is likely to precipitate musculoskeletal pain.

Breathlessness

Was the breathlessness sudden? A sudden onset of breathlessness with tachycardia and light-headedness caused by hypotension are suggestive of substantial pneumothorax or major pulmonary artery embolism.

Haemoptysis

Was there any haemoptysis? Haemoptysis occurs because of pulmonary infarction and strongly supports the diagnosis of PE.

Patients with pneumonia can cough up blood-stained sputum, but at presentation the cough is often dry and sputum is most typically produced only as recovery begins.

Fever

Has there been fever? It is probable that this woman has had a PE, but ask about fevers, sweats or rigors. Most patients with PE are feverish, but high fever (>38.5°C), sweats or rigors make the diagnosis of pneumonia more likely.

Other relevant history

A rapid screen of past medical history and functional enquiry will be appropriate, but particular issues to concentrate on are thromboembolic risk factors and contraindications to anticoagulation.

Thromboembolic risk factors

Establish the presence of any of the following risk factors.

- Previous thromboembolism.

- Recent surgery, particularly major abdominal, pelvic, hip or knee surgery.

- Cancer.

- Immobility, eg long-haul aeroplane flights.

- Pregnancy/puerperium/oral contraceptive.

- Thrombophilia: protein C, protein S or antithrombin III deficiency; factor V Leiden mutation; or a family history of thromboembolism.

- Smoking.

- Obesity.

Contraindications to anticoagulation

It is unlikely that this woman will have any contraindications to anticoagulation, but ask about

TABLE 17 CAUSES OF PLEURITIC CHEST PAIN

Incidence	Cause	Comment
Common	PE with pulmonary infarction	Haemoptysis Leg/calf pain Risk factors for thromboembolism
	Pneumonia with infective pleurisy	Fever and 'flu-like symptoms May have purulent sputum
	Musculoskeletal causes	History of trauma or osteoporosis
	Pneumothorax	Sudden onset
Less common	Malignant disease	Often a duller and steady pain of some duration
Rare	Autoimmune rheumatic disorder	Systemic lupus erythematosus Rheumatoid arthritis

PE, pulmonary embolism.

these (the most common being a history of gastrointestinal bleeding). It is probable that, unless any contraindications were exceedingly strong, you would still decide to anticoagulate someone proven to have PE, although in the presence of a relative contraindication you would advise particularly close monitoring and counsel the patient to report any problems immediately, eg a change in colour of bowel motions or any feeling of dizziness. If you really felt that you could not anticoagulate, you would consider trying to prevent further emboli by insertion of an inferior vena cava filter.

Examination

General features

Is the woman well, ill, very ill or nearly dead? Assess this on the basis of the following.

- Speech: is this normal, or can she say only a few words at a time?

- Accessory muscles: is she breathing comfortably or does she have to use them?

- Exhaustion: does she look tired? Do you think that she will be able to keep breathing like this for another 10 minutes?

- Cyanosis.

- Vital signs: pulse, respiratory rate and BP.

Check her temperature: if it is >38.5°C, then pneumonia is likely in this case. Also check pulse oximetry.

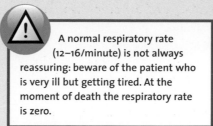

A normal respiratory rate (12–16/minute) is not always reassuring: beware of the patient who is very ill but getting tired. At the moment of death the respiratory rate is zero.

Cardiovascular system

Look for features to support a diagnosis of PE: high JVP, right ventricular heave, third heart sound over the right ventricle and loud P2.

Respiratory system

Is there a pleural rub, consistent with a diagnosis of PE or pneumonia? Signs of consolidation (dull percussion note and bronchial breathing) would suggest pneumonia. Pleural effusion can be found in PE or pneumonia. Reduced breath sounds on one side of the chest would be suspicious of pneumothorax (see *Acute Medicine*, Section 1.2.14, for discussion of tension pneumothorax).

Other signs

Look carefully at the legs for signs of deep venous thrombosis. Palpate the lymph nodes, breasts and liver and perform a rectal examination to look for malignancy.

Investigations

Chest radiograph

This may be normal, but common findings in PE are linear infiltrates, segmental collapse, raised hemidiaphragm and pleural effusion. Look for other causes of pleuritic chest pain, in particular pneumothorax, but also for pneumonic consolidation.

ECG

The most common abnormalities are tachycardia and non-specific ST/T-wave changes. Look for acute right heart strain with tall P waves, right-axis deviation and ST/T-wave changes in right ventricular leads (V1 and V2), and remember that the 'classical' S1Q3T3 pattern is seen in fewer than 10% of cases of proven PE.

Arterial blood gases

Occlusion of a pulmonary artery or its branches results in an area of lung that is ventilated but not perfused. This part of the lung does not then participate in gas exchange and hence results in wasted ventilation. Because of this ventilation–perfusion mismatching and hyperventilation, the arterial blood gases in PE frequently show arterial hypoxaemia, hypocapnia and respiratory alkalosis, although the Pao_2 can be normal.

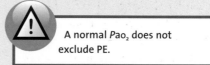

A normal Pao_2 does not exclude PE.

Plasma D-dimer

D-dimer is a breakdown product of cross-linked fibrin and is elevated in active venous thromboembolism. A normal value can be used to exclude thromboembolism, but the test is not useful when there is a high index of clinical suspicion, as in this case. A high value would be anticipated, but even if it was normal you would still need to pursue specific investigations in this case and hence measuring plasma D-dimer levels would not help the clinical decision-making process.

The patient who is cyanosed and looks exhausted is near death.

If an acutely breathless hypoxic patient has a normal CXR, then the diagnosis is PE until proved otherwise.

If there is a high index of clinical suspicion of PE, do not measure D-dimer but proceed directly to lung imaging.

Specific tests for PE

Ventilation–perfusion isotope scanning Ventilation scans are obtained using krypton-81m, technegas or xenon-133 and perfusion scans with intravenous ^{99m}Tc-labelled macroaggregates of albumin (Fig. 6). Scanning should ideally be performed within 24 hours of clinical suspicion as appearances can revert to normal within a few days, and 50% do so within a week. The scans are interpreted as being normal, or of low, intermediate or high probability: reports need to be interpreted in the clinical context.

Pulmonary angiography This is not routinely available in most hospitals in the UK. It is regarded by some as the gold standard for diagnosing PE, but it is invasive (with major or fatal complications in 0.5–1.3% of investigations, and minor complications in 2%) and interpretation is not always straightforward, particularly for those who do not perform the test regularly. The most common finding is a filling defect in the pulmonary artery as the radio-opaque dye flows around the embolus (Fig. 7). It has been largely superseded by spiral CT.

Spiral CT This can detect intravascular clot from the pulmonary trunk down to the segmental arteries, but unlike pulmonary angiography it cannot visualise emboli in the subsegmental arteries. In many centres this has become the investigation of choice, particularly for patients with pre-existing lung disease, which renders the interpretation of ventilation–perfusion scans difficult or impossible (Fig. 8).

Other investigations

Blood tests should include the following:

* FBC (platelets);

* clotting screen (prior to anticoagulation);

* inflammatory markers (expect very high C-reactive protein in pneumonia);

* creatinine, electrolytes, liver and bone function tests;

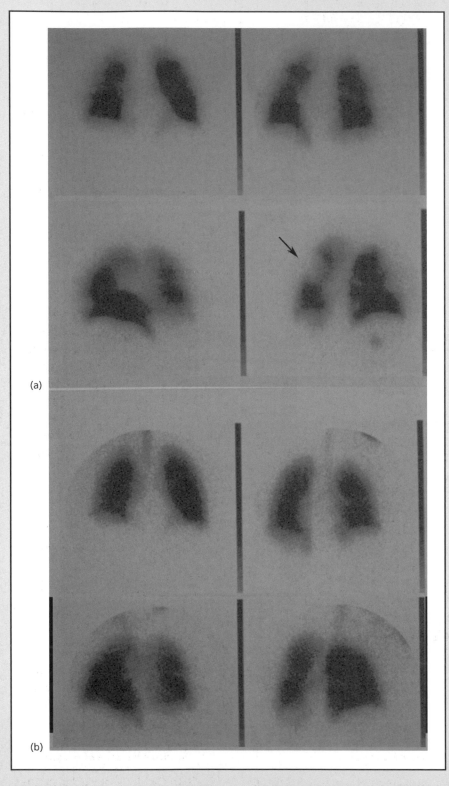

▲**Fig. 6** Ventilation–perfusion scan showing right mid-zone pulmonary embolism (arrow): (a) perfusion; (b) ventilation.

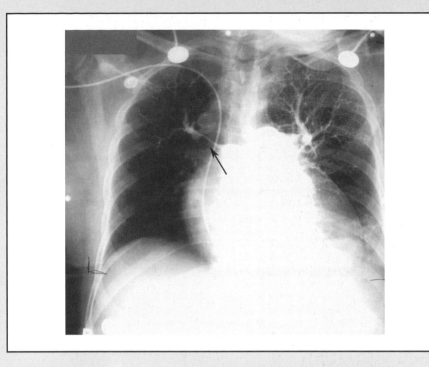

▲**Fig. 7** Pulmonary angiogram showing large right PE (arrow). There are also clear abnormalities of perfusion in the left middle and lower zones.

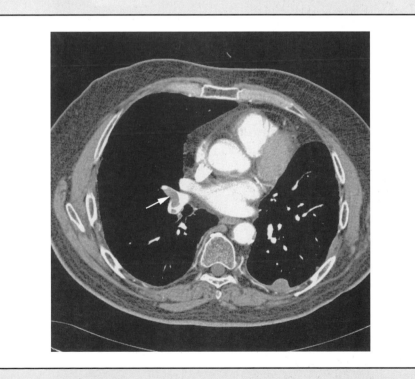

▲**Fig. 8** Spiral CT showing a large PE visible as a grey filling defect (arrow) against the white contrast in the pulmonary artery.

- blood cultures (if there is suspicion of pneumonia);

- autoimmune serology (eg rheumatoid factor and antinuclear

antibodies), although only in selected cases.

Echocardiography can be helpful in PE if a large embolus is suspected;

when there may be right ventricular dilatation and hypokinesis, pulmonary artery enlargement, tricuspid regurgitation or abnormal septal movement; and if the inferior vena cava fails to collapse during inspiration.

Treatment

Supportive

- Administer high-flow oxygen and intravenous fluids.

- If the patient is very unwell or nearly dead, immediately seek senior medical review/intensive care help.

Specific (for PE)

Anticoagulation reduces the incidence of fatal recurrent embolism, and heparin should be started immediately pending the results of investigations when there is high or intermediate clinical suspicion. Low-molecular-weight heparin is as effective as standard unfractionated heparin in non-life-threatening PE and has the advantages of rapid anticoagulation, simple once-daily administration and no need for laboratory monitoring.

> If the patient is likely to have had a PE and has no strong contraindication to anticoagulation, start treatment immediately. Do not wait for imaging.

Thrombolytic treatment is recommended for patients who are haemodynamically unstable. This is given peripherally, the doses used often being different from those used in myocardial infarction (refer to *British National Formulary*).

Warfarin should be started once the diagnosis is confirmed.

Pulmonary embolectomy is now reserved for patients who do not respond to thrombolysis or who have a contraindication to thrombolysis.

Inferior vena caval filters should be considered in patients at high risk of emboli in whom anticoagulation is contraindicated, and in those with recurrent embolism despite adequate anticoagulation.

Further comments

- Sudden unexplained dyspnoea is the most common and often the only symptom.

- The combination of dyspnoea plus tachypnoea is present in 90% of patients.

- Only 3% of patients do not have one of the following: dyspnoea, tachypnoea or pleuritic chest pain.

- An examination may be normal.

- Tachycardia is a consistent but non-specific finding.

In patients without a contraindication to warfarin it is reasonable to start this at the same time as heparin, even in patients in whom the diagnosis is unsure. It can be stopped if the diagnosis of PE is subsequently excluded. If PE is confirmed, then the patient may be able to return home earlier.

1.4.2 Unexplained hypoxia

Scenario

A 44-year-old man has been admitted with a 2-week history of non-specific symptoms of tiredness and being unwell. His CXR is reported as normal but he is found to be hypoxic with a Pao_2 of 8.4 kPa.

TABLE 18 PATHOPHYSIOLOGICAL PROCESSES LEADING TO HYPOXIA

Process	Example
Insufficient inspired oxygen	Altitude and anaesthetic mishaps
Right-to-left shunt	Anatomical (cardiac and pulmonary arteriovenous malformation) Physiological (eg resulting from atelectasis)
Ventilation–perfusion imbalance	Many causes, eg asthma, pneumonia, fibrosis, thromboembolic disease
Alveolar hypoventilation	Severe obstructive sleep apnoea and neurological/neuromuscular disease
Impaired diffusion	Fibrosis

Introduction

It is reasonable to assume that the patient has new-onset hypoxia, given that he is experiencing new symptoms. There are five physiological processes that can give rise to hypoxia (Table 18). In this case the finding of a normal CXR makes some of these causes less probable.

History of the presenting problem

As always in acute medicine it is vital to distinguish between genuinely new conditions and acute presentations of chronic conditions. With the CXR reported as normal, the main differential diagnoses in this case are shown in Table 19, and the history should pursue these possibilities.

Is the problem really acute?

Try to identify whether, with hindsight, the patient has had respiratory symptoms previously, perhaps on exercise. Has the patient had to stop doing anything or slow down recently?

If the problem seems to be long-standing, look for the following.

- Are there any respiratory or cardiac clues to the diagnosis? Clearly, any history of chest pain/tightness, cough, sputum or haemoptysis would be important clues.

- Are there features of untreated asthma (see Section 2.6)?

- Are there features of sleep-disordered breathing? If this is severe enough to cause daytime hypoxia, then it should be associated with excessive daytime somnolence (see Section 2.6).

- Is there anything to suggest that there might be a cardiac problem, eg report of a heart murmur is likely to be innocent, but could be relevant in this context.

- Is the patient at risk of interstitial lung disease? Enquire about hobbies and occupation (see Section 2.6).

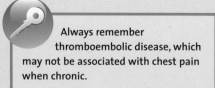

Always remember thromboembolic disease, which may not be associated with chest pain when chronic.

What acute conditions is the patient at risk of?

- PE may be suggested by recognised risk factors for thromboembolic disease.

TABLE 19 DIFFERENTIAL DIAGNOSIS OF HYPOXIA WITH A 'NORMAL' CXR

	Long-standing problem	New condition
Common	Chronic obstructive pulmonary disease (COPD) Diffuse parenchymal lung disease Obstructive sleep apnoea	Pulmonary embolism (PE) Acute upper airway obstruction Pneumonic process without CXR changes, eg atypical pneumonia, miliary tuberculosis (TB), *Pneumocystis carinii* pneumonia and acute aspiration
Rare	Neuromuscular disease Cardiac shunts Pulmonary arteriovenous malformation Pulmonary hypertension	Extrinsic allergic alveolitis

- The risk of atypical pneumonia is increased by exposure to air-conditioning systems (*Legionella*) or birds (*Chlamydia*).

- Miliary TB should be carefully considered in those at high risk, eg patients from particular ethnic groups.

- *Pneumocystis carinii* pneumonia (PCP) may present with isolated hypoxia, at which point risk factors for HIV should be recorded (see *Infectious Diseases*, Sections 1.3.20 and 2.11).

- Acute aspiration may present without radiographic changes initially and an appropriate history should be sought (eg risk factors for disordered swallow or reduced level of consciousness), although such a diagnosis could not explain this patient's 2-week history.

Examination

General features

- Does the patient have a fever or look toxic?

- Does the patient look as though he has lost weight? In this case weight loss might suggest miliary TB, or PCP as a complication of AIDS.

- Are there any other features to suggest AIDS, eg oral candidiasis?

- Is the patient likely to have obstructive sleep apnoea, eg is he obese or does he have a thick neck?

- Is the patient clubbed? This might suggest interstitial lung disease or a congenital cardiac shunt in this context.

Respiratory and cardiac

- Are there features of airways disease? Are there crackles in the chest? This might suggest interstitial lung disease in this context.

- Are there cardiac features to suggest PE? (See Section 1.4.1.)

- Are there any cardiac murmurs?

- Spirometry should form part of the clinical assessment: COPD is common and should not be overlooked.

Neuromuscular

Is there evidence of neuropathy or myopathy? In particular, does the patient's diaphragm move normally, ie does the abdomen move out as the patient breathes in? If in doubt, place your hand gently on the epigastrium and ask the patient to sniff: on doing so, the epigastrium should move out.

Investigations

Chest radiograph

Review the CXR carefully. Take it back to the radiologist for further scrutiny with additional clinical information.

- Is the cardiac silhouette really normal?

- Is there subtle evidence of airspace shadowing (Fig. 9)? This would suggest interstitial lung disease or a pneumonic process.

- Are both hemidiaphragms clearly visible? Check that you are not overlooking left lower lobe consolidation, which is easy to miss.

- Are both costophrenic angles clearly visible? A small pleural effusion might be caused by a pneumonic process or thromboembolism. Sampling of pleural fluid could be diagnostic (see Section 1.2.4).

Arterial blood gases

An increased $Paco_2$ (or the demonstration, by calculation, of a normal arterial–alveolar oxygen gradient) would suggest true alveolar hypoventilation. Comparison of arterial blood gases measured on room air and 100% oxygen enables calculation of the anatomical shunt, which in normal subjects is less than 5%.

Spirometry and flow–volume loop

These measurements should be abnormal if there is occult airways

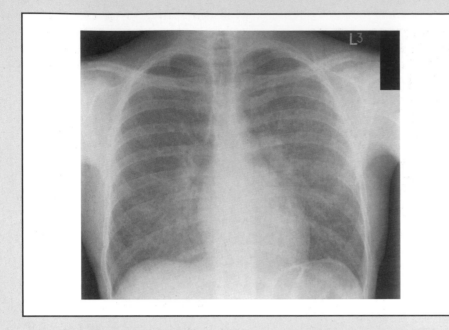

▲**Fig. 9** CXR of a 29-year-old homosexual man with a history of dyspnoea and weight loss. Diagnostic possibilities include PCP pneumonia.

disease of sufficient severity to cause hypoxia. In interstitial lung disease there is usually a restrictive defect. Upper airway obstruction is an unlikely diagnosis in this case, but would be revealed by the flow–volume loop (see Section 1.14).

Blood tests

Routine FBC, biochemistry and inflammatory markers are indicated because of the non-specific nature of symptoms in this case. Serum angiotensin-converting enzyme and calcium are indicated if sarcoid is possible. Atypical pneumonia titres or avian precipitins would be indicated if the history is appropriate, as might testing (after discussion) for HIV.

CT scan of thorax

This is likely to be a very helpful investigation, but the way in which the study is performed will depend on what is considered the most likely diagnosis. Discussion with the radiologist is required, not just an order form stating 'hypoxia – cause?'

- For suspected thromboembolic disease a CT pulmonary angiogram is required.

- For suspected interstitial lung disease a high-resolution scan gives the best images and is preferred. Significant pulmonary fibrosis may be invisible on a plain radiograph but seen on CT.

Bronchoscopy

Analysis of bronchial lavage fluid is indicated whenever PCP and miliary TB is suspected. If there is CT evidence of interstitial lung disease, then transbronchial biopsy is likely to be required. However, open lung biopsy may be preferred in selected patients.

Echocardiography

A contrast echocardiogram is the first-choice investigation if an anatomic shunt is identified (estimation of pulmonary artery pressure is a useful piece of extra data from this study, and should be specifically requested). If there is no cardiac shunt, then a CT scan will usually identify a pulmonary arteriovenous malformation.

Management

Oxygen should be administered to relieve hypoxia, but other aspects of management will depend on the underlying condition.

1.4.3 Haemoptysis and weight loss

Scenario

A 35-year-old man, who came as a political refugee to the UK 5 years ago, presents with haemoptysis and weight loss. He has been previously fit and well. His CXR is shown in Fig. 10.

Introduction

The presentation says nothing about the patient's ethnic background and travel history, details of which are clearly critical in this case. Tuberculosis (TB) must be the most likely diagnosis from the scanty information given, but causes of haemoptysis in a young person are shown in Table 20.

History of the presenting problem

The first thing to do is to confirm that the specific problem is indeed haemoptysis. Is the patient sure that the blood is in the sputum and not in vomit or coming from the throat or nose? Assuming haemoptysis is described, then for how long has the patient been coughing up blood?

Haemoptysis caused by TB

A detailed personal, social, family and travel history is required, with particular emphasis on the following.

- Has the patient been treated for TB in the past? If so, was he given anti-TB medication, and how many different drugs did this include? Few people remember the names of the tablets so ask for descriptions of them: combination

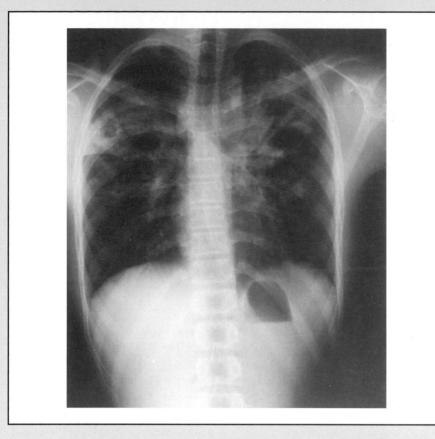

▲ **Fig. 10** CXR showing bilateral apical changes and a cavity in the periphery of the right upper lobe.

TABLE 20 CAUSES OF HAEMOPTYSIS IN A YOUNG PERSON

Classification	Examples
Common	Infection, eg pyogenic bacteria or *Mycobacterium tuberculosis*
Consider	Bronchiectasis Pulmonary emboli
Rare	Tumour (benign or malignant) Goodpasture's or other vasculitis

preparations that have distinctive colours and shapes are often used, eg Rifater and Rifinah.

- Have any of the patient's family members or close household contacts ever been treated for TB? Many patients deny this, particularly before a diagnosis has been made, because of the stigma surrounding the disease.

- Where was the patient born, and in which countries has he lived before coming to the UK? What sort of places has the patient lived in, eg refugee camps or hostels? The incidence of single drug-resistant and multidrug-resistant TB varies from region to region and this should be taken into consideration in any subsequent treatment. Remember also that some areas of West Africa have much higher rates of HIV infection than, say, Bangladesh.

- Where is the patient living now, and how many people is he living with? Many immigrants live in overcrowded housing, and from the point of view of contact tracing and subsequent screening it is important to know who the patient's close contacts are.

- Has the patient lost any weight? How is his appetite? Has he had any fevers or drenching night sweats, such that he needed to change the bedclothes? Weight loss, anorexia, fevers and sweats would all be expected in TB, and their absence would cast doubt on the diagnosis.

Other relevant history

- Bronchiectasis: is the patient producing any sputum? How much: teaspoonfuls or cupfuls? Ask about childhood respiratory infections, including TB and whooping cough, which would predispose to this condition (see Section 1.3).

- Pulmonary emboli: is the patient at risk from this? (See Section 1.4.1.)

- Malignancy: this is very unlikely in this case.

- Goodpasture's or other pulmonary vasculitides: these are also exceedingly unlikely in this case.

Examination: general features

How unwell is the man? Look for evidence of respiratory distress: inability to speak in sentences, abnormal respiratory rate and use of accessory muscles, and cyanosis. Also check for toxicity: is he hot and feverish? Check for clues to the underlying aetiology (Table 21).

Examination: respiratory system

The symptoms/signs picked up by your examination may give a good indication of the cause of the haemoptysis.

TABLE 21 GENERAL SIGNS POINTING TO THE CAUSE OF HAEMOPTYSIS IN A YOUNG PATIENT	
Diagnosis	**Signs**
TB	Lymphadenopathy BCG scar?
Bronchiectasis	Sputum pot Clubbing
Vasculitis	Splinter haemorrhages Vasculitic rash Bruising (steroid side effect) Inflammatory arthropathy Episcleritis Nasal bridge abnormality (eg collapse)
Malignancy	Sputum pot Hoarse voice Cachexia Tar staining of fingers Clubbing Jaundice (hepatic metastasis) Horner's syndrome (ptosis, miosis, anhydrosis and enophthalmos) Neck lymphadenopathy Superior vena cava obstruction Scar (from previous thoracic/breast surgery, CT-guided lung biopsy or pleural biopsy) Breast abnormalities (nipple retraction, deviation and mass)

BCG, bacilli Calmette-Guérin; TB, tuberculosis.

Tuberculosis

- Pleural effusion.

- Inspiratory crackles in upper zones that do not clear on coughing.

Bronchiectasis

- Coarse inspiratory crackles that clear on coughing.

- Dextrocardia (Kartagener's syndrome).

Pulmonary embolism

- Raised JVP.

- Right parasternal (ventricular) heave.

- Right ventricular gallop rhythm.

- Loud P2.

- Pleural effusion (small).

- Pleural rub.

Malignancy

- Signs of a pleural effusion/lobar collapse.

Investigations

Chest radiograph

Do not forget that TB can mimic many other pathologies, such as lung cancer, other bacterial infections and pneumonia. Do not forget to look for pleural thickening and evidence of calcification, and also for the unexpected (Fig. 11).

Sputum examination

Urgent (same day) examination for microscopy, culture and sensitivity and acid-fast bacilli (you will need to send at least three samples in total). Send a sample for cytology as well.

Bronchoscopy

Bronchial biopsies, if taken, must be sent for both histology (in formalin) and microbiology (in normal saline). It is good practice for bronchial lavage to be performed and sent for cytology (for malignant cells) and microbiology and virology. Silver staining is not indicated unless there are other reasons to suggest *Pneumocystis carinii* pneumonia.

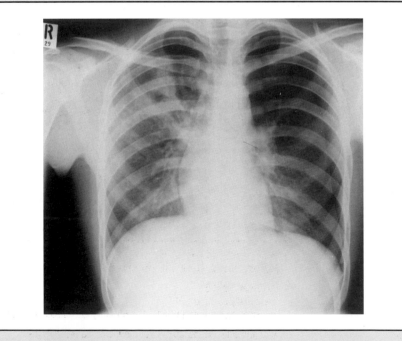

▲ **Fig. 11** CXR of a patient presenting with haemoptysis and later found to have TB: the unexpected left-sided pneumothorax was caused by coughing (and resolved spontaneously without intervention).

Other tests

It will be appropriate to check FBC (for anaemia and abnormal white cell count), electrolytes, renal function, liver function (prior to treatment with anti-TB drugs), blood cultures (for possible pyogenic pneumonia), inflammatory markers (to establish baseline) and (after appropriate counselling) HIV status. In selected cases, serological tests for autoimmune rheumatic and vasculitic diseases would be appropriate, as would CT scanning of the chest.

> In any patient presenting with TB, consider HIV and discuss testing with the patient.

Management

From the time of admission it must be assumed that this man has TB and he should be managed accordingly, in isolation from other patients. Definitive treatment will clearly depend on the diagnosis.

- TB: see *Infectious Diseases*, Section 2.6.1.

- Bronchiectasis: see Section 2.4.

- Pulmonary emboli: see *Cardiology*, Sections 1.4.6 and 2.18.1; and *Haematology*, Section 3.6.

- Malignancy (see Section 2.9).

1.4.4 Pleural effusion and fever

Scenario

A 45-year-old woman is admitted to the hospital with a history of fever for the last 7 days. Her CXR shows a right pleural effusion.

Introduction

Pleural effusion and fever is most likely due to an infective process, but there are other causes (Table 22).

Any pleural effusion associated with a bacterial pneumonia is called a parapneumonic effusion, which if not treated may progress to become an empyema (pus in the pleural space). Pleural infection can also develop without evidence of pneumonia (primary empyema).

History of the presenting problem

It is essential to establish that this effusion is related to an underlying infective process.

- Is there any history of cough with purulent phlegm?

- Is there any haemoptysis? This could indicate pneumonia, TB, malignancy and PE.

- Is there any history of weight loss? This could suggest TB or a malignancy.

- Has the patient travelled abroad recently? This could suggest pneumonia or PE.

- Is the patient a smoker? Remember that proximal malignancy can present with pneumonia.

- Is there any history of contact with TB or evening rise of temperature with night sweats? This would strongly indicate TB.

- Has there been any rash? This may suggest *Mycoplasma*.

It is also important to consider non-infective causes.

- Is there any history of joint pains, rash or red/painful eyes? Rheumatoid arthritis and systemic lupus erythematosus may present with an exudative pleural effusion.

- Any past history of extrathoracic malignancy (breast, ovaries or lymphoma)?

- Has there been any exposure to asbestos?

You should also consider the possibility that the cause of the pleural effusion may not be the same as the cause of the fever: is there a history of congestive cardiac failure or any of the other conditions discussed in Section 1.2.4?

Examination

General features

As always, note immediately how unwell the patient is and check the vital signs: temperature, pulse rate, respiratory rate and BP (watch out for septic shock). Establish if the patient is cyanosed: use pulse oximetry to record Sao_2.

Look for cachexia (suggesting TB or malignancy), clubbing (from malignancy), lymphadenopathy (from TB or malignancy) or any

TABLE 22 CAUSES OF PLEURAL EFFUSION AND FEVER

Frequency (in UK)	Condition
Common	Pneumonia: parapneumonic Empyema: secondary to pneumonia or (rarely) primary
Less common	Tuberculosis (TB) Pulmonary embolism (PE) Malignancy: primary bronchial, secondary and mesothelioma
Rare	Autoimmune rheumatic disorder, eg rheumatoid arthritis, systemic lupus erythematosus

features to suggest autoimmune rheumatic disorder (such as a rash or arthritis).

Respiratory system

- Look at the contents of any sputum pots.

- Palpation: check movements of both sides of the chest (reduced on the side of a large effusion) and look for mediastinal shift by palpating the trachea and the apex beat (both will be shifted away from a large effusion).

- Percussion: will be stony dull on the side of effusion.

- Auscultation: breath sounds will be reduced on the side of effusion, with bronchial breath sounds if it is consolidated or has a collapsed lung above it.

Investigations

Given that pleural effusion is confirmed on the CXR in this case, other appropriate investigations on admission would include the following.

- FBC: likely to show neutrophilia, with a very high neutrophil count ($>20 \times 10^9$/L), supporting the diagnosis of empyema.

- Erythrocyte sedimentation rate/ C-reactive protein: raised inflammatory markers are anticipated in bacterial infection.

- Blood cultures.

- Sputum for alcohol- and acid-fast bacilli and bacterial culture.

- Creatinine and electrolytes are required in any acutely ill patient: impaired renal function may be due to hypoperfusion of the kidneys.

- Liver function tests may be abnormal in Legionnaire's disease.

Regarding the pleural effusion itself.

- Thoracic ultrasound can differentiate pleural fluid from pleural thickening. Four patterns have been described: (i) anechoic effusion (may be transudate or exudate); (ii) complex non-septate effusion; (iii) complex septate effusion; and (iv) homogeneously echogenic effusion (the latter three are always exudative). Pleural aspiration can be done at the same time.

- Pleural aspiration: all patients with a pleural effusion in association with sepsis or a pneumonic illness require diagnostic pleural fluid sampling, as the pleural fluid characteristics will determine if there is a need for chest tube insertion. A chest tube should be inserted if the aspirate is purulent, microscopy and culture of pleural fluid is positive for bacteria, or the pH of pleural fluid is <7.2. See Section 1.2.4 for further discussion of pleural fluid sampling.

> In any patient with sepsis and a pleural effusion, a diagnostic pleural aspirate must be performed.

In some patients it may be appropriate to send blood for an atypical pneumonia screen, test urine for *Legionella* and pneumococcal antigens, and check serological tests for autoimmune rheumatic disorder.

Management

General

- Bed-rest.

- Oxygen if hypoxic.

- Ensure adequate hydration and nutrition.

- Prophylaxis against thromboembolism.

Specific

- Pleural effusion due to community-acquired pneumonia.

- Pleural effusion due to TB: see *Infectious Diseases*, Section 2.6.1.

- For details of chest drain insertion and its subsequent management: see Section 3.4.

- Antibiotics: the bacteriology of parapneumonic effusions and empyema is notably different from that of community-acquired pneumonia (Fig. 12). In particular,

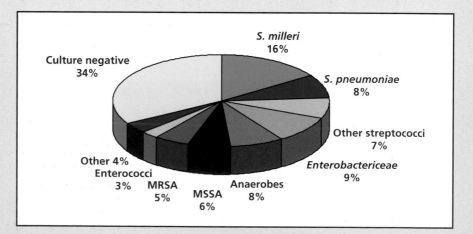

▲ **Fig. 12** Bacteriology of parapneumonic effusions (N = 430). (Adapted with permission from Maskell NA, Davies CDH and Nunn AJ. UK Controlled trial of intrapleural streptokinase for pleural infection. *N. Engl. J. Med.* 2005; 352: 865–74.)

so-called 'atypical' pathogens are rarely to blame, and anaerobes and Enterobacteriaceae are much more common. The choice of first-line antibiotic treatment should reflect this.

- Surgical intervention: patients with persistent sepsis and collections of pus despite antibiotics and appropriate chest tube insertion should be referred to the thoracic surgeons.

Further comments

Contrary to previous small trials, the UK controlled Trial of Intrapleural Streptokinase for Pleural Infection found that this treatment did not reduce mortality, the need for surgical drainage or the length of patient's hospital stay.

Most pleural effusions associated with pneumonia resolve without any specific therapy directed toward the pleural fluid, but about 10% require specific intervention.

1.4.5 Lobar collapse in non-smoker

Scenario

A 55-year-old woman is referred with a 10-day history of productive cough, gradually increasing shortness of breath and fever. Her symptoms have failed to resolve on oral antibiotics and her CXR shows right upper lobe collapse (Fig. 13).

Introduction

The causes of lobar collapse are shown in Table 23.

Is there any concomitant consolidation? If there is, then your initial concern must be to treat infection because a collapse of the lung may be caused by inflamed and swollen bronchial mucosa, and mucous plugging secondary to lobar pneumonia. Collapse alone, or collapse with concomitant consolidation that is slow to clear (say more than 6 weeks from onset of symptoms), requires investigation to exclude an endobronchial lesion causing mechanical obstruction.

History of presenting problem

It is important that you obtain as many specific details as possible regarding this patient's symptoms.

- When did the shortness of breath start? Was it before the illness that precipitated admission? If so, how long ago? A long history would clearly indicate underlying chronic lung disease, eg chronic obstructive pulmonary disease in a smoker who has now developed a chest infection or lung cancer.

- Did the shortness of breath start gradually or suddenly? If sudden, then is inhalation of a foreign body a possibility? Infants,

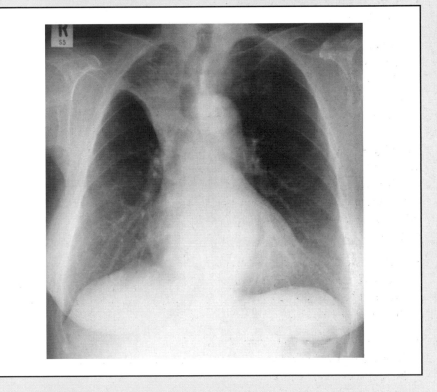

▲ **Fig. 13** Posteroanterior CXR showing right upper lobe collapse. Note the tenting of the right hemidiaphragm and the raised right hilum. (Courtesy of Dr I. Vlahos.)

TABLE 23	DIFFERENTIAL DIAGNOSIS OF LOBAR COLLAPSE
Classification	**Examples**
Common	Infection (pneumonia and pulmonary tuberculosis)
Other causes	Carcinoma of the lung
	Inhaled foreign body
	Asthma
	Allergic bronchopulmonary aspergillosis
	Bronchiectasis (particularly cystic fibrosis)
	Other lung tumours (eg carcinoid)

children and patients with learning difficulties or dementia are particularly at risk in such circumstances, as well as those with risk factors for reduced level of consciousness (eg epilepsy and alcoholism). Ask for a history of choking while eating food or losing a dental filling.

- How long has she had the fever? Pyogenic pneumonia will typically present with a shorter history than tuberculosis (TB).

- What is the colour of her sputum, and has she noticed any blood in it? Haemoptysis can occur in cases of infection, carcinoma of the lung and pulmonary embolism, although the latter is not a cause of lobar collapse.

- Has she had any associated pains in the chest? Severe pleurisy would be most likely in pneumonia, but pain can be a feature of TB or malignancy.

- Was there a preceding upper respiratory tract infection, which can sometimes precipitate pulmonary infection?

Other relevant history

- Is there any history of an underlying lung condition? Patients with chronic chest problems are particularly prone to infection. The thick tenacious sputum occurring in asthma, allergic bronchopulmonary aspergillosis and cystic fibrosis may cause mucous plugging resulting in lobar/subsegmental collapse.

- Has she ever smoked? If so, for how long and when did she quit? Lung cancer is relatively uncommon in patients who have never smoked, although some types are not smoking-related.

- Is there any history of weight loss? Consider carcinoma of the lung and pulmonary TB, as well as the possibility of pulmonary metastases from other primary sites (known or unknown).

- Is there any history of night sweats? Is there any previous history of TB/contact with TB? (See Section 1.4.3 for further discussion.)

- Are there any odd symptoms such as flushing, sweats or diarrhoea that might indicate carcinoid syndrome?

Examination

General features
A full general examination is needed, with particular attention to the following.

- Is the patient acutely unwell? Check her vital signs and note her ability to speak, use of accessory muscles and whether her breathing is laboured or she is cyanosed. Check pulse oximetry.

- Does she look chronically unwell? Evidence of weight loss would support the diagnosis of TB or malignancy, as would the presence of peripheral lymphadenopathy.

- Finger clubbing would most likely indicate lung cancer in this context.

Respiratory system
Check carefully for signs of consolidation (dullness to percussion and bronchial breathing) and for the features of lobar collapse described in Section 1.2.7.

Investigations
Given that lobar collapse is confirmed on the CXR in this case, other appropriate investigations on admission would include the following.

- Blood tests: for evidence of infection (raised white cell/neutrophil count or raised C-reactive protein) and to establish baseline creatinine, electrolytes, renal, liver and bone function tests (hypercalcaemia would suggest malignancy). Screen for allergic bronchopulmonary aspergillosis (raised eosinophil count, total and specific IgE, and precipitins) in (highly) selected cases.

- Sputum and blood cultures: for routine microbiology staining and cultures. If pulmonary TB is suspected, special sputum testing for acid-fast bacilli should be requested, as this is not performed routinely.

- Bronchoscopy: this should be performed if there is no/poor response to antibiotics, a high suspicion of endobronchial lesion or foreign body inhalation, or if collapse/consolidation persists. If an endobronchial lesion is seen, it should be biopsied and sent for histological examination. Bronchial washings and blind brushings should also be taken for cytological and microbiological examination (even if no endobronchial lesion was found).

- CT scan of the chest and upper abdomen: if there is suspicion of an intrapulmonary lesion you should proceed with a formal staging scan. This includes a search for potential metastases in the liver and adrenal glands, which is where carcinoma of the lung tends to metastasise, and will also sometimes detect the unexpected primary that has metastasised to the lung.

Management
Give oxygen if the patient's pulse oximetry and/or arterial blood gases

reveal hypoxaemia (Sao_2 <94%) together with, in the first instance unless an alternative diagnosis is readily apparent, appropriate antibiotics for community-acquired pneumonia. Further management will depend on the most likely initial diagnoses and response to treatment.

- Chest infection: arrange a repeat CXR in 6 weeks' time to ensure that radiological abnormalities have fully resolved.

- Carcinoma of the lung: see Section 2.9.1.

- Foreign body: this may be difficult to remove via fibreoptic bronchoscopy, in which case the patient should be given broad-spectrum antibiotics and referred for urgent rigid bronchoscopy in a specialist centre. Long-term occlusion of bronchi can lead to bronchiectasis, associated with chronic cough and repeated chest infections.

- Pulmonary tuberculosis: see Section 2.9.1.

1.4.6 Upper airway obstruction

Scenario

A 56-year-old woman presents with a 5-day history of stridor. She is obese, complains of recent hoarseness of voice and says that she is tired all the time.

Introduction

Stridor is a musical sound best heard on inspiration, in contrast to wheeze, which is heard on expiration. It is caused by the turbulence of air passing through a narrow glottis or trachea and indicates extrathoracic obstruction. The narrowing of the airway can be intrinsic or extrinsic (Table 10). Stridor should be investigated urgently as it may be life-threatening if it proceeds to occlude the airway, and may be due to an underlying malignancy.

Hoarseness of the voice that has lasted for more than 6 weeks is an indication for investigation for malignancy in its own right, but in general this is a less worrying symptom than stridor, although in this case they could clearly be due to the same thing.

History of the presenting problem

In taking the history, important issues to explore include the following.

- Does the patient have any other respiratory symptoms? Is she short of breath, and has she had any cough or haemoptysis?

- Although she is obese, has her weight changed? A loss of weight would suggest a malignancy, whilst a gain in weight might indicate hypothyroidism.

- Has she always been tired? Tiredness is a non-specific symptom, but along with a change in voice could point to hypothyroidism. Further support for this diagnosis would be obtained if the patient said that she was constipated, did not like the cold or had any other typical symptoms (see *Endocinology*, Section 2.3.1).

- Is there any history of dysphagia? This might be due to an underlying mediastinal tumour pressing on the oesophagus.

- Has the patient noticed any lymphadenopathy or had fevers? These would suggest lymphoma.

- Are there any features of myasthenia gravis? This could be indicated by diplopia or dysphagia.

Relevant past history

- Has the patient ever had any thyroid disorder/surgery?

- Stridor can be due to tracheal stenosis secondary to intubation. Has she ever been intubated, had an operation or been on a breathing machine?

- Has she ever suffered from a lymphoma?

- Does she smoke or has she smoked in the past?

Examination

General features

- Is she acutely unwell? Check vital signs and note her ability to speak, use of accessory muscles and whether her breathing is laboured or she is cyanosed. Check pulse oximetry.

- Does she look chronically unwell? Evidence of weight loss would support the diagnosis of malignancy, as would the presence of peripheral lymphadenopathy.

- Are there any signs of superior vena cava (SVC) obstruction? Swelling of the face and arms, dilated chest wall veins or raised venous pressure would indicate intrathoracic disease pressing on the SVC.

- Could she be hypothyroid? Look at and palpate for the thyroid gland. Look carefully for the clinical features of sallow complexion, puffy hands and face, and dry skin as well as checking for the most reliable clinical sign of hypothyroidism: slow relaxation of the tendon jerks.

Respiratory system

Confirm the presence of stridor. Note if the trachea is deviated, but remember that there will be no abnormal signs in the chest itself if the problem is confined to the upper airway.

Investigations

> If a patient with stridor is having difficulty breathing, then the first priority must be to protect the airway. This is easier said than done. Urgent advice from anaesthetic, ear/nose/throat and/or respiratory specialists is required. Cricothyroidotomy or tracheostomy may be needed.

If the patient is well enough, the following tests would be appropriate.

Flow–volume loop
The standard method of showing that there is functional upper airway obstruction (Fig. 14).

Bronchoscopy or laryngoscopy
One of these tests is mandatory in cases of undiagnosed upper airway obstruction.

Chest radiograph
This may show a mediastinal mass (including thymoma) or lymphadenopathy.

CT
This is only helpful if intrathoracic disease is identified, or for the staging of localised head and neck disease.

Other tests
Thyroid function tests, FBC, serum calcium, and renal and liver function tests; use acetylcholine receptor antibodies if there is suspicion of myasthenia. Thyroid scans can be used to look for retrosternal goitre. A tensilon test is indicated in suspected myasthenia gravis with underlying thymoma.

Treatment
Definitive management depends, as always, on the diagnosis.

- Laser therapy or stenting can be used for post-intubation stenosis.

- If the problem is at the level of the vocal cords, then tracheostomy can be helpful if the problem itself cannot be treated.

- If there is tracheal stenosis that cannot be treated, the use of a helium–oxygen mixture (which has low resistance to flow) may provide palliation.

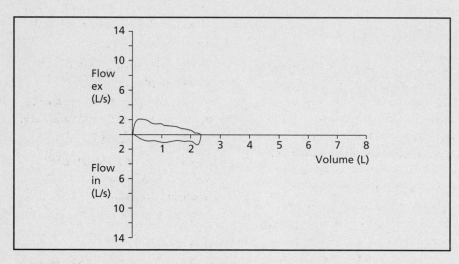

▲**Fig. 14** Flow–volume loop of a patient complaining of exertional dyspnoea. Diagnosis: tracheal stenosis.

2.1 Upper airway

2.1.1 Sleep apnoea

The term 'sleep-related apnoea' has been defined as periods of complete absence of breathing during sleep. Based on the analysis of breathing patterns, three types of sleep apnoea have been described.

1. Obstructive apnoea: cessation of airflow through the nose or mouth with persistence of diaphragmatic and intercostal muscle activity.

2. Central apnoea: cessation of airflow without any diaphragmatic or intercostal muscle activity.

3. Mixed apnoeas: an initial episode of central apnoea followed by a period of obstructive apnoea.

Hypopnoea is defined as a decrease in airflow at the mouth and nose along with a decreased respiratory effort. Some investigators define hypopnoea as a one-third reduction in tidal volume associated with a 4% reduction of oxygen saturation.

Obstructive sleep apnoea syndrome

This is the most common sleep disorder seen in sleep clinics. The prevalence of obstructive sleep apnoea syndrome (OSAS) among middle-aged men and women is estimated to be 1–4% and 1.2–2.5%, respectively. The prevalence increases with age, partly due to a gain in weight.

OSAS is associated with:

- obesity;

- hypertension (the prevalence of OSAS is greater than 25% in hypertensive patients, and in untreated cases of severe OSAS the prevalence of hypertension may be as high as 50%);

- gastro-oesophageal reflux disease (GORD);

- smoking.

OSAS results from the narrowing and closure of the upper airway during sleep. The pharynx, which lacks supporting cartilage and bone, is the site of the occlusion, which can occur at the level of the velopharynx, oropharynx or hypopharynx. Owing to the relative hypotonia that occurs during sleep there is airway closure and the patient then attempts to breathe without success, resulting in oxygen desaturation. This results in arousal (lightening of sleep) and reopening of the airway. Such episodes occur many times each hour during sleep. Arousals can be detected on the electroencephalogram (EEG) and frequent such arousals at the cortical level results in fragmented sleep and excessive daytime somnolence. Conditions causing a narrow upper airway that predispose to OSAS include the following.

- Mucosal oedema and inflammation, for example in rhinitis.

- Anatomical deformities such as micrognathia and retrognathia.

- Enlarged tongue, soft palate or uvula: present in Down's syndrome and hypothyroidism.

- Infiltration of pharyngeal tissue: obesity and Prader–Willi syndrome.

- Structural lesions: enlarged tonsils and adenoids.

- Cranial base abnormalities: achondroplasia and rheumatoid arthritis.

- Weakness of pharyngeal and laryngeal dilator muscles: congenital myopathies, muscular dystrophies, medullary lesions and vocal-cord paralysis.

- Increased airway compliance: Marfan's syndrome, tracheomalacia and laryngomalacia.

Symptoms

It is essential to take a history from the bed partner as most symptoms occur during sleep:

- snoring;

- apnoeic episodes during sleep;

- snorting, gasping and choking sounds during sleep;

- restless sleep due to arousals;

- nocturnal sweating;

- nocturia;

- excessive daytime somnolence;

- morning headaches;

- mood disturbances;

- reduced libido;

- personality change;

- forgetfulness;
- symptoms of GORD.

Signs

- Obesity: BMI (body weight in kg divided by height in m^2) of 25 or more.
- Collar size: men with a collar size of more than 17 inches (43 cm) and women with one of more than 16 inches (41 cm) are at risk of OSAS.
- Features of hypothyroidism.
- Anatomical facial deformities.
- Enlarged tonsils.
- Large oedematous uvula.
- Hypertension.
- Congestive cardiac failure.

Diagnosis

In order to obtain as accurate a diagnosis as possible, make sure you do the following.

- Take an appropriate history from the patient and bed partner.
- Assess subjective sleepiness using the Epworth Sleepiness Scale.

Confirmatory tests

Overnight pulse oximetry This may be normal and so in a patient with a good history and evidence of daytime sleepiness without any other reason, either polysomnography should be requested or a trial of nasal continuous positive airways pressure (nCPAP) initiated.

Polysomnography This is the investigation of choice. It records the EEG, electrooculogram, submental electromyelogram, airflow at the nose and mouth, and thoracic and abdominal wall movement (respiratory effort). At the same time, Sao_2, ECG, leg

movements and snoring sounds can be recorded. Additional sensors can be used to assess the patient's body position (more apnoeas occur in the supine position) and oesophageal pH (respiratory effort against an obstructed airway is associated with gastro-oesophageal reflux). Simultaneous video recording can help in diagnosing apnoeic spells with restless sleep due to arousals. Polysomnography helps to determine the presence and type of apnoea, and its relation to sleep stage and body position: more apnoeas occur in the supine position and during rapid eye movement (REM) sleep. The severity of an obstructive sleep apnoea (OSA) is determined by the frequency and duration of apnoeas and hypopnoeas (mild 5–15/hour, moderate 15–30/hour and severe >30/hour).

The Epworth Sleepiness Scale

How likely are you to doze off or fall asleep in the following situations, in contrast to just feeling tired? Using the following scale, choose the most appropriate response for each situation.

Scale

0 = would never doze
1 = slight chance of dozing
2 = moderate chance of dozing
3 = high chance of dozing

Situation

1. Sitting and reading
2. Watching TV
3. Sitting inactive in a public place
4. As a passenger in a car for an hour without a break
5. Lying down to rest in the afternoon
6. Sitting and talking to someone
7. Sitting quietly after a lunch without alcohol
8. In car while stopped for few minutes in traffic

If your score adds up to 10 or more, you may have significant sleep deprivation or a sleep disorder.

Treatment

There are three reasons to treat OSA:

- to relieve symptoms;
- to reduce the risk of comorbidities associated with OSA;
- to provide relief from the effects of OSA on others.

Weight reduction

When appropriate weight loss should be encouraged. Obese individuals may develop two distinct but often-related disorders of nocturnal ventilation: OSA and obesity hypoventilation syndrome (OHS). Patients with the OHS have daytime hypercapnia and hypoxemia and may eventually develop pulmonary hypertension, right heart failure and polycythaemia.

Nasal continuous positive airway pressure

Nasal continuous positive airway pressure (nCPAP), introduced in 1981, is now the treatment of choice. The mask covers the nose and the continuous positive airway pressure delivers pressurised air to keep the upper airway open. The pressure is titrated to achieve the optimum pressure needed to reduce the apnoeas. Once a patient is on nCPAP, regular follow-up with the sleep laboratory is needed to monitor compliance, assess the effect on symptoms, and for regular machine servicing and mask/tubing replacement.

Dental appliances

In patients who are not able or are unwilling to use nCPAP, dental devices that advance the tongue or the mandible and hence open the airway are used.

Tracheostomy

Prior to nCPAP, this was the treatment of choice. The tube

stays capped during the daytime and the person breathes and speaks normally. During the night-time when the person is about to retire to bed, the plug is removed allowing the lungs to breathe directly through the tube. This bypasses any previous obstruction in the upper airway, thereby rectifying the problem.

Systemic effects of OSA

Cognitive and psychosocial function
Complaints of poor memory or impaired attention are common in OSA. These improve with treatment.

Nocturnal hypoxaemia
Nocturnal hypoxaemia is common in OSA and is usually more severe in REM sleep. It leads to increased sympathetic activity, vasoconstriction, raised BP and cardiac arrhythmias.

Cardiac function
Bradycardia, common during apnoeas, is a result of increased vagal tone caused by fluctuations in intrathoracic pressure and stimulation of the carotid body receptors by hypoxaemia.

Cerebral perfusion
Intracranial pressure may exceed 50 mmHg during obstructive apnoeas. This is associated with a reduction in cerebral perfusion pressure. Subsequent arousals lower intracranial pressure and hence increase perfusion. This fluctuation in cerebral blood flow can contribute to chronic vascular stress and stroke.

Renal function
OSA is associated with increased release of atrial natriuretic peptide during sleep because of atrial distension. This results in increase in urine output causing nocturia and enuresis.

Endocrine function
- Reduced nocturnal growth hormone secretion occurs in children with OSA and contributes to growth retardation.

- Dysmenorrhoea and amenorrhoea can occur in women with OSA and may improve with treatment.

- In some patients with OSA, hyperinsulinaemia can occur. Treatment of OSA improves insulin responsiveness in some patients with OSA.

Complications of OSA

- Accidents: in the UK, patients must inform the Driver and Vehicle Licensing Agency (DVLA) once OSA has been diagnosed. For group I license holders (private cars), driving must cease until satisfactory control of symptoms has been achieved. For group II license holders (heavy goods vehicles), driving must cease until satisfactory control of symptoms has been achieved with ongoing compliance with treatment that has been confirmed by a specialist.

- Increased risk of stroke.

- Increased risk of myocardial infarction.

- Increased risk of hypertension.

- Anaesthetic complications: due to narrow airway, there may be difficulty in intubation.

2.2 Atopy and asthma

2.2.1 Allergic rhinitis

Aetiology
Allergic rhinitis is defined as a symptomatic nasal disorder brought about by IgE-mediated inflammation of the membranes of the nose following allergen exposure. The classification of allergic rhinitis is based on symptoms and quality-of-life parameters. It is subdivided according to duration and severity into 'intermittent' or 'persistent', and 'mild' or 'moderate–severe' (Fig. 15).

There is a strong pathophysiological relationship between allergic rhinitis and asthma, with both conditions commonly coexisting. Patients with allergic rhinitis have inflammation of the lower airways and in patients with asthma, the presence of allergic rhinitis is common. Both allergic rhinitis and asthma represent allergic conditions with shared components of airway hyperresponsiveness. Moreover, patients who suffer from both allergic rhinitis and asthma far exceed the overall prevalence of asthma in the general population. Indeed, allergic rhinitis is known to precipitate and exacerbate asthma. Therefore, both allergic rhinitis and asthma represent a spectrum of allergic airway disease extending from the nose to the lung, the so-called unified airway.

Known triggers of allergic rhinitis include the following.

- Aeroallergens: domestic animals, house-dust mites, insects, moulds, plants and pollens.

- Pollutants: automobile contaminants, diesel exhaust, domestic allergens, gas pollutants, oxides of nitrogen, ozone, sulphur dioxide and tobacco smoke.

- Drugs: aspirin and NSAIDs.

- Occupational factors.

- Latex allergy.

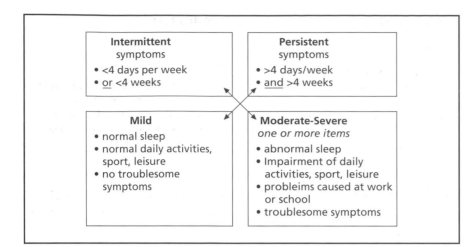

▲**Fig. 15** Classification of allergic rhinitis.

Clinical presentation

Patients present with sneezing, itching, watery rhinorrhoea and nasal obstruction.

Physical signs

Look for nasal polyps that can both cause and exacerbate rhinitis.

Investigations

The majority of patients are treated with success empirically; for patients who are refractory to therapy consider the differential diagnosis (below) and also consider occupational history, skin-prick testing, FBC and eosinophil count.

Differential diagnosis

Other non-allergic causes of rhinitis include infection, nasal polyps, foreign bodies or anatomical variants, nasal tumours, granulomatous diseases, and vasomotor (secondary to 'over-the-counter' medication) and idiopathic factors.

Treatment

- Allergen avoidance, although this is not always possible.

- Topical (nasal) steroids are often very effective. Side effects are local irritation and nose-bleeds. Check for compliance and technique if there is failure to improve.

- Oral antihistamines: warn the patient about the sedative side effects of some preparations and interactions with other drugs, eg terfenadine with erythromycin results in prolonged QT interval.

- Cromoglycates: no major side effects, but require frequent use. Eye drops are particularly effective in allergic conjuctivitis.

- Oral leukotriene receptor antagonists.

- Immunotherapy: desensitisation is sometimes possible in selected patients. The technique must be performed in specialist centres.

FURTHER READING

Bousquet J, Van Cauwenberge P and Khaltaev N. Allergic rhinitis and its impact on asthma. *J. Allergy Clin. Immunol.* 2001; 108: S147–S334.

2.2.2 Asthma

Aetiology

Asthma is defined as reversible airway obstruction associated with airway inflammation and bronchial hyperresponsiveness. The hyperresponsiveness of the airways is caused by a variety of local stimuli including histamine, leukotrienes and prostaglandins. This produces the reversible airflow obstruction that leads to the characteristic symptoms of shortness of breath, chest tightness and wheeze. Risk factors include:

- genetic predisposition;

- family or personal history of atopy;

- maternal smoking and ethnicity;

- socioeconomic status.

The role of other factors such as diet and pollution (black smoke, fine particulate matter, ozone and sulphates) remains controversial. While not directly linked to an increased prevalence of the disease, they certainly exacerbate asthmatic symptoms and there is increased asthma mortality in areas of high industrial pollution. Other precipitants of asthma attacks include house-dust mites, pollens, moulds, fungi, cat and dog dander, aspirin and NSAIDs in sensitive patients (approximately 10–20%), and occupational exposure.

Epidemiology

The prevalence of asthma continues to rise worldwide, particularly in developed countries. Approximately 15% of the adult population in the UK have asthma and, despite effective medication, there are still approximately 1,500 deaths from the disease each year. This continued morbidity and mortality highlights the importance of education for both patients and their doctors, with emphasis on adequate treatment regimens, good compliance and rapid access to medical help when deterioration occurs.

 Patients are at particular risk of dying from asthma if they:

- are taking more than three classes of drugs;
- have required hospital admission in the last year;
- have psychosocial problems;
- have ever had life-threatening asthma.

Clinical presentation

- Severe acute attacks: acute breathlessness and wheeze; also hypoxia and/or carbon dioxide retention can lead to stupor and/or confusion.

- Chronic asthma: shortness of breath, wheeze and a chronic cough, particularly at night when associated with a disturbed sleep pattern. Symptoms may be produced by exposure to cold air or exercise.

An isolated dry cough is perhaps the most overlooked symptom of mild asthma (especially in children). Particularly after colds and 'flu, patients may be left with an annoying dry cough and are frequently referred to specialists for further investigation. Bronchial hyperresponsiveness is often the cause and responds to a course of low-dose inhaled steroids. Patients should be warned, however, that their symptoms may persist or return with a subsequent cold or chest infection.

Physical signs

Life-threatening asthma

- Peak flow <33% of predicted or personal best.

- Silent chest.
- Cyanosis.
- Altered level of consciousness, confusion or even coma.
- Exhaustion and inability to speak.
- Hypotension or bradycardia.

Severe acute attack

- Peak flow <50% of predicted or personal best.
- Tachycardia.
- Increased respiratory rate (>25/minute).
- Patient cannot complete sentences in one breath.
- Use of accessory muscles of respiration and intercostal recession (especially children).
- Increased pulse rate (>110 bpm).

Moderate

- Peak flow 50–70% of predicted or personal best.
- Wheeze.
- Dyspnoea.
- Chest tightness.

The British Guidelines on Asthma Management are invaluable, but remember that the patient in front of you is an individual. If you are worried in any way about someone with asthma, especially at night, admit him or her. This is particularly the case for those who have an attack that has been going on for some time, if they live alone, do not have a telephone or would find it difficult to return to hospital. Do not feel pressurised by the patient, nursing staff or the hospital's bed state to send them home.

Investigations

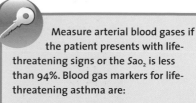 **Measure arterial blood gases if the patient presents with life-threatening signs or the Sao_2 is less than 94%. Blood gas markers for life-threatening asthma are:**

- normal or high $Paco_2$ (normal range 4.5–6.0 kPa/35–35 mmHg);
- low pH;
- severe hypoxia despite oxygen treatment (Pao_2 <8 kPa/60 mmHg).

Chest radiograph

In outpatients, a CXR helps exclude other causes of wheeze, such as infiltrates resulting from eosinophilia or fibrosis. For patients presenting acutely, a pneumothorax should be excluded and evidence of infection looked for.

Peak flow

This can be used diagnostically to look for morning dips. Motivated chronic asthmatics can also monitor their progress at home. In patients who clearly do not take measurements on a daily basis, make sure they know their best peak flow and encourage them to at least monitor when they get coughs or a cold.

All patients should be given a management plan based on deterioration of their peak flow: credit-card-sized self-management plans are produced by the National Asthma Campaign (Fig. 16).

Lung function tests

These should be performed before and after bronchodilator (eg salbutamol). They are not helpful acutely, but are important as a diagnostic tool to look for evidence of reversibility and to monitor chronic asthmatics.

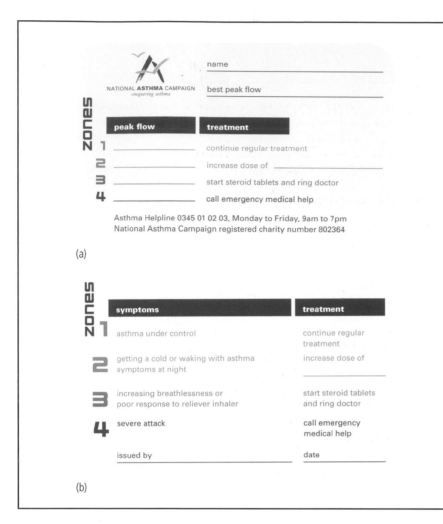

(a)

(b)

▲ Fig. 16 Credit-card-sized self-management plan produced by the National Asthma Campaign: (**a**) front; (**b**) back. These cards are available free on request from their offices. (Reproduced with permission of the National Asthma Campaign.)

In acute severe asthma (Fig. 18), the patient should not be left sitting in a side room in the Emergency Department. He or she should be in the resuscitation room and monitored for cardiac rhythm and oxygen saturation. The most senior member of the medical team in the hospital (usually the Medical Registrar) should be informed of the patient's condition and urgent anaesthetic and intensive care review should be requested if the patient does not improve rapidly or if the presenting symptoms appear life-threatening. Anaesthetists would rather be called to a sick patient than one who has suffered a respiratory arrest.

Allergy testing

Skin-prick tests can help identify allergens that may precipitate asthma attacks, although in practice many of these are not easily avoided.

Differential diagnosis

This includes chronic obstructive pulmonary disease, congestive heart failure, upper airway obstruction (ie foreign body, tumour), pneumothorax, bronchiectasis, pulmonary eosinophilia, Wegener's granulomatosis and Churg–Strauss syndrome.

Treatment

The stepwise approach to the treatment of chronic asthma remains the gold standard (Fig. 17).

For all steps following step 1, inhaled steroids are advocated for controlling airway inflammation and therefore chronic asthma.

Management can be divided into:

- 'relievers' (short-acting β agonists);

- 'preventers' (inhaled steroids);

- 'controllers' (long-acting β agonists and leukotriene receptor antagonists).

It is important to explain to patients that preventers and controllers must be taken regularly, while relievers are helpful for acute symptomatic relief. Oral preparations include oral steroids, aminophylline and the leukotriene receptor antagonists.

Newer treatments for asthma

The leukotriene receptor antagonists are the most recent drugs to be added to the therapeutic armamentarium for asthma. They include montelukast and zafirlukast and work by reducing the production of leukotrienes, which cause bronchoconstriction, mucus hypersecretion and airway oedema. They may have an anti-inflammatory action. Side effects include abdominal discomfort, diarrhoea and headaches. Their position in the stepwise treatment of asthma has yet to be decided; they may be useful for chronic asthmatics who cannot achieve control with inhaled steroids (step 3), as well as in cases of exercise-induced and aspirin-sensitive asthma. They have no place in the treatment of acute severe asthma.

A single dose of intravenous magnesium sulphate may be considered in patients with acute severe life-threatening or near-fatal asthma who fail to respond to initial therapy. A consultant must be involved in the decision to use intravenous magnesium sulphate. The use of repeated dosing with

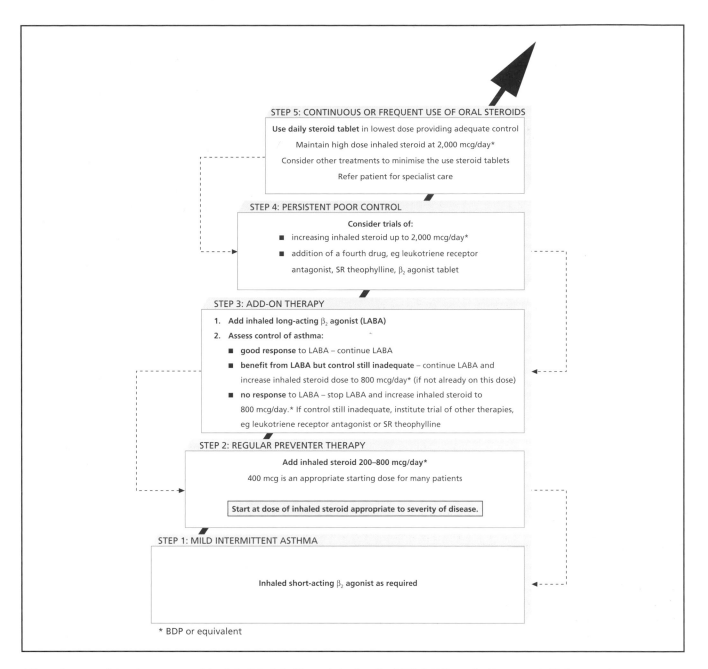

STEP 5: CONTINUOUS OR FREQUENT USE OF ORAL STEROIDS

Use daily steroid tablet in lowest dose providing adequate control

Maintain high dose inhaled steroid at 2,000 mcg/day*

Consider other treatments to minimise the use steroid tablets

Refer patient for specialist care

STEP 4: PERSISTENT POOR CONTROL

Consider trials of:

■ increasing inhaled steroid up to 2,000 mcg/day*

■ addition of a fourth drug, eg leukotriene receptor antagonist, SR theophylline, β_2 agonist tablet

STEP 3: ADD-ON THERAPY

1. **Add inhaled long-acting β_2 agonist (LABA)**
2. **Assess control of asthma:**

   ■ **good response** to LABA – continue LABA

   ■ **benefit from LABA but control still inadequate** – continue LABA and increase inhaled steroid dose to 800 mcg/day* (if not already on this dose)

   ■ **no response** to LABA – stop LABA and increase inhaled steroid to 800 mcg/day.* If control still inadequate, institute trial of other therapies, eg leukotriene receptor antagonist or SR theophylline

STEP 2: REGULAR PREVENTER THERAPY

Add inhaled steroid 200–800 mcg/day*

400 mcg is an appropriate starting dose for many patients

Start at dose of inhaled steroid appropriate to severity of disease.

STEP 1: MILD INTERMITTENT ASTHMA

Inhaled short-acting β_2 agonist as required

* BDP or equivalent

▲**Fig. 17** Summary of stepwise management in adults. (Adapted with permission from the *British Guideline on the Management of Asthma*, 2005).

intravenous magnesium sulphate is discouraged as it can potentially lead to muscle weakness and respiratory failure.

Omalizumab, a recombinant humanised anti-IgE monoclonal antibody, has been developed for the treatment of patients with persistent allergic asthma. However, the role of omalizumab in the stepwise management of asthma is currently uncertain.

FURTHER READING

British Thoracic Society/Scottish Intercollegiate Guidelines Network. *British Guidelines on the Management of Asthma*, November 2005. Available at http://www.enterpriseportal2.co.uk/filestore/bts/asthmaupdatenov05.pdf

Jarad NA. Occupational asthma. *J. R. Coll. Physicians Lond.* 1999; 33: 537–40.

Lipworth BJ. Leukotriene-receptor antagonists. *Lancet* 1999; 353: 57–62.

Rees J and Kanabar D, eds. *ABC of Asthma*, 4th edn. London: BMJ Publications, 2000.

Features of acute severe asthma
- Peak expiratory flow (PEF) 33%–50% of best (use % predicted if recent best unknown)
- Can't complete sentences in one breath
- Respirations ≥25 breaths/min
- Pulse ≥110 beats/min

Life threatening features
- PEF < 33% of best or predicted
- SpO_2 < 92%
- Silent chest, cyanosis, or feeble respiratory effort
- Bradycardia, dysrhythmia, or hypotension
- Exhaustion, confusion, or coma

If a patient has any life threatening feature, measure arterial blood gases. No other investigations are needed for immediate management.

Blood gas markers of a life threatening attack:
- Normal (4.6–6 kPa, 35–45 mmHg) $PaCO_2$
- Severe hypoxia: PaO_2 < 8 kPa (60 mmHg) irrespective of treatment with oxygen
- A low pH (or high H^+)

Caution: Patients with severe of life threatening attacks may not be distressed and may not have all these abnormalities. The presence of any should alert the doctor.

Near fatal asthma
- Raised $PaCO_2$
- Requiring IPPV with raised inflation pressures

IMMEDIATE TREATMENT
- Oxygen 40–60% (CO_2 retention is not usually aggravated by oxygen therapy in asthma)
- Salbutamol 5 mg or terbutaline 10 mg via an oxygen-driven nebuliser
- Ipratropium bromide 0.5 mg via an oxygen-driven nebuliser
- Prednisolone tablets 40–50 mg or IV hydrocortisone 100 mg or both if very ill
- No sedatives of any kind
- Chest radiograph only if pneumothorax or consolidation are suspected or patient requires IPPV

IF LIFE THREATENING FEATURES ARE PRESENT:
- Discuss with senior clinician and ICU team
- Add IV magnesium sulphate 1.2–2 g infusion over 20 minutes (unless already given)
- Give nebulised β_2 agonist more frequently, eg salbutamol 5 mg up to every 15–30 minutes or 10 mg continuously hourly

SUBSEQUENT MANAGEMENT
IF PATIENT IS IMPROVING continue:
- 40–60% oxygen
- Prednisolone 40–50 mg daily or IV hydrocortisone 100 mg 6 hourly
- Nebulised β_2 agonist and ipratropium 4–6 hourly

IF PATIENT NOT IMPROVING AFTER 15–30 MINUTES:
- Continue oxygen and steroids
- Give nebulised β_2 agonist more frequently, eg salbutamol 5 mg up to every 15–30 minutes or 10 mg continuously hourly
- Continue ipratropium 0.5 mg 4–6 hourly until the patient is improving

IF PATIENT IS STILL NOT IMPROVING:
- Discuss patient with senior clinician and ICU team
- IV magnesium sulphate 1.2–2 g over 20 minutes (unless already given)
- Senior clinician may consider use of IV β_2 agonist or IV aminophylline or progression to IPPV

MONITORING
- Repeat measurement of PEF 15–30 minutes after starting treatment
- Oximetry: maintain SpO_2 > 92%
- Repeat blood gas measurements within 2 hours of starting treatment if:
  – initial PaO_2 < 8 kPa (60 mmHg) unless subsequent SpO_2 > 92%
  – $PaCO_2$ normal or raised
  – patient deteriorates
- Chart PEF before and after giving β_2 agonist and at least 4 times daily throughout hospital stay

Transfer to ICU accompanied by a doctor prepared to intubate if:
- Deteriorating PEF, worsening or persisting hypoxia, or hypercapnea
- Exhaustion, feeble respirations, confusion or drowsiness
- Coma or respiratory arrest

DISCHARGE
When discharged from hospital, patient should have:
- Been on discharge medication for 24 hours and have had inhaler technique checked and recorded
- PEF >75% of best or predicted and PEF diurnal variability <25% unless discharge is agreed with respiratory physician
- Treatment with **oral and inhaled steroids** in addition to bronchodilators
- Own PEF meter and **written asthma action plan**
- GP follow up arranged within 2 working days
- Follow up appointment in respiratory clinic within 4 weeks

Patients with severe asthma (indicated by need for admission) **and adverse behavioural or psychological features are at risk of further severe or fatal attacks**
- Determine reason(s) for exacerbation and admission
- Send details of admission, discharge and potential best PEF to GP

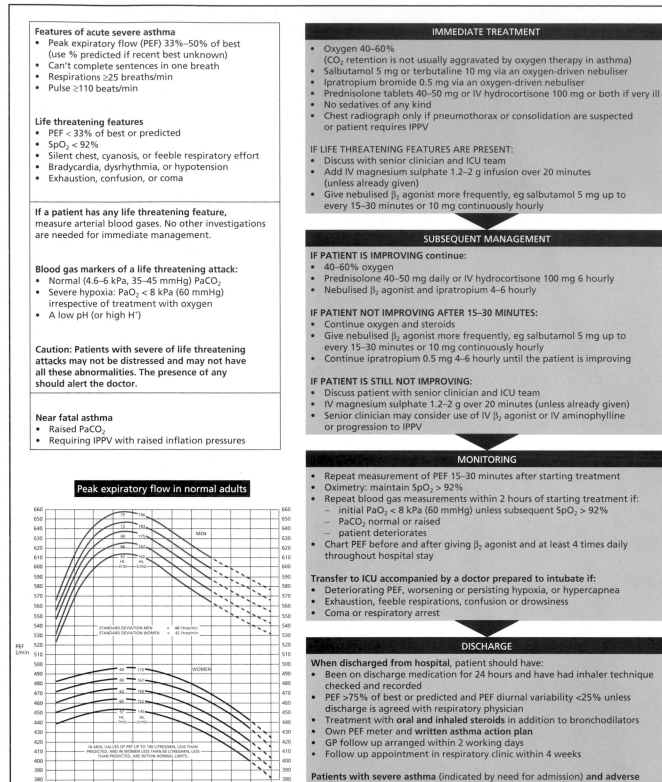

Peak expiratory flow in normal adults

MEN

STANDARD DEVIATION MEN   = 48 litres/min
STANDARD DEVIATION WOMEN = 42 litres/min

WOMEN

IN MEN, VALUES OF PEF UP TO 100 LITRES/MIN, LESS THAN PREDICTED, AND IN WOMEN LESS THAN 85 LITRES/MIN, LESS THAN PREDICTED, ARE WITHIN NORMAL LIMITS.

PEF L/min

AGE IN YEARS

Nunn AJ, Gregg I. New regression equations for predicting peak expiratory flow in adults. *BMJ* 1989; 298: 1068–70.

▲**Fig. 18** Management of acute severe asthma in adults in hospital (reproduced with permission from British Thoracic Society and Scottish Intercollegiate Guidelines Network. *British Guideline on the Management of Asthma: a National Clinical Guideline*, revised ed. BTS and SIGN, 2007).

2.3 Chronic obstructive pulmonary disease

Aetiology

Tobacco smoking is responsible for 80% of the risk of developing chronic obstructive pulmonary disease (COPD). Other common risks include occupational exposure to environmental dust (eg coal miners), organic antigens (eg farm workers) and α_1-antitrypsin deficiency. Smokers vary in their susceptibility to COPD, only 15–20% developing clinically significant disease.

Pathophysiology

COPD is characterised by airflow obstruction that is usually progressive, not fully reversible and does not change markedly over several months. Airflow obstruction is due to a combination of airway and parenchymal damage that result from an abnormal inflammatory response of the lungs to noxious particles or gases. It also produces significant systemic consequences.

Epidemiology

The prevalence of COPD among adults is approximately 4–6%.

Clinical presentation

COPD is frequently diagnosed as a result of:

- recurrent respiratory infections or exertional dyspnoea;

- an incidental finding during medical assessment for other reasons (eg elective surgery) or during a GP's 'screening' of smokers;

- patients presenting with polycythaemia, cor pulmonale or respiratory failure, although this is rare.

Physical signs

- May be none in the early stages, but look for prolonged expiration, signs of hyperinflation, bilaterally reduced breath sounds and widespread wheezes.

- In instances of advanced disease look for use of accessory respiratory muscles of the neck and shoulder girdle, paradoxical inward movement of the intercostal muscles on inspiration (Hoover's sign), expiration through pursed lips, cyanosis, cor pulmonale and weight loss.

Investigations

Spirometry

This is essential for establishing the diagnosis (see Section 3.6.2) and assessing the severity of COPD (Table 24). Airflow obstruction is defined as a reduced forced expiratory volume in 1 second (FEV_1) below 80% predicted and a reduced FEV_1/forced vital capacity ratio below 70%.

- Spirometry is the only method of early diagnosis of COPD in asymptomatic patients and should be performed in all patients over the age of 35 who have a risk factor (generally smoking).
- Always confirm clinical suspicion of COPD by spirometry.
- Do not rely on peak expiratory flow, which in COPD may be misleadingly high while FEV, is already significantly reduced.

Reversibility testing

Not necessary in most patients, as a response to long-term therapy is not predicted by acute reversibility testing. Over-reliance on a single bronchodilator reversibility test may be misleading unless the change in FEV_1 is greater than 400 mL. Oral corticosteroid reversibility is no longer recommended, as it does not predict response to inhaled corticosteroid therapy.

Chest radiograph

Conduct to exclude other pathologies that can mimic COPD, eg signs of hyperinflation (increased lung height, flat diaphragm, increased retrosternal airspace and narrow heart shadow), parenchymal areas of hypoattenuation and bullae (Fig. 19).

Blood tests

Perform FBC to identify polycythaemia. Measure α_1-antitrypsin level if early onset, and take a minimal smoking history or family history of COPD.

Arterial/earlobe gases

Perform if FEV_1 is <40% of predicted, Sao_2 is <92% and there are signs of right heart failure or respiratory failure in order to assess the indication for long-term oxygen therapy.

Body mass index

Decreasing body mass (observed in 20% of patients with severe COPD) is associated with increasing mortality.

TABLE 24 ASSESSMENT OF SEVERITY OF AIRFLOW OBSTRUCTION USING FEV$_1$ (AS PERCENTAGE OF PREDICTED VALUE)

Severity	FEV$_1$
Mild airflow obstruction	50–80% of predicted
Moderate airflow obstruction	30–49% of predicted
Severe airflow obstruction	<30% of predicted

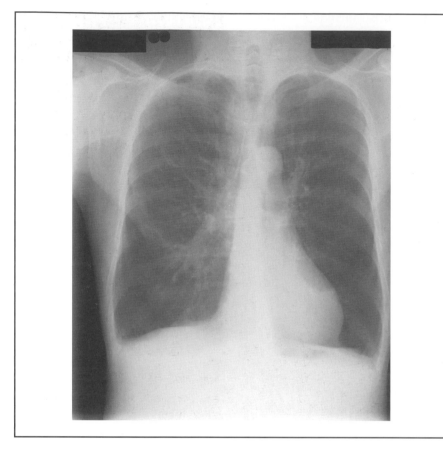

▲ Fig. 19 CXR of a patient with emphysema. Note hyperinflation (low flat diaphragms).

Transfer factor for carbon monoxide

Check if the patient's symptoms are disproportionate to the spirometric impairment.

High-resolution CT scan

A CT scan of the chest should be performed if symptoms are disproportionate to the spirometric impairment, if there are unexpected abnormalities on the CXR or to assess suitability for surgery.

ECG and echocardiogram

If features of cor pulmonale are apparent.

Differential diagnosis

A major differential diagnosis is asthma and this should be considered if a patient shows an exceptionally good response to treatment. Serial domiciliary peak expiratory flow measurements may be required if diagnostic doubts remain. Other common conditions presenting with similar symptoms, signs and spirometry include bronchiectasis, congestive cardiac failure and lung cancer. Bear in mind that as well as mimicking COPD, these conditions may also coexist in a patient with COPD.

Emergency treatment

See *Acute Medicine*, Section 1.2.12.

Treatment of stable patients

Smoking

All patients regardless of age should be encouraged to stop smoking and offered help (eg nicotine replacement therapy, bupropion and smoking cessation clinics) at every opportunity.

Inhaled therapy

Short-acting bronchodilators (β₂ agonists and/or anticholinergics) Initial treatment, as required, for the relief of exertional dyspnoea.

Long-acting inhaled bronchodilators (β₂ agonists and/or anticholinergics) If symptoms persist despite the use of short-acting bronchodilators.

Inhaled corticosteroids Prescribe as follows.

- A trial of 6 weeks to 3 months should be offered to all patients to identify those with airflow limitation responsive to inhaled corticosteroid treatment. If there is no improvement in symptoms or airflow obstruction inhaled corticosteroids should be discontinued.

- These should be added to long-acting bronchodilators to decrease frequency of exacerbations in patients with FEV_1 ≤50% predicted, who have had two or more exacerbations requiring treatment with antibiotics or oral corticosteroids in a 12-month period.

 Maintenance use of oral corticosteroid therapy in COPD is not normally recommended.

Theophylline (slow-release formulations)

This should only be considered after a trial of short-acting bronchodilators and long-acting bronchodilators.

Mucolytic therapy

Consider in patients with a chronic productive cough. Continue if there is symptomatic improvement (eg reduction in frequency of cough and sputum production).

Pneumococcal and influenza vaccination

This should be offered to all patients with COPD.

Nutritional supplementation

For malnourished patients.

Antidepressant treatment

Depression should be considered in patients who are hypoxic (Sao_2 <92%), have severe dyspnoea or are admitted to hospital for exacerbation of COPD.

Pulmonary rehabilitation

This should be offered to all patients who consider themselves functionally disabled by COPD.

Long-term oxygen therapy

See Section 2.12.1.

Non-invasive ventilation

See Section 2.12.3.

Surgery

- Bullectomy: for breathless patients who have a single large bullae on a CT chest scan and FEV_1 <50% predicted.

- Lung-volume reduction surgery: consider if the patient is experiencing marked restrictions in activities of daily living despite maximal medical therapy (including rehabilitation), if FEV_1 >20% of predicted, carbon monoxide transfer factor >20% of predicted and $Paco_2$ <7.3 kPa, and if there is upper lobe-predominant emphysema.

- Lung transplantation: consider if FEV_1 <25% of predicted, $Paco_2$ >7.3 kPa or cor pulmonale is present (see Section 2.13).

Complications

- Common: infection (bacterial and viral) and side effects of corticosteroid treatment.

- Uncommon: pneumothorax, cor pulmonale and respiratory failure.

Prognosis

In general this is inversely related to age and post-bronchodilator FEV_1. The 5-year survival rate in patients admitted with a hypercapnic exacerbation is 28%.

> **FURTHER READING**
>
> British Thoracic Society. BTS Guidelines for the management of chronic obstructive pulmonary disease. *Thorax* 2004; 59: S1–S232.

National Collaborating Centre for Chronic Conditions. *Chronic Obstructive Pulmonary Disease: Management of Chronic Obstructive Pulmonary Disease in Adults in Primary and Secondary Care (NICE Guideline 12).* London: National Institute for Health and Clinical Excellence, 2004. Available at www.nice.org.uk.

2.4 Bronchiectasis

Aetiology

Bronchiectasis is a condition characterised by the permanent dilatation of bronchi (Figs 20 and 21) due to a variety of reasons (Table 25). No definite cause of bronchiectasis is found in over 50% of patients.

Pathology

Recurrent bacterial colonisation and infection lead to progressive airway injury that is mediated by neutrophils, T lymphocytes and

TABLE 25 CAUSES OF BRONCHIECTASIS

Causes	Examples
Idiopathic	
Post-infectious	Respiratory infection in childhood (measles, whooping cough or bronchiolitis), pneumonia, pulmonary tuberculosis (TB), non-TB mycobacteria (eg *Mycobacterium avium* complex)
Bronchial obstruction	Inhaled foreign body, endobronchial tumour, extrinsic lymph node/tumour compression, middle lobe syndrome
Mucociliary clearance defects	Genetic: cystic fibrosis (CF) and primary ciliary dyskinesia (Kartagener's syndrome)
	Acquired: Young's syndrome (azoospermia and sinusitis) and toxic gas inhalation
Immune deficiency	Hypogammaglobulinaemia and HIV
Congenital	α_1-Antitrypsin deficiency, Williams–Campbell syndrome (bronchial cartilage deficiency), McLeod's syndrome (unilateral emphysema), pulmonary sequestration (non-functioning lung with blood supply from the aorta)
Immunological over-response	Allergic bronchopulmonary aspergillosis (ABPA) and post-lung transplantation
Others	Gastro-oesophageal reflux disease (GORD), rheumatoid arthritis, Sjögren's syndrome, systemic lupus erythematosus (SLE), sarcoidosis, yellow-nail syndrome, ulcerative colitis, Marfan's syndrome, Ehlers–Danlos syndrome

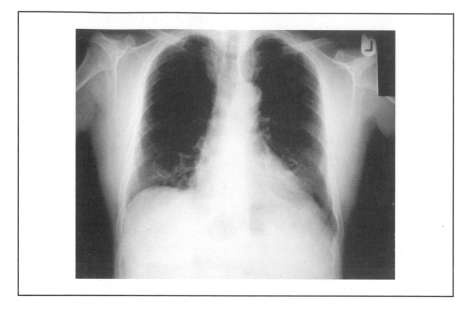

▲ **Fig.20** Plain CXR showing tramlines in the right lower lobe consistent with bronchiectasis.

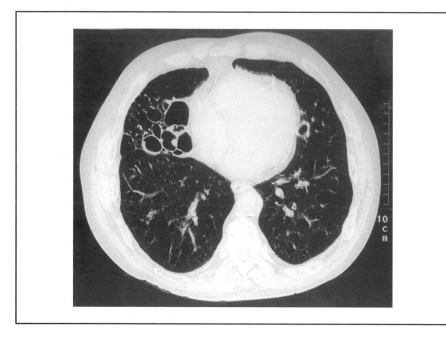

▲ **Fig. 21** High-resolution CT chest scan: gross bilateral bronchiectasis, more prominent in the right lung with a classic 'signet ring' appearance generated by an enlarged bronchus and a neighbouring vessel.

TABLE 26 SYMPTOMS OF BRONCHIECTASIS (FREQUENCY OF OCCURRENCE IN PARENTHESES)	
Common	Cough (90%)
	Daily sputum production (76%)
	Dyspnoea (72%)
	Haemoptysis (50%)
	Recurrent pleuritic pain (46%)
Uncommon	Chronic sinusitis

monocyte-driven cytokines. Released inflammatory mediators, elastase and collagenase lead in turn to the inflammation and then destruction of the elastic and muscular components of the bronchial walls, resulting in permanent bronchial wall dilatation.

Clinical presentation

Symptoms

The classic clinical manifestations of bronchiectasis are a cough and daily production of mucopurulent and tenacious sputum: less than 10 mL per day suggests mild bronchiectasis, whereas more than 150 mL per day indicates severe bronchiectasis. Other complaints are listed in Table 26.

Signs
See Table 27.

Investigations
Investigations are carried out to confirm clinical suspicion of bronchiectasis, identify any potentially treatable underlying causes, and assess any functional impairment and the extent of the bronchiectasis (Table 28).

Treatment

- Postural drainage is the cornerstone of treatment. It should be performed at least twice daily.

- Antibiotics: for acute infections, treatment failure or repeated symptomatic episodes over a short period of time following sputum sampling for culture and sensitivity.

- Bronchodilators: if there is evidence of airflow obstruction.

- Suppressive/preventive antibiotic treatment for *Pseudomonas aeruginosa* colonisation (one representative definition of colonisation requires the same

TABLE 27 SIGNS OF BRONCHIECTASIS (FREQUENCY OF OCCURRENCE IN PARENTHESES)

Common	Coarse crackles: early inspiratory and late expiratory (70%) Wheezes (44%) Finger clubbing (30%)
Uncommon	Halitosis Syndrome specific (eg discoloured nails/lymphoedema/pleural effusion in yellow-nail syndrome and situs inversus in Kartagener's syndrome)

TABLE 28 INVESTIGATIONS IN BRONCHIECTASIS

Test type	Description	Possible findings/indications
Generic	Chest radiograph	In combination with clinical presentation, this may be sufficient to establish the diagnosis, although it is not always abnormal. Look for 'tramlines' (parallel thickened lines representing dilated thickened bronchial walls), ring opacities, band shadows (fluid- or mucous-filled bronchi), crowded bronchial markings resulting from atelectasis and the 'finger in glove' appearance that results from impacted central bronchi
	High-resolution CT scan (sensitivity 97%)	Indicated if there is clinical suspicion of bronchiectasis but a normal CXR, if there are other abnormalities on a CXR that need clarification, or if surgery may be contemplated. A central (perihilar) distribution suggests ABPA and upper lobe distribution suggests CF/previous pulmonary TB
	Lung function tests	Obstructive pattern
	Arterial blood gases	Hypoxia and/or hypercapnia in advanced disease
	Sputum cultures	*Haemophilus influenzae, Streptococcus pneumoniae, Staphylococcus aureus* (if recurrent this may indicate atypical presentation of CF), *Pseudomonas aeruginosa*
	Bronchoscopy	To exclude foreign body/endobronchial lesion or for assessing and localising the source of haemoptysis
Specific for underlying disease	Serum immunoglobulins	IgG, specific IgG (to pneumococcus and *H. influenzae*), IgA
	Sweat sodium concentration	CF
	Eosinophils/ABPA screen	ABPA
	ACE/calcium	Sarcoidosis
	RhF/ANA/ANCA	Rheumatoid arthritis/SLE/vasculitis

ACE, angiotensin-converting enzyme; ANA, antinuclear antibodies; ANCA, antinuclear cytoplasmic antibodies; RhF, rheumatoid factor.

low-dose administration of an antibiotic to which the organism is sensitive, or as cyclical antibiotics. There is of course no evidence to support the use of either.

- Bronchoscopy: for extraction of mucus (bronchial toilet) if physiotherapy has failed.

- Bronchial artery embolisation: to control severe haemoptysis.

- Surgery: for the treatment of symptomatic localised disease (it is *essential* to exclude a systemic disease that may result in bronchiectasis affecting the remaining lung, eg immunodeficiency or aspiration) or massive haemoptysis. Perform lung transplantation for end-stage bilateral disease (see Section 2.13).

Specific treatments

- Immunoglobulin replacement in hypogammaglobulinaemia.

- Oral steroids and itraconazole in ABPA. There are no data on the efficacy of voriconazole or other imidazole agents in ABPA.

- Gastric acid suppression and prokinetics for recurrent aspiration associated with GORD.

- Recombinant human DNase (rhDNase) in CF.

Complications

- Common: recurrent infectious episodes, recurrent pneumonias and cor pulmonale.

- Uncommon: massive haemoptysis, amyloidosis and brain abscess.

Prognosis

Depends on severity, bacterial colonisation (eg *Pseudomonas* colonisation might be associated with a poorer outcome) and the

organism to be isolated on at least two occasions separated by 3 months within 1 year). Options include nebulised antibiotics (colistin/tobramycin) and macrolide antibiotics (daily or three times weekly). Long-term antibiotics may also be considered in cases of colonisation by other organisms, either as long-term

underlying cause. Deterioration may be due to recurrent and worsening sepsis, or to hypoxia and cor pulmonale.

Prevention

- Vaccination against measles, pertussis, influenza and TB.

- Prompt treatment of bronchopulmonary infections and ABPA.

- Early removal of foreign body and obstructing lesion.

> - If there is no obvious cause for bronchiectasis, diagnostic evaluation for an underlying cause should be performed, as the results may lead to treatment that may slow or halt progression of disease.
> - It is *essential* that the patient's sputum is sent for routine bacterial as well as mycobacterial microscopy and culture prior to starting antibiotics for exacerbations, although treatment should not be deferred pending results.

FURTHER READING

Rosen MJ. Chronic cough due to bronchiectasis: ACCP evidence-based clinical practice guidelines. *Chest* 2006; 129: 204S–205S.

2.5 Cystic fibrosis

Aetiology

Cystic fibrosis (CF) is an autosomal recessive disease caused by a defect in the gene encoding an epithelial cell transmembrane protein termed the cystic fibrosis transmembrane conductance regulator (CFTR). The gene is located on the long arm of chromosome 7 and the most common mutation in the UK is ΔF508. The function of this protein is to serve as a chloride channel and also as a regulator of an epithelial sodium channel; however, the exact mechanism by which defects in CFTR-mediated ion transport cause the phenotype of CF is unknown.

The lungs of CF patients are thought not to be infected at birth, but endobronchial bacterial colonisation occurs within the first months of life and usually progresses to colonisation with *Pseudomonas aeruginosa*. Lung destruction follows, with the development of an obstructive respiratory defect and eventually respiratory failure.

Epidemiology

Prevalence in Europeans is 1 in 2,500; it is rare in Afro-Caribbeans (1 in 17,000) and very rare in Orientals (1 in 90,000).

Clinical presentation

Presentations of CF are shown in Table 29. The average age of newly diagnosed patients is 4.8 years, but may be up to 65 years. The prevalence of diabetes in cases of CF increases with age, affecting 9% of children and 43% of those over 30 years of age.

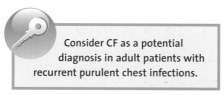

> Consider CF as a potential diagnosis in adult patients with recurrent purulent chest infections.

Physical signs

These will depend on the presentation and stage of disease. An adult patient with CF is likely to be clubbed with signs of hyperinflation. Crackles and/or wheeze may be audible. In advanced disease there may also be cyanosis or respiratory distress. The patient may appear undernourished (see below) and hepatosplenomegaly may be present.

Investigations

The diagnosis of CF is based on one or more clinical features consistent with the CF phenotype (see above) plus one of:

- two CF gene mutations;

- a positive sweat test;

- abnormal nasal potential differences.

Gene mutations

In excess of 800 mutations are recognised: most UK laboratories only screen for 12 of these, covering an estimated 93% of UK patients. Thus, it is possible for a patient to have CF without routine genotyping identifying a mutation. Conversely, the finding of one mutation does not diagnose CF because the carrier frequency of the single gene is 1 in 25.

Sweat test

This should be performed at least twice.

TABLE 29 PRESENTATIONS OF CF	
Classification	**Example**
Respiratory disease (40%)	Frequent infections, recurrent bronchitis/bronchiolitis
Malabsorption (30%)	Failure to thrive, rectal prolapse, intussusception, fatty diarrhoea
Meconium ileus (20%)	
Rare	Infertility (men), cirrhosis or portal hypertension, nasal polyps, adult bronchiectasis
CF, cystic fibrosis.	

Nasal potential difference

Although this test can be useful for patients with a borderline sweat test, it should not be considered diagnostic in isolation outside of specialist centres.

> Investigations relevant to the management of an acutely unwell CF patient would depend on clinical presentation. In specialist CF centres all patients would undergo annual review. As well as symptomatic enquiry and a physical examination this would include, from a physician's perspective:
>
> - CXR (Fig. 22);
> - full lung function tests;
> - FBC, along with urea and electrolytes, calcium and liver function tests;
> - sputum microbiology;
> - ECG.

Differential diagnosis

This is the differential diagnosis of the presenting symptom.

Treatment

The best care of the CF patient requires multidisciplinary team work between physician, nurse, social worker, physiotherapist, nutritionist, GP and genetic counsellor. In CF centres all patients undergo annual review, which enables assessment by this multidisciplinary team as well as the physician (see above).

Respiratory system

Respiratory symptoms should be managed aggressively with the aim being to defend pulmonary function.

- Standard therapy comprises antibiotics (both for acute infection and in colonised patients) and physiotherapy.

- Sputum clearance may be enhanced in some patients by the administration of nebulised recombinant DNase.

- Bronchodilators and anti-inflammatory drugs are also often helpful.

Gastrointestinal disease

The majority (90%) of CF patients have pancreatic insufficiency and benefit from replacement of enzymes and fat-soluble vitamins. Professional dietetic assessment is indicated for all patients.

There is no specific therapy for CF liver disease, but supportive management is as for other causes of cirrhosis/portal hypertension.

Transplantation

In an advanced case of the disease, lung transplantation (see Section 2.13) offers the best chance of survival. For patients awaiting a transplant, non-invasive positive-pressure ventilation can be a useful bridge; endotracheal ventilation of patients with advanced CF is almost always unsuccessful.

Broadly speaking, patients may be considered suitable for transplantation if the forced expiratory volume in 1 second (FEV_1) is <30% predicted. Other features favouring transplantation are the development of ventilatory failure and increasing hospitalisations. Because cadaveric organs are in short supply, there is increasing interest in living donor bilateral lobar lung transplantation.

> In advanced CF, respiratory failure as a result of overwhelming infection is a common cause of death. Endotracheal ventilation does not alter the outcome in this situation and hence this treatment is not usually offered.

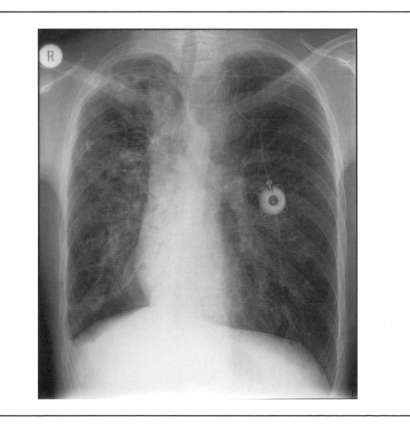

▲ **Fig. 22** CXR of an adult patient with CF. Hyperinflation and cystic change (most obvious in the right upper lobe) is evident. A Portacath is seen over the left lung field.

Complications

Of pulmonary disease

The more severe complications occur in more advanced disease:

- sinusitis and nasal polyps;

- bacterial respiratory infection;

- pneumothorax;

- haemoptysis;

- aspergillosis;

- respiratory failure and pulmonary hypertension.

Of gastrointestinal disease

Adults with CF may have abdominal pain, but the cause is seldom appendicitis or other surgically remediable problems. Although surgical advice should be sought where appropriate, most experts prefer to have a high threshold for abdominal surgery. Other complications include:

- obstruction;

- malabsorption;

- glucose intolerance/diabetes;

- cirrhosis and portal hypertension.

Other/iatrogenic

The total list of possible complications of CF is enormous but includes:

- infertility in men;

- pregnancy (represents a hazard if FEV_1 <40–50% of predicted or if there is pulmonary hypertension);

- ototoxicity from repeated aminoglycosides;

- Portacath complications.

Prognosis

The median survival of newborns with CF is now estimated to be about 40 years; this compares with 14 years in 1969. The 5-year survival rate after transplantation is around 50%.

Prevention

For parents who are CF gene carriers (eg because a sibling with CF is already identified), prenatal diagnosis is possible. The risks of chorionic villous sampling are roughly equal to those of amniocentesis but with the advantage of an earlier result.

Therapy aimed at preventing the phenotypic expression of CF by gene replacement is not yet a practical clinical option.

FURTHER READING

Scientific Background to Medicine 1, Cell Biology..

Rosenstein BJ and Zeitlin PJ. Cystic fibrosis. *Lancet* 1998; 351: 277–82.

Shapiro B, Veerarghaven S and Barbers RG. Lung transplantation for cystic fibrosis: an update and practical considerations for referring candidates. *Curr. Opin. Pulm. Med.* 1999; 5: 365–70.

Stern M and Alton E. The pathogenesis of cystic fibrosis and progress towards gene therapy. *J. R. Coll. Physicians Lond.* 1999; 33: 434–9.

Varlotta L. Management and care of the newly diagnosed patient with cystic fibrosis. *Curr. Opin. Pulm. Med.* 1998; 4: 311–18.

2.6 Occupational lung disease

2.6.1 Asbestosis and the pneumoconioses

Aetiology and pathology

The pneumoconioses are occupational lung diseases caused by inhalation of a variety of industrial dusts. Strictly speaking, asbestosis is a subtype of the pneumoconioses but, because of its relative prevalence, it tends to be considered separately. Likewise, coal worker's pneumoconiosis (CWP) merits its own discussion.

CWP aside, the pneumoconioses can be divided into two subgroups (further details in Table 30).

- Benign forms tend to be asymptomatic. They can be recognised by the CXR appearances that they produce: small round opacities caused by perivascular collections of dust.

- Fibrotic forms produce, as the name suggests, pulmonary fibrosis associated with a restrictive lung defect. They may cause symptoms and sometimes progress to respiratory failure.

Asbestosis

The interstitial fibrosis produced by asbestos exposure is dose related, with length and level of exposure relating directly to the development and severity of symptoms. There is often a lag of 20–30 years between exposure and the development of symptoms. The fibrosis tends to be in the lower lobes and is frequently associated with pleural thickening and the appearance of pleural plaques on CXR. Asbestos exposure can also lead to mesothelioma and lung cancer, particularly adenocarcinoma.

Coal worker's pneumoconiosis

CWP is seen in workers exposed to coal dust and accounts for 90% of pneumoconiosis claims for industrial compensation that are not related to asbestos exposure. The condition is generally divided into two groups.

- Simple CWP: based on the CXR appearances of small round

TABLE 30 INDUSTRIAL SUBSTANCES WHOSE DUSTS CAUSE PNEUMOCONIOSIS

Disease type	Causative agent (disease name)
Benign disease	Iron (siderosis) Tin (stannosis) Barium (bariosis) Antimony
Fibrotic disease	Asbestos Silica (silicosis) Beryllium (berylliosis) Aluminium ores (Shaver's disease or aluminosis)

opacities that represent small fibrous nodules in the lung, predominantly in the upper lobes.

- Complicated CWP (progressive massive fibrosis, PMF): a patient is said to have advanced to PMF when these fibrous lesions have reached more than 3 cm in diameter. Histologically, these larger lesions commonly undergo necrosis and cavitation.

CWP associated with rheumatoid arthritis is known as Caplan's syndrome. It is also worth noting that silicosis can also progress to PMF, and has also been associated with rheumatoid arthritis.

Clinical presentation
This may include:

- breathlessness;
- cough;
- jet-black sputum production (CWP only).

Physical signs
There will be few in the early stages of the disease, but later the patient may exhibit:

- decreased chest expansion;
- inspiratory crackles;
- wheeze (in CWP);

- clubbing (asbestosis, but not silicosis; rarely in CWP).

Investigations

Chest radiograph
The International Labour Office has produced a method of classification for the radiographic changes seen in pneumoconiosis. These classifications are largely based on the size and number of opacities seen on the CXR and are used by medical panels when discussing compensation claims.

- For benign pneumoconiosis, small round opacities are diagnostic of the disease.

- Asbestos can produce a number of changes, including pleural thickening, pleural (holly leaf) plaques, fibrosis and evidence of tumours (Fig. 23).

- Silicosis produces classical eggshell calcification around the hilar lymph nodes, as well as peripheral nodules.

- For CWP, see above.

Lung function tests
These show a restrictive picture with decreased forced vital capacity, total lung capacity, residual volume and gas transfer.

High-resolution CT scan
Prone and supine films will help reveal the extent of the disease, and are particularly helpful when extensive pleural disease masks the lung parenchyma (Fig. 23).

Treatment
A priority is avoidance of further dust exposure. The employers of the patient should, if necessary, consider a review of the protective equipment used by their other employees in the workplace. The benign pneumoconioses require no other treatment.

Fibrotic disease is normally considered resistant to therapy, except berylliosis, where high-dose prednisolone can produce clinical improvement. Occasionally, courses of steroids are tried in patients with asbestosis who are showing rapid deterioration of lung function. Treatment of CWP is largely supportive.

Complications
These may include:

- respiratory failure;
- right heart failure;
- tuberculosis in silicosis.

Compensation
Through the Industrial Injuries Scheme, workers in the UK can claim compensation for the following diseases: mesothelioma, pneumoconiosis (including CWP, silicosis and asbestosis), diffuse pleural thickening, primary carcinoma of the lung (only if accompanied by asbestosis or diffuse pleural thickening) and byssinosis. Potential claimants should be advised to contact their local Citizens Advice Bureau when a diagnosis is made.

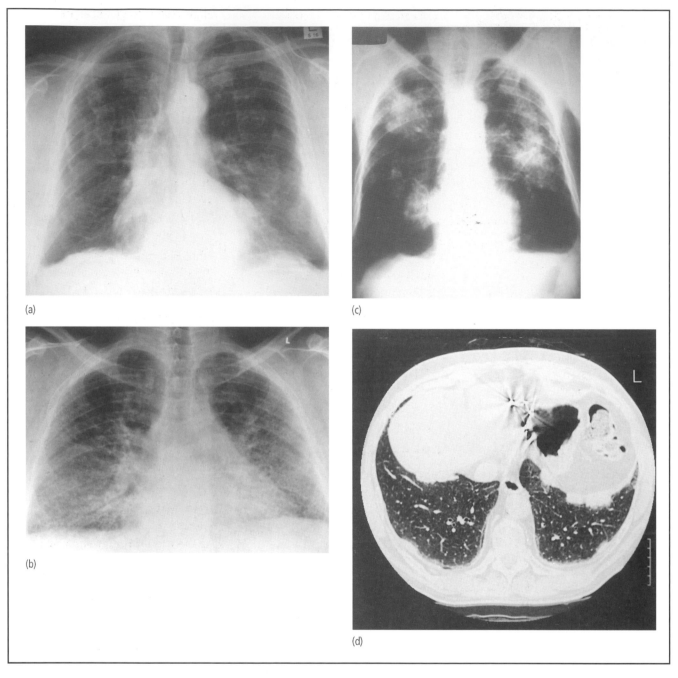

▲ **Fig. 23** (**a**) CXR of a patient with previous asbestos exposure who has extensive pleural plaques. (Courtesy of Dr J. Moore-Gillon.) (**b**) CXR showing widespread pulmonary fibrosis secondary to asbestos exposure. (Courtesy of Dr R. Rudd.) (**c**) CXR showing progressive massive fibrosis of CWP in a coal miner. (Courtesy of Dr R. Rudd.) (**d**) CT scan of the thorax: note the posterior changes, with pleural thickening, and the adjacent early changes of asbestosis. (Courtesy of Dr J. Moore-Gillon.)

FURTHER READING

Jarad NA. Asbestos-related disease. *J. R. Coll. Physicians Lond.* 1999; 33: 537–40.

- - - - - - - - - - - - - - - - - - -

Morgan WKC and Gee JBL. Asbestos-related disease. In: Morgan WKC and Seaton A, eds. *Occupational Lung Diseases*, 3rd edn. Philadelphia: WB Saunders, 1995: 308–73.

- - - - - - - - - - - - - - - - - - -

Morgan WKC and Gee JBL. Coal worker's pneumoconiosis, and other pneumoconiosis. In: Morgan WKC and Seaton A, eds. *Occupational Lung Diseases*, 3rd edn. Philadelphia: WB Saunders, 1995: 374–406.

- - - - - - - - - - - - - - - - - - -

Morgan WKC, Elmes P and McConnochie K. Pneumoconiosis. In: Brewis RAL, Corrin B, Geddes DM and

Gibson GJ, eds. *Respiratory Medicine*, 2nd edn. London: WB Saunders, 1998: 570–604.

- - - - - - - - - - - - - - - - - - -

Rudd RM. Asbestos-related disease. In: Brewis RAL, Corrin B, Geddes DM and Gibson GJ, eds. *Respiratory Medicine*, 2nd edn. London: WB Saunders, 1998: 545–69.

- - - - - - - - - - - - - - - - - - -

Waldron HA. *Lecture Notes on Occupational Medicine*, 4th edn. Oxford: Blackwell Scientific Publications, 1990.

2.7 Diffuse parenchymal lung disease

The classification of diffuse parenchymal lung disease (DPLD) has recently been updated and is summarised in Table 9. Most of the subtypes are very rare and the domain of specialist physicians. The most commonly seen in routine practice are summarised below.

2.7.1 Usual interstitial pneumonia

This was previously known as cryptogenic fibrosing alveolitis.

Aetiology

Not known, but it is more common in cigarette smokers.

Pathology

For many years the gold standard for diagnosis of cryptogenic fibrosing alveolitis was histopathological evidence from lung biopsy, which in the majority of cases shows features of usual interstitial pneumonia (UIP). With developments in high-resolution CT scanning, which can diagnose UIP with a high degree of certainty, lung biopsy is now indicated only when diagnostic doubt remains after radiological assessment. When a tissue diagnosis is required, video-assisted thoracoscopic lung biopsy or open lung biopsy is necessary, as transbronchial biopsy does not usually provide an adequate sample

to make a confident diagnosis of UIP.

Epidemiology

Most patients are between 40 and 70 years of age at the time of presentation. The incidence of UIP increases with age from 2.7 per 100,000 among adults aged 35–44 years old to 175 per 100,000 among those over 75 years old.

Clinical presentation

Insidious onset of breathlessness often with a dry cough and fatigue. Sputum production is unusual. Haemoptysis is uncommon and suggests malignancy (see below).

Physical signs

- Bibasilar late-onset inspiratory crackles: these may be present in the absence of radiographic abnormalities on the CXR.

- Finger clubbing occurs in 50% of cases.

- Look for non-pulmonary features that would suggest alternative diagnoses, eg skin rashes, arthritis or lymphadenopathy.

Investigations

Pulmonary function tests

Look for restrictive pattern and/or decreased diffusing capacity of the lung for carbon monoxide (D_{LCO}). As a high proportion of patients with UIP are smokers, in practice a mixed restrictive and obstructive pattern may be present.

Chest radiograph

Check for peripheral bilateral basilar irregular linear opacities often with fine nodules, evidence of volume loss and, in severe cases, honeycombing. In the small proportion of cases subsequently shown to have UIP, the CXR may be normal.

High-resolution CT scan of the chest

Look for peripheral and basal subpleural distribution, honeycombing, irregular linear opacities, septal and intralobular thickening, minimal ground-glass opacities and traction bronchiectasis.

Arterial blood gases

These may be normal at rest, or may reveal hypoxaemia and respiratory alkalosis. Normal resting P_{aO_2} or S_{aO_2} does not rule out significant hypoxaemia during exercise or sleep, which is common in DPLD.

Differential diagnosis

UIP is a diagnosis of exclusion. Other known causes that may show similar high-resolution CT appearances to UIP must be excluded, such as asbestosis, drug reaction, chronic hypersensitivity pneumonia, chronic sarcoidosis and cryptogenic organising pneumonia.

Treatment

There have been no prospective, placebo-controlled, randomised trials. Only a minority respond to treatment, and the pros and cons of immunosuppressive therapy should be discussed with each patient. Options for treatment include the following.

- First-line treatment: oral prednisolone 0.5 mg/kg with or without azathioprine (2–3 mg/kg daily), with reassessment at 1 month. In severely ill patients intravenous methylprednisolone may be used. A response (1–3 months) or stability should be followed by a slow tapering of prednisolone to a maintenance dose of 10 mg daily for 1 year. A further slow reduction may be considered subsequently. Objective response rates are poor.

- Second-line treatment: cyclophosphamide (1–2 mg/kg) if azathioprine is not tolerated.

- Single lung transplantation: for end-stage disease (see Section 2.13).

- Palliative treatment: oxygen, diuretics and opiates.

Complications

- Cor pulmonale and respiratory failure.

- Ten-fold increased risk of lung maligancy.

Prognosis

Poor: median survival is 3 years; 10-year survival rate is 5–10%.

FURTHER READING

Diffuse Parenchymal Lung Disease Group. The diagnosis, assessment and treatment of diffuse parenchymal lung disease in adults. *Thorax* 1999; 54: S1–S14.

Joint Statement of the American Thoracic Society (ATS) and the European Respiratory Society (ERS). ATS guidelines: Idiopathic pulmonary fibrosis: diagnosis and treatment. *Am. J. Respir. Crit. Care Med.* 2000; 161: 646–64.

2.7.2 Cryptogenic organising pneumonia

Previously known as bronchiolitis obliterans organising pneumonia.

Aetiology

Not known. Possibly results from viral infection, cryptic antigens or capsid proteins. Cryptogenic organising pneumonia (COP) may be a manifestation of, or be associated with, various medical conditions. This is predominantly connective tissue disease, but other reported conditions include infection (viral, *Mycoplasma pneumoniae* and HIV), vasculitis, drug toxicity, toxic fume inhalation or smoke inhalation, post radiation, aspiration and transplantation.

Pathology

Bronchiolar and alveolar fibrous plugging. Lung architecture is preserved (no fibrosis).

Epidemiology

COP occurs most commonly in the fifth and sixth decades of life, and has no gender preference.

Clinical presentation

Typically there is a subacute (6–10 weeks) onset with 'flu-like illness (fever, malaise and weight loss), persistent cough and breathlessness. Occasionally there is a fulminant presentation with rapidly progressive severe disease.

Physical signs

Inspiratory crackles are heard in up to 74% of cases, but physical examination may be normal.

Investigations

- Blood tests: neutrophilic leucocytosis in 50% of patients and elevated inflammatory markers (erythrocyte sedimentation rate and C-reactive protein).

- CXR: patchy, bilateral and variable-sized areas of consolidation predominantly in the lower lobes, often peripherally. The infiltrates may be migratory. Unilateral changes occur in 5% of cases.

- High-resolution CT scan: bilateral, patchy and asymmetric areas of airspace consolidation with ground-glass opacities. These are mainly in the lower zones with a subpleural or peribronchial distribution.

- Pulmonary function tests: restrictive defect with reduced D_{LCO}.

- Arterial blood gases: resting or exercise hypoxaemia in 80% of patients.

- Video-assisted thoracoscopic lung biopsy: this is the most helpful examination. A wedge biopsy is required to avoid sampling and interpretation errors related to patchy interstitial changes. As COP often requires lengthy corticosteroid treatment, histopathological confirmation is strongly recommended, if clinically feasible.

Differential diagnosis

A variety of other disorders may have a similar presentation, such as infections (including opportunistic), pulmonary lymphoma (beware, as this may initially improve with corticosteroids), usual interstitial pneumonia, bronchoalveolar carcinoma, chronic eosinophilic pneumonia and sarcoidosis.

Treatment

Oral corticosteroids are usually very effective. The optimal regimen is uncertain, but usually high-dose prednisolone (1.0–1.5 mg/kg daily) is recommended, gradually tapering to zero over several months. Most patients improve within several weeks to 3 months.

Prognosis

Excellent in the majority of patients. However, relapses are common (58%), especially within the first 12 months, so close monitoring with CXR and pulmonary function test is recommended. Patients with frequent recurrences (more than three episodes) may require low-dose maintenance corticosteroid therapy.

 Although COP is uncommon, it should be included in the differential diagnosis in any patient with bilateral airspace radiological changes that are unresponsive to antibiotics.

FURTHER READING

Cordier JF. Cryptogenic organizing pneumonia. *Clin. Chest Med.* 2004; 25: 727–38.

Schlesinger C and Koss M. The organizing pneumonias: an update and review. *Curr. Opin. Pulm. Med.* 2005; 11: 422–30.

2.7.3 Bronchiolitis obliterans

Do not confuse bronchiolitis obliterans (BO) with cryptogenic organising pneumonia (COP). Both conditions differ clinically, radiologically and histologically and in their responsiveness to steroid treatment.

Aetiology

BO is characterised by mainly irreversible airflow obstruction that is usually progressive. It occurs mainly in lung and heart–lung allograft recipients, and is the major cause of lung allograft rejection. The most common cause of non-transplant BO is connective tissue disease (especially rheumatoid arthritis); other less common causes include toxic fume inhalation, infection (viral and *Mycoplasma pneumoniae*), drugs (penicillamine), radiation and ulcerative colitis.

Pathology

The hallmark of BO is submucosal bronchiolar fibrosis that is preceded by bronchiolar inflammation resulting in epithelial necrosis. As a result of this the bronchiole becomes plugged by granulation tissue. Subsequently, collagen is formed, which may completely obliterate the airway lumen.

Clinical presentation

This is often non-specific and insidious. The most common complaint is exertional dyspnoea, often accompanied by a chronic productive cough. Lung and heart–lung allograft recipients may present with a decline in their forced expiratory volume in 1 second (FEV_1) (see Section 2.13).

Physical signs

These are often unremarkable in the early stages. In more advanced stages there are signs of hyperinflation, end-inspiratory crackles, squeaks and wheezes.

Investigations

- Pulmonary function tests: to look for an obstructive defect.

- CXR: initially normal or may show hyperinflation. As the disease progresses, subsegmental atelectasis, loss of volume and/or fibrosis may be found.

- High-resolution CT scan of the chest: radiological appearances are quite distinct from those of COP and reflect underlying airway obstruction. For example, bronchial wall thickening of the segmental and subsegmental bronchi with mosaic perfusion is clearly demonstrated on CT scan carried out during expiration.

- Lung biopsy: the only method of definite diagnosis of BO. However, this may be difficult because the diagnostic yield of transbronchial biopsy in BO varies between 15 and 82%, due to the patchy nature of BO and the small size of biopsy samples obtained during the procedure. Video-assisted thoracoscopic lung biopsy should be considered if transbronchial biopsy is inconclusive or atypical.

- Arterial blood gases: hypoxaemia and hypercapnia develop in end-stage disease only.

Differential diagnosis

Consider asthma, emphysema, desquamative interstitial pneumonia and hypersensitivity pneumonia.

Treatment

There is no reliable therapy. Unlike patients with COP, those with BO usually respond poorly to corticosteroids. Various immunosuppressive regimens are used to slow the rate of decline in FEV_1.

Prognosis

BO has a variable course. Some patients present with a rapid decline in FEV_1 and are likely to die within a year of diagnosis, whereas others show progressive slow deterioration. Overall mortality varies from 25 to 56%, and most patients die of infection or respiratory failure.

FURTHER READING

Chan A and Allen R. Bronchiolitis obliterans: an update. *Curr. Opin. Pulm. Med.* 2004; 10: 133–41.

2.8 Miscellaneous conditions

2.8.1 Extrinsic allergic alveolitis

Aetiology

Extrinsic allergic alveolitis (EAA), also known as hypersensitivity pneumonia, is caused by hypersensitivity to inhaled organic dusts. The best-known type is farmer's lung, but an enormous range of agents has been reported to cause the condition (Table 31).

Epidemiology

EAA accounts for 2% of all occupational lung disease: half of these cases occur in farmers.

Pathology

Histological material is rarely available, but the condition begins as a non-specific diffuse pneumonia that later develops the characteristic feature of epithelioid non-caseating granulomas. Fibrosis and obstruction/obliteration of bronchioles arises in parallel with inflammatory changes. Honeycombing occurs in advanced cases.

Acute form of EAA

Clinical presentation

This can occur weeks to years after a sensitising period of exposure. The patient develops recurrent 'flu-like illness (malaise, fever, headache, and general aches and pains) with a cough and breathlessness, usually starting about 6 hours after exposure to the relevant organic dust. Wheeze can occur but is not a typical feature. Breathing difficulty can range from trivial to life-threatening.

Physical signs

- Fever.

- Respiratory distress.

- Basal crackles.

- Clubbing is rare.

Investigations

- Unless the patient has recently been exposed to the precipitant, pulmonary function tests are likely to be normal.

- The CXR may be normal, but it characteristically reveals diffuse interstitial shadowing. This is particularly the case in lower and mid zones, resolving within 24–48 hours after exposure has ceased.

- The history is often diagnostic, but it may be necessary, particularly in circumstances not known to be associated with EAA, to make industrial hygiene measurements (eg with personal samplers) so that respirable agents can be identified.

- The demonstration of a serum IgG antibody response to the inducing organic dust is the most widely used method of confirming hypersensitivity: a negative test effectively excludes EAA (to that antigen), but false positives are common.

- When the diagnosis is in doubt, inhalational challenge tests are sometimes used in specialist centres.

Differential diagnosis

A single episode must be distinguished from other acute parenchymal lung disorders associated with systemic symptoms, the most common of these being infection. Distinction of recurrent episodes from organic dust toxic syndrome (usually caused by fungal toxins) and nitrogen dioxide pneumonia (silo-filler's disease) can be extremely difficult in those at risk of all these conditions.

Treatment

In an acute episode, spontaneous recovery begins within 12–24 hours of removing the sensitising antigen. Steroids can hasten improvement, but there is a concern that they may increase the risk of recurrence. Respiratory support (oxygen and, rarely, mechanical ventilation) may be needed in severe cases.

Prevention

Avoidance of exposure is the counsel of perfection, but is easier said than done in many cases. Patients may be unwilling to put their livelihood (eg farming) or hobbies (eg pigeons) at risk. Exposure can be reduced by changing work practices or the use of industrial respirators. If monitoring suggests that disease is progressive despite these manoeuvres, then exposure must cease. An affected worker may be entitled to compensation.

	Source	Antigen
TABLE 31 AETIOLOGY OF EAA		
Farmer's lung	Mouldy hay	*Micropolyspora faeni*
Pigeon fancier's lung	Pigeons, parakeets, budgerigars, etc.	Avian or animal proteins
Malt worker's lung	Mouldy malt	*Aspergillus clavatus*
Cheese worker's lung	Cheese mould	*Penicillium casei*
Bagassosis	Mouldy sugar cane	*Thermoactinomyces sacchari*

Prognosis

Continuing exposure and repeated acute exacerbations can lead to permanent impairment of lung function, but this is relatively uncommon.

Occupational aspects

The environment that has caused illness in one individual may pose a risk to others. It may be necessary to survey the exposed population at risk, eg with questionnaires about respiratory symptoms and serological tests.

Chronic form of EAA

Clinical presentation

This presents as a gradual reduction in exercise tolerance because of worsening breathlessness. There is no systemic upset, except sometimes weight loss, and no acute exacerbations. It most often occurs in those exposed continuously to a low level of antigen, eg a patient who keeps a single budgerigar (parakeet) at home, rather than someone exposed intermittently to high levels of antigen.

Physical signs

Respiratory distress. Widespread crackles, as in other forms of diffuse parenchymal lung disease, but in contrast clubbing is uncommon. Signs of pulmonary hypertension and right heart failure may develop.

Investigations

- Pulmonary function tests reveal restricted ventilation (forced vital capacity diminished in proportion to forced expiratory volume in 1 second), increased residual volume and impaired carbon monoxide transfer factor.

- The CXR can show a range of patterns, including diffuse interstitial shadowing,

honeycombing and fibrotic changes (in the upper lobes particularly).

- High-resolution CT scanning is more sensitive than the CXR, again showing a range of appearances, with a mosaic pattern being most characteristic.

- Bronchoscopy/bronchoalveolar lavage is useful in excluding other diagnoses, and a lung biopsy may be needed to distinguish from other causes of diffuse parenchymal lung disease in some cases.

Differential diagnosis

The main differential diagnosis in many cases is sarcoidosis, as well as other granulomatous lung conditions.

Treatment/prevention

Avoidance of exposure, as indicated above for acute EAA. Steroids are again thought to hasten improvement, but the optimum dose and duration of treatment is not known and, as for acute EAA, their use may be associated with relapse.

Complications/prognosis

Many patients continue their antigenic exposure despite medical advice to the contrary. Some cases develop respiratory failure, but this is relatively uncommon.

Occupational aspects

As for acute EAA.

FURTHER READING

Hendrick DJ, Faux JA and Marshall R. Budgerigar fancier's lung: the commonest variety of allergic alveolitis in Britain. *BMJ* 1978; 2: 81–4.

- - - - - - - - - - - - - - - - - -

Grammar LC. Occupational allergic alveolitis. *Ann. Allergy Asthma Immunol.* 1999; 83: 602–6.

2.8.2 Sarcoidosis

Aetiology

Sarcoidosis is a multisystem non-caseating granulomatous disorder of unknown cause. It may result from an exaggerated cellular immune response to some antigens. Other points include the following.

- Genetic factors: familial cases are described and some patterns of disease are more prevalent in certain racial groups.

- Increased incidence in black patients with human leucocyte antigen (HLA)-Bw15.

- Epstein–Barr virus has been implicated.

- *Mycobacterium tuberculosis* may be a trigger.

Pathology

Accumulation of T-helper (CD4) lymphocytes and mononuclear phagocytes in the affected organs, driven by unknown antigens, is followed by the formation of granulomas with accumulation of macrophages and multinucleated giant cells in active disease. The alveolar macrophages in the lungs release platelet-derived growth factor and fibronectin. These stimulate fibroblast proliferation and result in fibrosis, which is almost always irreversible.

Epidemiology

- Sarcoidosis is a common disease and occurs worldwide, but there is great geographical variation. The incidence in the UK is 19 per 100,000, whereas it is much less common in Japan.

- Maximum incidence is between 30 and 40 years of age.

- It is more common in females.

TABLE 32 COMMON CLINICAL FEATURES OF SARCOIDOSIS

Body system involved	Symptoms	Signs
Respiratory	Cough, dyspnoea, wheeze	Crackles
Skin	Painful dusky blue nodules and shiny raised purple eruption on nose, face, hands or feet	Erythema nodosum, lupus pernio
Eyes	Gritty painful eyes, photophobia	Keratoconjunctivitis, uveitis, iridocyclitis, chorioretinitis
Musculoskeletal	Swollen digits, joint pains, proximal myopathy	Phalangeal bone cysts, proximal muscle weakness
Cardiological	Dyspnoea (cardiac failure), palpitations	Irregular pulse/rhythm disturbance, crackles at lung bases
Neurological	Headache, paraesthesia	Bell's palsy, mononeuritis, aseptic meningitis
Gastrointestinal	Abdominal pain, disordered LFTs	Pancreatitis, hepatomegaly
Endocrine/metabolic	Polyuria, polydipsia, confusion (caused by hypercalcaemia)	Splenomegaly
Renal	Renal colic caused by calculi	Parotid enlargement
Haematological	Lymphadenopathy	
Exocrine	Parotid gland enlargement	

LFT, liver function test.

- In the USA, it is 10–17 times more common in black people than white people.

Clinical presentation

The symptoms and signs depend on the organ(s) involved (Table 32). In over 90% of the patients the lungs are affected. Pulmonary involvement may be asymptomatic and detected by a routine CXR. Acute or subacute sarcoidosis may develop over a period of weeks.

Investigations

Chest radiograph

The International Congress on Sarcoidosis established four stages of sarcoidosis based on the CXR (Fig. 24).

Serum angiotensin-converting enzyme

- Raised levels in 41–80% of patients only.
- Raised levels also seen in hepatitis, miliary tuberculosis (TB), HIV and histoplasmosis.
- If it is raised, it may be a useful contributing factor in monitoring disease progression and treatment.

Serum calcium

Sarcoid tissue produces an abnormal hydroxylating enzyme that converts vitamin D precursors to active 1,25-dihydroxycholecalciferol leading to hypercalcaemia and hypercalciuria, which respond to corticosteroids.

Heaf or tuberculin test

Very often the main differential diagnosis is TB, either because of the finding of mediastinal lymphadenopathy or because a biopsy obtained elsewhere (eg the liver) has unexpectedly shown granuloma. In this case the finding of anergy in response to Heaf or tuberculin testing would favour sarcoid. The problems with this approach are:

- prior BCG makes interpretation difficult;

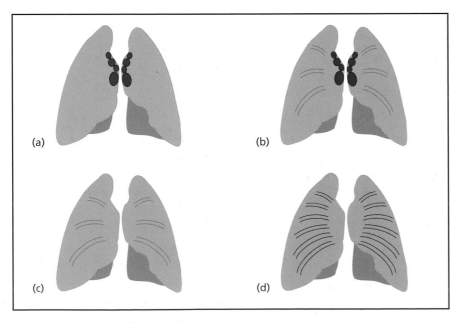

(a)

(b)

(c)

(d)

▲**Fig. 24** Stages of sarcoidosis: (**a**) stage I, hilar lymph node enlargement only; (**b**) stage II, lymph node enlargement and diffuse pulmonary disease; (**c**) stage III, diffuse pulmonary disease without lymph node enlargement; (**d**) stage IV, pulmonary fibrosis. (Note that stage 0 is a normal CXR.)

- patients with overwhelming TB can be anergic, particularly if they also have HIV.

Transbronchial biopsy

Transbronchial biopsy reveals granuloma in 85–90% of patients and these may also be seen in endobronchial specimens. In cases that are clinically clear-cut, biopsy is not required. However, it is essential to obtain histological material if there is diagnostic doubt.

Tests of disease activity

These will depend on the parameters that were originally abnormal. Good examples might be:

- Kco if there is pulmonary disease;

- liver function tests;

- serum angiotensin-converting enzyme, erythrocyte sedimentation rate, calcium.

Differential diagnosis

The differential diagnosis depends on the distribution of organ involvement, but might include:

- TB;

- lymphoma;

- eosinophilic granuloma;

- berylliosis;

- interstitial fibrosis from other causes.

Treatment

Corticosteroids

The beneficial effects of corticosteroids were first reported in 1951, but many patients do not need treatment: stage 0 and 1 disease commonly resolve spontaneously. Stage 2 disease without any symptoms should be monitored for at least 6 months, with treatment offered if symptoms develop (dyspnoea and cough).

Oral prednisolone (0.5 mg/kg daily) is the treatment of choice, given for 4 weeks and then reduced in a stepwise pattern to a maintenance dose of 5–15 mg/day. The disease should be monitored by the patient's symptoms, CXR and carbon monoxide transfer factor (see Section 3.6.2). Relapse is common and is usually treated with an increase in dose.

Inhaled corticosteroids

Inhaled budesonide may have a role as maintenance treatment once disease activity has been suppressed by oral steroids. Topical steroids may be used for cutaneous sarcoid, and systemic steroids for ocular sarcoid.

Immunosuppressants and other therapies

- Chloroquine, chlorambucil, methotrexate, azathioprine, cyclophosphamide, ciclosporin and pentoxifylline have been tried in sarcoidosis, often as steroid-sparing agents.

- Oxygen for hypoxaemia.

- Lung transplantation (see Section 2.13).

Complications

These relate to the distribution of organ involvement.

- Pulmonary fibrosis with hypoxaemia resulting in cor pulmonale.

- Mycetoma: may grow within a lung cavity and cause severe haemoptysis.

- Hypercalcaemia, which can provoke renal failure.

- Complications related to affected organ.

Prognosis

- Stage 0 and 1 disease are usually self-limiting.

- Stage 2 disease: 60–70% of patients show complete radiographic clearance within 5 years.

- Stage 3 disease is unlikely to clear and often leads to cor pulmonale if untreated.

FURTHER READING

British Thoracic Society. The diagnosis, assessment and treatment of diffuse parenchymal lung disease in adults. *Thorax* 1999; 54: S1–S14.

Crystal RG. Sarcoidosis. In: Wilson JD, Braunwald E, Isselbacher KJ, *et al. Harrison's Principles of Internal Medicine*, 12th edn. New York: McGraw-Hill, 1991: 1463–9.

Fanburg BL and Lazarus DS. Sarcoidosis. In: Murray JF and Nadel JA, eds. *Textbook of Respiratory Medicine*, 2nd edn. Philadelphia: WB Saunders, 1994: 1873–88.

Flenley DC. *Respiratory Medicine*, 2nd edn. London: Baillière Tindall, 1989: 277–84.

2.8.3 Respiratory complications of rheumatoid arthritis

Aetiology

The association of rheumatoid arthritis with lung disease may be due to:

- rheumatoid-associated lung disease;

- drug-related lung disease secondary to drugs used to treat rheumatoid arthritis;

- infection secondary to immunosuppression;

- coexistent medical conditions.

Epidemiology

Although rheumatoid arthritis is more common in women, rheumatoid lung disease occurs more frequently in men who have long-standing rheumatoid disease, a positive rheumatoid factor and subcutaneous nodules.

Pulmonary involvement is one of the most frequent extra-articular manifestations of rheumatoid arthritis. The most common lung diseases associated with rheumatoid arthritis are interstitial lung disease (ILD) and pleural effusion. Approximately 30–40% of patients with rheumatoid arthritis demonstrate either radiological or pulmonary function abnormalities indicative of interstitial fibrosis or restrictive lung disease.

Although rheumatoid arthritis disease activity is important, smoking is the most consistent independent predictor of radiological and physiological abnormalities suggestive of ILD in rheumatoid arthritis.

Clinical presentation

The range of pulmonary problems is wide.

Rheumatoid nodules

Rheumatoid nodules are the only pulmonary manifestation specific to rheumatoid arthritis. They are typically benign but can lead to pleural effusion, pneumothorax, haemoptysis, secondary infection and bronchopulmonary fistula.

Caplan's syndrome

This is the combination of rheumatoid arthritis with pneumoconiosis related to mining dust. Look for rapid development of multiple basal peripheral nodules in the rheumatoid arthritis patient who has a history of exposure to mining dusts. This can progress to progressive massive pulmonary fibrosis.

Interstitial lung disease

Radiographic findings of ILD occur in 2–5% of patients, while diffusion capacity abnormalities occur in 40%. High-resolution CT scans and histology have shown even higher rates, but clinically significant disease probably occurs in 5–10% of rheumatoid patients.

Bronchiolitis

- Bronchiolitis obliterans with organising pneumonia: bilateral parenchymal opacities, often with preserved lung volumes. Typically presents as a relapsing, non-resolving pneumonia that does not respond to antibiotics. Steroids can be curative.

- Obliterative bronchiolitis: rare, usually fatal condition. Associated with penicillamine, gold and sulfasalazine treatment. Presents with rapid-onset dyspnoea and dry cough. Fever is uncommon.

Bronchiectasis

About 10% of patients may show radiographic signs of bronchiectasis and it may occur in the absence of ILD. Rheumatoid arthritis patients with this complication are more likely to be heterozygous for the transmembrane conductance regulator mutation seen in cystic fibrosis.

Arteritis

Arteritis of the pulmonary artery and lung is rare. Signs of systemic vasculitis are usually present.

Infection

Respiratory infections account for 15–20% of deaths in rheumatoid patients.

Pleural effusions

These are common in rheumatoid arthritis, are exudative and have a low glucose. Occasionally an empyema may develop.

Lung cancer

Lung cancer is more common in patients with rheumatoid arthritis than in normal control subjects.

Other diseases

Patients with rheumatoid arthritis can develop apical fibrobullous disease (apical fibrotic cavity lesions similar to ankylosing spondylitis), thoracic cage immobility causing restrictive lung disease and, rarely, primary pulmonary hypertension. Secondary pulmonary hypertension (due to ILD) is more common.

Methotrexate pneumonia

Methotrexate pneumonia is an unpredictable and life-threatening side effect that may occur in 1–5% of patients given this drug. Presentation is often subacute, with symptoms of cough, dyspnoea and fever often present for several weeks or months before diagnosis. Progression to respiratory failure can be rapid. Early diagnosis, cessation of methotrexate and treatment with corticosteroids and/or cyclophosphamide are important in management. There is a high rate of recurrence of lung injury after a rechallenge with methotrexate.

Penicillamine and gold can also cause pulmonary complications.

FURTHER READING

Rheumatology and Clinical Immunology, Section 2.3.3.

2.8.4 Pulmonary vasculitis

Aetiology

This is a group of conditions characterised by the prescence of antineutrophil cytoplasmic antibodies (ANCA). These antibodies are split into two types on the basis of the pattern of immunofluorescence:

- c-ANCA directed against proteinase-3;

- p-ANCA directed against myeloperoxidase.

Some ANCA-positive patterns do not fit into either category. Many, but not all, have associated evidence of systemic vasculitis. The exact pathophysiology of vasculitides is unknown but one current hypothesis is that primed neutrophils release lysosomal enzymes and reactive oxygen species that cause endothelial damage.

Vasculitides are classified by size of vessel (see *Rheumatology and Clinical Immunology*, Section 2.5).

Large-vessel vasculitis

Temporal arteritis and Takayasu's arteritis cause large-vessel vasculitis. These do not generally cause pulmonary disease, except where there is involvement of the thoracic aorta.

Medium-vessel vasculitis

Churg–Strauss syndrome, polyarteritis nodosa and Kawasaki's disease cause medium-vessel vasculitis. Churg–Strauss syndrome involves both small and medium-sized arteries. Polyarteritis nodosa can involve bronchial arteries.

Small-vessel vasculitis

Wegener's granulomatosis, Churg–Strauss syndrome and Henoch–Schönlein syndrome (the latter rarely involves the lung) cause small-vessel vasculitis. In Wegener's granulomatosis, involvement of the respiratory tract occurs by definition. Wegener's granulomatosis is c-ANCA positive in >90% of patients. p-ANCA has an association with Churg–Strauss syndrome.

For practical purposes the two conditions of greatest relevance to the lung are Wegener's granulomatosis and Churg–Strauss syndrome. Some cases of Churg–Strauss syndrome have been described in patients treated for asthma with leukotriene antagonists. Opinion is divided as to whether Churg–Strauss syndrome has been caused by these drugs or simply uncovered because of the reduction in steroid dose permitted by their use.

Epidemiology

- Wegener's granulomatosis: mean age at presentation 41 years. No gender predominance. Median time to diagnosis 5 months.

- Churg–Strauss syndrome: mean age of onset of asthma is 35 years and of vasculitis is 38 years.

Clinical presentation

Wegener's granulomatosis

The majority (90%) of sufferers present with upper or lower respiratory tract symptoms; 73% of cases involve nasal, sinus or tracheal airways. Respiratory symptoms include:

- cough (in 46%);

- haemoptysis (in 30%);

- pleuritis (in 28%).

Other presentations are seen: 77% develop glomerulonephritis within 2 years of onset; 52% develop ocular symptoms during their illness (eg proptosis); 67% experience arthralgia. Fever is present in 50% during the course of the illness. Skin involvement, mononeuritis multiplex and pericarditis are other recognised features.

Churg–Strauss syndrome

This has three distinct phases:

1. prodromal phase of asthma/rhinitis;

2. blood and tissue eosinophilia;

3. characterised by systemic vasculitis.

In the final phase, cardiac (48%) and skin (67%) lesions are characteristic. Glomerulonephritis, mononeuritis, arthropathy and conjunctivitis are also recognised.

Physical signs

These depend on the clinical presentation (see above) but could include the following.

- Wegener's granulomatosis: pulmonary signs could include those of consolidation or pleural effusion. Upper airway ulceration may be visible on physical examination.

- Churg–Strauss syndrome: in the prodromal phase wheeze and reduced peak flow are evident. Later, skin lesions (erythema, purpura with or without nodules) and signs of cardiac failure can be seen.

> **Consider Churg–Strauss syndrome in patients with asthma whose disease becomes more aggressive and steroid dependent.**

Investigations

FBC

In Wegener's granulomatosis there may be a normochromic anaemia

(73%) with leucocytosis and thrombocytosis. A normochromic anaemia may also occur in Churg–Strauss syndrome, but the characteristic abnormality is eosinophilia. The erythrocyte sedimentation rate is usually high in both conditions.

Antineutrophil cytoplasmic antibodies

- Approximately 90% of patients with Wegener's granulomatosis are c-ANCA positive.

- Of those with Churg–Strauss syndrome, 48% are p-ANCA positive.

Histology

Except in clinically clear-cut cases, histological confirmation of diagnosis is required. However, the yield of diagnostic histology by transbronchial biopsy in patients with Wegener's granulomatosis is low (approximately 10%). Alternative possibilities include:

- biopsy of upper airway lesions;

- renal biopsy (if there is evidence of nephritis);

- open lung biopsy.

Other investigations

- Screening blood tests: renal and liver function tests, antinuclear antibodies, rheumatoid factor, angiotensin-converting enzyme and autoantibodies.

- Urine: look for proteinuria, haematuria and cellular casts as evidence of renal involvement.

- CXR: may show pulmonary infiltrates, nodules, haemorrhage or a combination of these abnormalities (in 45% of patients).

- High-resolution CT scan: may be a useful adjunct to diagnosis and for monitoring disease progression.

Differential diagnosis

The differential diagnosis depends on the nature of the presenting symptom. The more difficult differential can be of eosinophilia. Where there is significant diagnostic doubt, the case for obtaining biopsy material is strengthened.

Treatment

- Wegener's granulomatosis: steroids with or without cyclophosphamide with or without plasmapheresis. Septrin may have a role for patients with disease confined to the upper airway. Azathioprine is often used to maintain remission.

- Churg–Strauss syndrome: steroids with or without cyclophosphamide with or without plasmapheresis.

Complications

- Wegener's granulomatosis: chronic renal insufficiency (in 42%, of whom one-quarter will require dialysis), hearing loss (in 35%), nasal deformities (in 28%), tracheal stenosis (in 13%) and visual loss (in 8%).

- Churg–Strauss syndrome: essentially a more benign condition than Wegener's granulomatosis, but myocardial damage and gastrointestinal tract involvement are recognised.

Prognosis

- Wegener's granulomatosis: 13% mortality.

- Churg–Strauss syndrome: 11% morbidity in long-term follow-up.

FURTHER READING

Nephrology, Sections 1.4.3 and 2.7.6.

Rheumatology and Clinical Immunology, Sections 1.1.7 and 2.5.

Burns A. Pulmonary vasculitis. *Thorax* 1998; 53: 220–7.

Guillevin L, Cohen P, Gayraud M, *et al.* Churg–Strauss syndrome. Clinical study and long-term follow up of 96 patients. *Medicine (Baltimore)* 1999; 78: 26–37.

Hoffman GS, Kerr GS, Leavitt RY, *et al.* Wegener granulomatosis: an analysis of 158 patients. *Ann. Intern. Med.* 1992; 116: 488–98.

Schnabel A, Holl-Ulrich K, Dalhoff K, *et al.* Efficacy of transbronchial biopsy in pulmonary vasculitides. *Eur. Respir. J.* 1997; 10: 2738–43.

Stirling RG and Chung KF. Leukotriene antagonists and Churg–Strauss syndrome: the smoking gun. *Thorax* 1999; 54: 865–6.

2.8.5 Pulmonary eosinophilia

Aetiology/pathology

Pulmonary eosinophilia is the term used for a group of disorders of different aetiology, characterised by peripheral blood eosinophilia and eosinophilic pulmonary infiltrates. The causes of pulmonary eosinophilia include:

- allergic bronchopulmonary aspergillosis;

- drug-induced pulmonary eosinophilia;

- tropical pulmonary eosinophilia;

- Löffler's syndrome;

- Churg–Strauss syndrome;

- hypereosinophilic syndrome;

- eosinophilic pneumonia.

Allergic bronchopulmonary aspergillosis

This is mainly caused by *Aspergillus fumigatus*, but may be caused by other *Aspergillus* species and *Candida*. Inhaled spores are deposited in secretions and then proliferate, resulting in mucous plugging of the airways. There is production of IgE and IgG antibodies and eosinophilic infiltration of the lungs. Proximal bronchiectasis occurs as the result of a local immune reaction.

Drug-induced pulmonary eosinophilia

Various drugs can cause pulmonary infiltrates, eosinophilia, fever and pulmonary symptoms such as wheeze and cough:

- aspirin;
- methotrexate;
- sulphonamides;
- captopril;
- naproxen;
- tetracycline;
- carbamazepine;
- nitrofurantoin;
- tolazamide;
- chlorpropamide;
- penicillamine;
- bleomycin;
- chlorpromazine;
- penicillin;
- gold;
- imipramine;
- phenytoin;
- sulfasalazine.

Tropical pulmonary eosinophilia

The common causes include:

- *Wuchereria bancrofti*;
- *Brugia malayi*;
- *Ancylostoma duodenale*;

- *Strongyloides stercoralis*;
- *Toxocara canis*.

Hypereosinophilic syndrome

This is characterised by marked blood eosinophilia and eosinophilic infiltration of the heart, lungs, skin, central nervous system and other organs. It usually affects men in the fourth decade and has high morbidity and mortality.

Chronic eosinophilic pneumonia

This is characterised by blood eosinophilia with pulmonary eosinophilic infiltration for which there is no obvious cause.

Epidemiology

- Allergic bronchopulmonary aspergillosis: the most common cause of eosinophilia. Occurs worldwide and at any age.

- Drug-induced pulmonary eosinophilia: dependent on local patterns of drug use.

- Tropical pulmonary eosinophilia: commonly seen in Asia, Africa and South America.

- Chronic eosinophilic pneumonia: mainly affects middle-aged women with a history of asthma.

Clinical presentation

- Allergic bronchopulmonary aspergillosis: most patients present with asthma; 10% have night sweats, fever or malaise.

- Drug-induced pulmonary eosinophilia: cough, dyspnoea and fever may start within hours of taking the drug.

- Tropical pulmonary eosinophilia: most patients are young adults and present with cough, mainly nocturnal. Breathlessness, chest pain, fever, weight loss and anorexia may occur. If untreated,

symptoms may persist or remit spontaneously and recur later.

- Hypereosinophilic syndrome: patients present with fever, anorexia and weight loss along with symptoms secondary to the organ affected. In 60% of cases the heart is affected with arrhythmias and heart failure. In 50% of cases the lungs are involved and the patient complains of cough.

- Chronic eosinophilic pneumonia: patients present with cough, dyspnoea, fever and weight loss.

Physical signs

- Allergic bronchopulmonary aspergillosis: there may be signs of consolidation or simply wheeze.

- Drug-induced pulmonary eosinophilia: wheeze and respiratory distress.

- Tropical pulmonary eosinophilia: wheeze.

- Hypereosinophilic syndrome: signs of mitral and tricuspid valve incompetence. Pulmonary consolidation and pleural effusions can occur.

Investigations

Allergic bronchopulmonary aspergillosis

- Blood eosinophilia is moderate ($0.5-2.0 \times 10^9$/L).

- All patients show positive immediate skin-prick test to *A. fumigatus*.

- IgG precipating antibodies to *A. fumigatus* are found in over 90% of patients.

- Total serum IgE is elevated during acute episodes, and serum IgE can be used to monitor treatment.

- A CXR may show segmental or lobar collapse, or bronchiectasis. In the acute phase, transient pulmonary infiltrates may be seen.

Drug-induced pulmonary eosinophilia

A CXR may show transient pulmonary infiltrates.

Tropical pulmonary eosinophilia

- Blood eosinophilia is high ($5-60 \times 10^9$/L).

- IgE is markedly elevated.

- Antifilarial antibodies are present in high titre.

- A CXR may be normal, but more typically it will show diffuse mottling with lesions 1–3 mm in diameter.

Chronic eosinophilic pneumonia

- There is likely to be peripheral eosinophilia, anaemia, raised erythrocyte sedimentation rate and elevated IgE.

- Lung function tests show a restrictive or mixed defect.

- CXR shows peripheral pulmonary densities that have been described as 'photograph negative of pulmonary oedema'.

Treatment

Allergic bronchopulmonary aspergillosis

Treatment is with oral corticosteroids during acute episodes. Response to treatment can be monitored by radiologic clearing, resolution of eosinophilia or serum IgE levels.

Drug-induced pulmonary eosinophilia

Withdrawal of the drug results in resolution of the symptoms, which can be hastened by corticosteroids.

Tropical pulmonary eosinophilia

- Treatment of filarial disease is with diethylcarbamazine (not available in the UK), building up to a dose of 6 mg/kg daily for 3 weeks. Any marked delay in treatment is associated with a poor clinical response and development of pulmonary fibrosis.

- Mebendazole, albendazole or pyrantel pamoate are used if *Ascaris* or *Necator* are the cause.

- Thiabendazole is the drug of choice for *Strongyloides stercoralis*.

Hypereosinophilic syndrome

Treatment is with corticosteroids. In resistant cases, hydroxycarbamide (hydroxyurea) may be helpful.

Chronic eosinophilic pneumonia

This responds rapidly to corticosteroids, and failure to respond within 48–72 hours raises the possibility of an alternative diagnosis such as bronchiolitis obliterans and organising pneumonia (now known as cryptogenic organising pneumonia, see Section 2.7.2). The dosage of corticosteroids is gradually tapered as relapses are common. Most patients regain normal lung function, although a few may develop a persistent obstructive defect, and in rare instances pulmonary fibrosis may occur.

FURTHER READING

See *Infectious Diseases*, Section 1.21.

- - - - - - - - - - - - - - - - - - - -

Douglas NJ and Goetzl EJ. Pulmonary eosinophilia and eosinophilic granuloma. In: Murray JF and Nadel JA, eds. *Textbook of Respiratory Medicine*, 2nd edn. Philadelphia: WB Saunders, 1994: 1913–32.

- - - - - - - - - - - - - - - - - - - -

Muers MF. Eosinophilic lung diseases. *Medicine* 2004; 32: 121–3.

2.8.6 Iatrogenic lung disease

Aetiology

A number of respiratory conditions may be precipitated by standard medical therapy, either by damage to the lung parenchyma or by disturbing pulmonary physiology. These effects must be remembered when prescribing such treatments, and highlight the importance of taking a thorough past medical and drug history when interviewing patients. Potential mechanisms include:

- bronchoconstriction;

- alveolitis/pneumonia;

- fibrosis.

Bronchoconstriction

Some of the drugs that can produce bronchoconstriction include:

- aspirin and the other NSAIDs;

- penicillins;

- tetracyclines;

- cephalosporins;

- cromoglycate;

- beta-blockers;

TABLE 33 DRUGS THAT CAN AFFECT THE LUNG PARENCHYMA

Drug type	Drug name
Cardiac	Amiodarone Procainamide Quinidine
Antibiotics	Nitrofurantoin Sulphonamides Penicillins
Anti-inflammatory	Sulfasalazine Penicillamine Gold
Cytotoxics	Bleomycin Mitomycin Busulfan Chlorambucil Cyclophosphamide Methotrexate Carmustine

- anticholinesterases;

- opiates;

- iodine contrast media;

- *N*-acetylcysteine.

⚠ Remember that drugs do not have to be given systemically to produce problems. Even eye drops such as timolol can produce wheeze and chest tightness, particularly in elderly patients.

Alveolitis

Some of the drugs that can affect the lung parenchyma are listed in Table 33. Some of these effects are potentially reversible on withdrawal of the treatment, while others may produce irreversible damage.

Radiotherapy

Radiation, prescribed with a view to eradicating tumour cells, also damages healthy tissue. When given to the thorax for the treatment of lymphoma, breast or lung cancer, it can produce a pneumonia in the underlying lung. The risk of damage is proportional to the dose of radiotherapy.

Clinical presentation

The clinical presentation will be determined by the nature of the underlying pathophysiology. In general:

- bronchoconstriction presents with wheezing after drug administration;

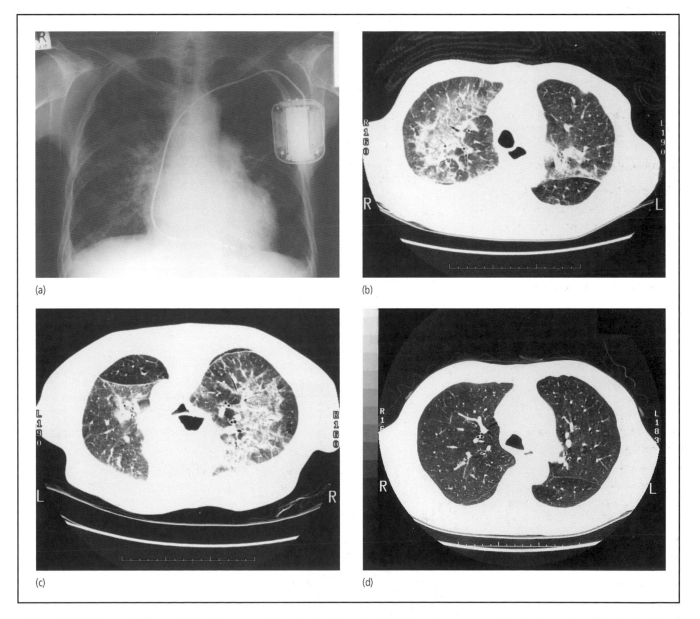

▲ **Fig. 25** (a) CXR of a man with ischaemic heart disease showing an implantable cardiac defibrillator and pulmonary shadowing; he was thought to have heart failure. CT scans of the same patient (b) supine and (c) prone were taken the next day. The pulmonary shadowing does not change in position and therefore is more consistent with fibrosis secondary to amiodarone. (d) CT scan of the same patient 2 years later showing complete resolution of the fibrosis; amiodarone had been stopped soon after the results of the first scan and he was given a 6-month course of oral steroids.

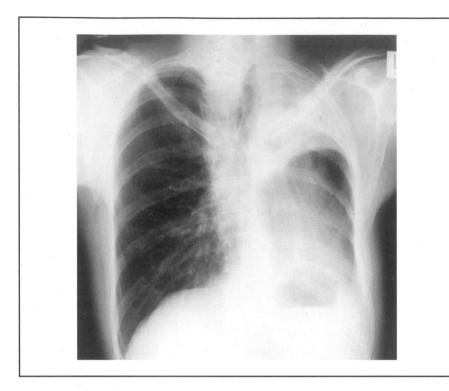

▲ **Fig. 26** CXR of a woman who had received mantle radiation for Hodgkin's lymphoma 30 years previously. The left upper lobe shows extensive tethering and fibrosis. On the basis of this radiograph she was referred to the chest physicians for bronchoscopy, with no reference to previous films. The changes had been present for many years.

- pneumonia or alveolitis is likely to have a slower onset, with exertional dyspnoea and fine inspiratory crackles being prominent.

Investigations

In bronchoconstriction, monitoring peak flow is worthwhile to see if this improves after a couple of days. It is then worth requesting lung function testing before and after a bronchodilator challenge to see if mild asthma or chronic obstructive pulmonary disease has been unmasked.

In alveolitis there should be radiological changes visible on plain CXR or high-resolution CT (Fig. 25), as well as appropriate changes in pulmonary function tests (reduced lung volumes with a reduced KCO).

Radiotherapy produces more localised fibrosis that may progress to cause lung contraction. The edge is often sharply defined (Fig. 26).

> Ensure that patients with radiation fibrosis are told that they have an abnormal CXR, especially if the changes are persistent. This can save them unnecessary investigations in the future.

Treatment

For all suspected drug side effects it is necessary to stop the offending medication and replace with another class of drug if necessary.

Patients with bronchoconstriction may also require a bronchodilator, at least in the short term until their symptoms improve, as well as a short course of corticosteroids.

In alveolitis some patients will respond to steroid therapy; in others the damage will be irreversible, but non-progressive. Baseline and serial KCO measurements are recommended by some authorities for patients taking amiodarone and other agents that are particularly associated with alveolitis.

FURTHER READING

Seaton A. Drug-induced lung disease, oxygen toxicity and related syndromes. In: Seaton A, Seaton D and Leitch AG, eds. *Crofton and Douglas's Respiratory Disease*, 5th edn. Oxford: Blackwell Scientific Publications, 1995: 1475–95.

2.8.7 Smoke inhalation

Historically, smoke inhalation was described as early as the first century AD, when Pliny reported the execution of prisoners by exposure to the smoke of greenwood fires.

Aetiology

Smoke inhalation includes potential exposure to a wide array of substances because of the complex chemistry of heat decomposition and pyrolysis. Cytotoxic anoxia from carbon monoxide, cyanide and oxidants is a major cause of morbidity, and a number of irritant chemical pyrolysis products have the potential to cause pulmonary damage. Smoke inhalation may cause the following.

Thermal injury

Thermal injury to the respiratory tract is limited to the upper airways, with laryngeal oedema presenting as a major medical management problem. This is due to the poor conductivity of air and the high amount of dissipation that occurs in the upper airways. Animal experiments have shown that if air at 142°C is inhaled, then by the time it reaches the carina it will have cooled to 38°C. Steam, volatile gases, explosive gases and the aspiration of hot liquids provide some exceptions, as moist air has a much greater heat-carrying capacity than dry air.

Irritant injury

Irritants can cause direct tissue injury, acute bronchospasm and activation of the body's inflammatory response system. Activated leucocytes and/or humoral mediators, such as prostanoids and leukotrienes, produce oxygen radicals and activate proteolytic enzymes. Some studies have shown that the administration of the cyclooxygenase inhibitor ibuprofen reduces lung lymph flow in animals with smoke inhalation. The direct injury is a consequence of the size of the particle, its solubility in water and its acid–base status. Ammonia produces alkaline injury, whereas sulphur dioxide and chlorine gas lead to acid injuries. Other chemicals act via different mechanisms; for instance, acrolein causes free radical formation and protein denaturation. The location of injury depends on the solubility of the substance in water. Highly soluble substances such as acrolein, sulphur dioxide, ammonia and hydrogen chloride cause injury to the upper airway. Substances with intermediate solubility, such as chlorine and isocyanates, cause upper and lower respiratory tract injury. Phosgene and oxides of nitrogen have low water solubility and cause diffuse parenchymal injury.

Asphyxiation

Tissue hypoxia can occur secondary to several mechanisms. Combustion utilises oxygen, decreasing the ambient concentration of oxygen to as low as 10–13%. The decrease in fraction of inspired oxygen

leads to hypoxia, despite adequate circulation and oxygen-carrying capacity. Combustion of plastics, polyurethane, textiles (silk, nylon and wool), rubber and paper products can lead to the production of cyanide gas. Hydrogen cyanide (HCN) is a colourless gas, with a bitter almond odour to the 40% of the population able to detect it. It is 20 times more toxic than carbon monoxide (CO) and can cause immediate respiratory arrest. Consider cyanide toxicity in all patients with smoke inhalation who have central nervous system or cardiovascular findings. Cyanide interferes with cellular metabolism, subsequently halting cellular respiration. As a consequence of the cessation of the electron transport system, anaerobic metabolism ensues, with corresponding high lactate acidosis and decreased oxygen consumption.

Diagnosis

The diagnosis of smoke inhalation is easy as the injury occurs in the presence of smoke and/or a fire. It is very important to find out if any chemicals were involved (eg from factory fires). It is equally important to determine the exact time of exposure and if other people have been involved. Patients with poor respiratory reserve may be seriously ill.

Smoke inhalation injury can range from an immediate threat to a patient's airway and respiratory status to only minor mucosal irritation.

Assessment of the patient

- First, assess the airway. Maintain cervical immobilisation in any patient who is unresponsive, has been involved in a significant mechanism of injury, has bony tenderness or complains of neck symptoms.

- Identification of impending respiratory failure is paramount.

- Assess breathing by respiratory rate, chest wall motion and auscultation. Wheeze and the use of the accessory muscles of respiration indicates respiratory distress.

- Assess circulation by level of consciousness, pulse rate, BP and capillary refill, and by symmetry and strength of pulses.

- A brief neurological evaluation should include determination of score on the Glasgow Coma Scale, pupil size and reactivity, and any focal findings.

- Remove all clothes to expose traumatic injuries/burns and to prevent ongoing thermal injury from smouldering clothes.

- Hoarseness, a change in voice, complaints of throat pain and odynophagia indicate an upper airway injury that may be severe.

- Assess patient for any other trauma (eg fractures).

Investigations

- Arterial blood gases: look for hypoxia and respiratory acidosis.

- Lactate levels: metabolic acidosis secondary to cyanide, methaemoglobinaemia, CO or hypoxia.

- Urea and creatinine: should be obtained for baseline renal function in patients in shock or rhabdomyolysis. Patients with large cutaneous burns, crush injuries or prolonged immobilisation should have serum creatine kinase measured and, if appropriate, urine myoglobin.

- Carboxyhaemoglobin and methaemoglobin: the pulse oximeter can be misleading in the setting of CO exposure or methaemoglobinaemia as it detects oxygenated and deoxygenated haemoglobin only and not any other form of haemoglobin. Co-oximeters are capable of detecting methaemoglobin and carboxyhaemoglobin in addition to haemoglobin and oxyhaemoglobin.

- Chest radiology: in smoke inhalation, most CXRs are normal. However, atelectasis, pulmonary oedema and acute respiratory distress syndrome may occur.

- ECG: this may show myocardial ischaemia, as the oxygen-carrying capacity of blood is impaired in the presence of carboxyhaemoglobin and methaemoglobin.

- Pulmonary function test: this may show a reversible obstructive airway pattern.

- Single-photon emission CT (SPECT): in patients with severe CO toxicity, the most common finding on SPECT in acute and delayed CO encephalopathy is ischaemia and necrosis of the basal ganglion. This finding is highly specific for CO insult.

- Bronchoscopy: can be diagnostic as well as therapeutic.

Management

- Correct hypoxia.

- Maintain clear airway: consider intubation, as the risk of developing laryngeal oedema is high.

- Maintain adequate circulation.

- Hyperbaric oxygen in CO toxicity: the half-life of CO is 320 minutes on room air, 90 minutes on 100% oxygen, and 23 minutes in a

hyperbaric chamber at 303 kPa (3 atmospheres). Elimination of CO depends primarily on the law of mass action, so alveolar Po_2, rather than alveolar ventilation, is the critical factor in its removal.

- Methaemoglobinaemia in smoke inhalation is relatively rare and rarely requires treatment with methylene blue. This antidote is reduced by the NADP methaemoglobin reductase enzyme, and in return reduces methaemoglobin to normal haemoglobin. Indications for treatment are a change in mental status, acidosis, ECG changes, and ischaemic chest pain. Levels lower than 30% may not require treatment, depending on the patient's cardiorespiratory reserve.

- Bronchodilators in patients with bronchospasm.

- Antibiotics if sepsis is present.

2.8.8 Sickle cell disease and the lung

Aetiology

Patients with sickle cell anaemia frequently develop acute pulmonary complications of their illness. The major pulmonary problems that occur in sickle cell disease include asthma, infection, thromboembolism, acute chest syndrome, chronic pulmonary fibrosis and pulmonary hypertension.

Epidemiology

Acute and chronic pulmonary complications of sickle cell anaemia are common but often underappreciated by healthcare providers. These conditions have clearly emerged as major threats to the well-being and longevity of patients with sickle cell disease, with more than 20% of adult patients

likely to have fatal pulmonary complications of sickle cell anaemia.

Acute chest syndrome is the most common cause of death and the second most common cause of hospitalisation of adults with sickle cell anemia.

Mortality rates for children with sickle cell anaemia have declined because of penicillin prophylaxis, vaccination for *Haemophilus influenzae* and *Streptococcus pneumoniae*, widespread implementation of newborn screening programmes for early detection, and improvements in parental education.

Despite significant improvements in the life expectancy of patients with sickle cell disease, the median age at death is 42 years for men and 48 years for women.

Clinical presentation

Any patient with sickle cell disease presenting with fever, pleuritic chest pain and shortness of breath should be carefully assessed and admitted for observation.

 Aggression and/or confusion should not be mistaken for a psychotic or 'drugged-up' individual; the patient may well be hypoxic and septic.

The acute chest syndrome is defined as a new pulmonary infiltrate on a CXR accompanied by fever, chest pain and a variety of respiratory symptoms including coughing, wheezing and tachypnoea. Acute chest syndrome often develops after vaso-occlusive crisis.

Multiple factors may contribute to the respiratory distress associated with the acute chest syndrome, including infection, pulmonary fat embolism, iatrogenic fluid overload, hypoxaemia, atelectasis secondary to splinting from painful rib and sternal infarctions, and pulmonary vascular obstruction.

Physical signs
Fever, confusion, dyspnoea, crackles in lung fields and evidence of consolidation.

Investigations

Emergency
For acutely ill patients obtain the following.

- FBC: severe anaemia may require transfusion or exchange tranfusion.

- Urea and electrolytes: ensure the patient is not dehydrated.

- CXR: look for pulmonary shadowing, consolidation and opacities (Fig. 27).

- Arterial blood gases: look for hypoxia; acidosis is a marker of severity of the illness.

- ECG: check for signs of acute/chronic right heart strain.

Short term
Aimed at identifying reversible disease:

- ventilation–perfusion scan or spiral CT looking for emboli and infarction;

- sputum for microscopy, sensitivity and culture;

- echocardiographic assessment of pulmonary hypertension.

Long term

- Lung function tests: note that sickle cell patients often have reduced indices even when in relatively good health.

- Most patients with sickle cell anaemia develop abnormal pulmonary function characterised by airway obstruction, restrictive lung disease, reduced gas transfer and hypoxaemia.

Treatment

Emergency
Try to reassure the patient while administering:

- broad-spectrum intravenous antibiotics and fluids;

- high-flow oxygen, humidified if possible;

- adequate analgesia;

- anticoagulants as for pulmonary emboli if veno-occlusion is suspected.

> Hypoxia in sickle cell disease is often ascribed to co-administration of analgesics and/or sedatives. This could be a dangerous assumption and you can check it by measuring $Pa\text{co}_2$. Reduction of respiratory drive should not affect the arterial–alveolar gradient.

Short to long term
Close cooperation between haematologist and respiratory physician is helpful. Prophylactic antibiotics will help reduce episodes of infection. The patient may require lifelong anticoagulation.

Complications
Repeated pulmonary emboli and infarction may lead to pulmonary hypertension, cor pulmonale and right heart failure in relatively young patients.

FURTHER READING

Haematology, Sections 1.4.1 and 2.1.2.

- - - - - - - - - - - - - - - - - -

Sergeant GR. Pulmonary system. In: Sergeant GR, ed. *Sickle Cell Disease*. Oxford: Oxford University Press, 1992: 150–67.

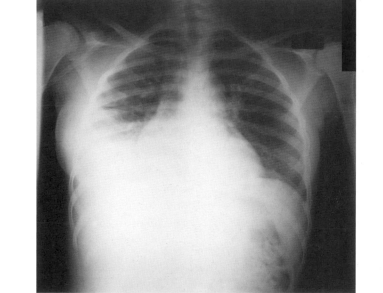

▲ **Fig. 27** CXR of a patient with sickle cell disease; there is right middle and lower lobe collapse and consolidation caused by pneumonia. Also note the cardiomegaly and small spleen. Less obvious are the surgical clips from a previous cholecystectomy. (Courtesy of Dr I. Vlahos.)

2.8.9 Human immunodeficiency virus and the lung

Aetiology/epidemiology

Lung pathology is common in patients with HIV infection and particularly in those with low $CD4^+$ T-cell counts. Like the immunocompetent, they are prone to the common viral and bacterial infections; but they are also at risk of atypical infections such as *Pneumocystis carinii* pneumonia (PCP). PCP was a common cause of death in AIDS patients until the introduction of Septrin prophylaxis in those with $CD4^+$ T-cell counts below 200×10^6/L. It now tends to be seen as a first presentation of the disease in previously undiagnosed HIV.

Tuberculosis (TB) is a major cause of mortality and morbidity in HIV patients, particularly in developing countries, and non-tuberculous mycobacteria including *Mycobacterium avium intracellulare* ($CD4^+$ T-cell count $<100 \times 10^6$/L), *M. kansasii* and *M. chelonae* are also seen. Multidrug-resistant TB started to become a substantial problem in the early 1990s, with a mortality between 80 and 100%. The relative numbers of patients infected with multidrug-resistant TB in Western countries remains small, but the plight of the developing world is uncertain.

Cytomegalovirus (CMV) pulmonary infection rarely occurs alone; if it is found, its presence does not affect the outcome of other lung infections. Fungal infections, eg *Cryptococcus neoformans*, tend to be seen as part of a disseminated syndrome.

Tumours such as Kaposi's sarcoma (KS) commonly occur in the lung as well as the skin, although lymphoma tends to arise in extrapulmonary sites in HIV patients.

Clinical presentation

The management of HIV patients with pulmonary symptoms can be difficult. Do not forget that acute shortness of breath can be caused by bacterial pneumonia, asthma or pulmonary emboli, just as in the immunocompetent. However, patients with HIV more commonly present with a history of gradually increasing breathlessness, fever, mild to moderate sputum production or just a dry cough, and occasionally with haemoptysis.

Physical signs

- How unwell is the patient? Is he or she hypoxic?

- Look for clubbing.

- Look closely in the mouth and on the skin for KS as well as other stigmata or evidence of immunodeficiency.

- Note any intercostal recession.

- Listen for crackles and wheezing.

Investigations

Chest radiograph

This may be virtually diagnostic (Fig. 28); on the other hand, it may appear normal, especially in early cases of PCP and KS.

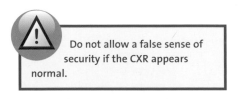

Do not allow a false sense of security if the CXR appears normal.

Oxygen saturation

Check both before and after exercise. Low post-exercise oxygen saturation is typical of PCP.

Arterial blood gases

Hypoxia demands explanation even if the CXR seems normal.

Bronchoscopy

Because of the wide range of respiratory pathology seen in the immunosuppressed, bronchoscopy is required in this group of patients if there are new respiratory symptoms and the diagnosis is not obvious. Make sure that samples are sent for the regular investigations, but in particular:

- cytology to look for PCP;

- microscopy to look for acid-fast bacilli;

- virology to look for CMV.

Intrapulmonary KS is unusual without cutaneous KS, but not impossible.

Sedation in HIV disease

Some newer antiretroviral agents – notably indinavir, efavirenz, nelfinavir, ritonavir and saquinavir – may greatly slow the metabolism of hypnotic agents by interaction with cytochrome P450. Check what your patient is taking, or he or she may stay sleepy for several hours or longer.

CT scan of chest

Useful when other investigations are negative or disease is slow to resolve. Not essential in all patients but can be useful in unexplained hypoxia or fever (you may see lymphadenopathy).

Treatment

Pneumocystis pneumonia

- High-dose intravenous Septrin, oxygen and steroids (if Pao_2 <9.3). Do not forget to monitor blood tests carefully, including FBC and liver function. Second-line

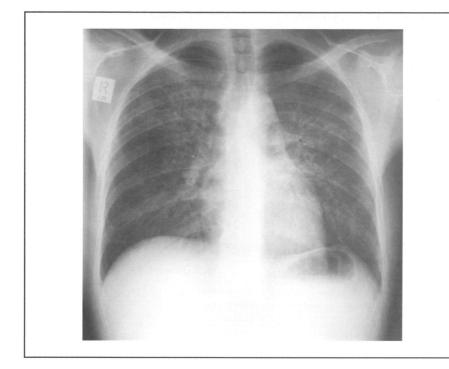

▲ **Fig. 28** CXR of a young man who presented with progressive shortness of breath, dry cough and a fever; note the classic bilateral perihilar appearance of the interstitial shadowing that is highly suggestive of PCP, which was later proved on bronchoscopic lavage to be the diagnosis. (Courtesy of Dr I. Vlahos.)

treatment in those unable to tolerate Septrin (co-trimoxazole) is pentamidine or dapsone and trimethoprim.

- Because of the improved overall prognosis of HIV patients, full supportive care (including intubation and mechanical ventilation) is usually recommended if indicated on physiological grounds.

 In severe PCP large cysts may form. Pneumothorax could explain a sudden deterioration.

Kaposi's sarcoma

KS may improve in patients with a high viral load who are started on antiviral drugs. Otherwise, refer to an oncologist for intravenous chemotherapy.

Tuberculosis

The frequency of atypical presentations is increased but management is along conventional lines. Interactions with new-generation antivirals are a problem; specialist advice is required.

⚠ Do not forget that drug regimens are different for atypical mycobacteria and multidrug-resistant TB.

FURTHER READING

Infectious Diseases, Sections 2.6.1 and 2.11.

Breen R and Johnson M. Respiratory infections in patients with HIV. *J. R. Coll. Physicians Lond.* 1999; 33: 430–3.

Miller R. AIDS and the lung. In: Adler MW, ed. *ABC of AIDS*. London: BMJ Publishing Group, 1999: 26–33.

Miller R. Respiratory manifestations of AIDS. In: Mindel A and Miller R, eds. *AIDS, A Pocket Handbook of Diagnosis and Management*, 2nd edn. New York: Arnold, 1995: 70–93.

Pozniak AL, Miller R and Ormerod LP. The treatment of TB in HIV-infected persons. *AIDS* 1999; 13: 435–45.

2.9 Malignancy

2.9.1 Lung cancer

Aetiology/pathology

Smoking remains the chief cause, although other aetiological factors include asbestos, arsenic and some heavy metals. Various histological types are recognised (Table 34).

Epidemiology

Bronchial carcinoma is one of the leading causes of mortality in the UK with around 35,000 deaths per year. It is more common in men, although the incidence in women continues to increase (male to female ratio 2:1).

Clinical presentation

Common

Any abrupt change in respiratory symptoms in a past or current smoker merits investigation:

- cough;
- haemoptysis;
- shortness of breath (may represent an effusion or lobar collapse);
- chest pain.

TABLE 34 COMMON HISTOLOGICAL CELL TYPES OF LUNG CANCER

Histological classification	Types
Non-small-cell lung cancer (NSCLC)	Squamous cell Adenocarcinoma Large cell
Small-cell lung cancer (SCLC)	Synonym: oat cell

Uncommon

See Table 35. Rarer presentations reflect the vagaries of anatomy or distribution of metastases:

- wheeze or stridor;

- dysphagia as a result of oesophageal compression by enlarged mediastinal nodes;

- nerve involvement, eg hoarseness secondary to recurrent laryngeal nerve palsy;

- Horner's syndrome;

- neuralgic pain as a result of tumour spread, eg Pancoast's syndrome and rib involvement;

- loss of power and/or numbness in a limb or confusion resulting from brain metastasis;

- facial swelling caused by superior vena cava obstruction (SVCO);

- confusion secondary to hypercalcaemia;

- confusion secondary to hyponatraemia caused by syndrome of inappropriate secretion of antidiuretic hormone (SIADH);

- cushingoid features and/or increased pigmentation (ectopic adrenocorticotropic hormone secretion).

Physical signs

Examination is often made with the benefit of a CXR.

Common

Look for:

- clubbing;

- tobacco-stained fingers;

- cachexia;

- pallor.

Uncommon

- Lymphadenopathy: feel carefully, including behind the sternomastoids and deep behind the medial clavicle.

- Evidence of consolidation or pleural effusion on percussion and auscultation.

- Liver edge secondary to metastases.

- Bone pain caused by metastases.

- Facial swelling and collateral venous circulation.

Rare

- Stridor secondary to tracheal or main bronchus involvement.

- Horner's syndrome.

- Pigmentation.

- Skin metastases.

Investigations

Chest radiograph

Posteroanterior and lateral views help to localise the lesion, especially for the bronchoscopist (Figs 29 and 30).

Bronchoscopy

If there is a visible lesion:

- biopsy for histology;

- washings and brushing to cytology;

- washings to microbiology for microscopy, sensitivity and culture, and acid-fast bacilli (remember that infection can mimic carcinoma).

The surgeon will want to know the endobronchial anatomy.

CT scan

For staging the tumour the scan needs to include the thorax, liver and adrenals to look for metastases, as well as the brain if there is evidence of neurological involvement (Fig. 31).

Percutaneous biopsy under CT guidance

This is useful when bronchoscopy does not establish the diagnosis. The patient should be warned that there is a 10% chance of pneumothorax

TABLE 35 NON-METASTATIC MANIFESTATIONS OF LUNG CANCER

Syndrome	Mechanism
Cushing's syndrome	Ectopic adrenocorticotropic hormone
SIADH	Ectopic antidiuretic hormone
Hypercalcaemia	Parathyroid hormone-like peptide
Hypertrophic pulmonary osteoarthropathy	Unknown
Eaton–Lambert syndrome	Unknown

SIADH, secretion of antidiuretic hormone.

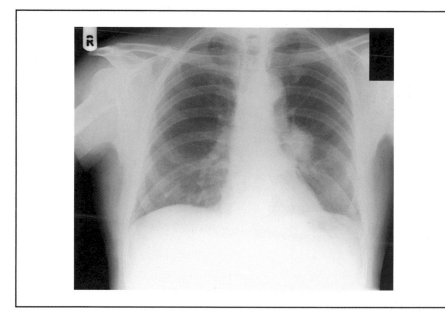

▲ **Fig. 29** CXR of a 56-year-old man presenting with cough, haemoptysis and weight loss. Note the large left hilar mass. Bronchoscopic biopsy revealed a large-cell carcinoma.

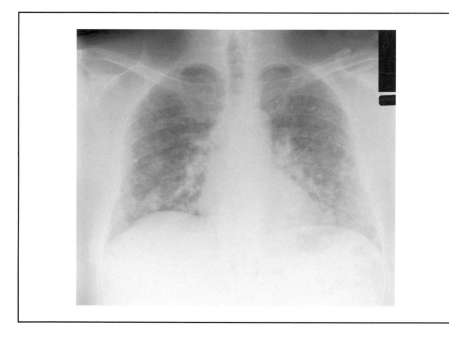

▲ **Fig. 30** CXR of a man with widespread nodular shadowing caused by diffuse adenocarcinoma of the lung.

and must be fit enough to tolerate such a complication.

Mediastinoscopy

Mediastinal nodes shown to be enlarged on CT/MRI are biopsied. This helps differentiate hyperplastic lymphadenopathy from tumour invasion. This can alter tumour staging and therefore operability. In some centres the nodes are sampled and analysed under frozen section before proceeding.

Positron emission tomography scans

These are becoming a useful tool in identifying tumour involvement of mediastinal nodes as well as other local spread.

Sputum cytology

This is mainly useful in patients who would not tolerate a bronchoscopy.

Blood tests

These are not diagnostic but can identify complications.

- FBC: anaemia may indicate progression of disease and/or bone marrow involvement.

- Urea and electrolytes: decreased sodium may indicate SIADH, increased urea dehydration.

- Liver function tests: if deranged may indicate metastatic disease.

Differential diagnosis

This is of the presenting problem but could include:

- infection (consolidation from a pneumonia or tuberculosis);

- lung abscess;

- bronchial adenoma.

Complications

The vigour with which complications are treated will depend on the patient's general performance status and local expertise (Table 36).

Treatment

Emergency

- Radiotherapy (DXT) for SVCO or tracheal/bronchial obstruction (see *Oncology*, Section 1.4.3).

- Laser bronchoscopy or stenting of tracheal or main bronchial obstruction: requires swift referral to a specialist centre.

- Pain control: early referral to Macmillan/palliative care team.

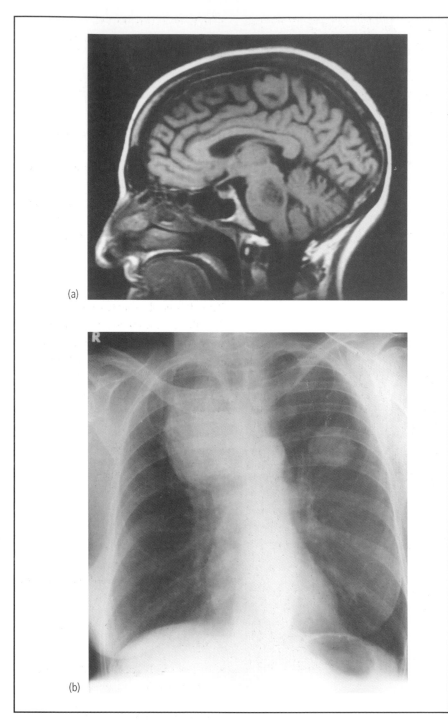

▲ **Fig. 31** This woman presented with incoordination in her left arm associated with mild loss of sensation. (a) MRI of her brain revealed a pontine lesion and (b) a CXR revealed left upper lobe mass associated with right paratracheal lymphadenopathy. She had a diagnosis of squamous cell carcinoma of the lung and was given palliative radiotherapy to the brain.

your local cardiothoracic surgeon, as in most cases resection is the only treatment likely to be curative. Make sure the patient comes back to see you immediately if turned down for surgery.

Non-surgical treatment
Radiotherapy High-dose DXT with curative intent may be given to patients with NSCLC without metastases who decline surgery. Patients with extrathoracic spread are generally given a palliative dose to control local symptoms as high-dose DXT has not been shown to alter prognosis, but can lead to considerable morbidity.

Prophylactic cranial DXT in SCLC has been shown to improve prognosis; however, postoperative DXT following resection does not improve prognosis.

Chemotherapy Oral and/or intravenous treatment is given with DXT in small-cell disease. Trials continue to evaluate its usefulness in NSCLC and before or after lung resection.

Pain and symptom control
It is essential to introduce patients and family to support teams as soon as appropriate.

Prognosis
Overall 5-year survival is 5.5%.

Prevention

Smoking cessation
Never underestimate your ability to counsel patients about smoking cessation: your words may be just the crucial encouragement the patient needs. Particularly if you have never smoked, do not appear distant and virtuous; imagine your worst habit, even if it is not life-threatening, and how difficult it would be to give up.

Short term
Surgery The most important step is to decide whether the patient is a candidate for surgery. Age should not be a barrier for referral. Those with solitary peripheral lesions should always be referred. In general, patients presenting with central lesions, metastases or SCLC are not candidates for thoracotomy. If in any doubt, always make a swift referral to

TABLE 36 COMPLICATIONS ASSOCIATED WITH LUNG CANCER

Problem	Treatment
Dyspnoea	DXT, endobronchial DXT, laser or cryotherapy, stenting and opiates
Bone metastases	DXT and non-steroidal analgesics. Prophylactic surgery is recommended if a lesion is found in a non-fractured weight-bearing bone
Brain metastases	Palliative DXT and steroids. Excision occasionally recommended for single metastasis
SVCO	DXT and stenting
Haemoptysis	DXT and laser bronchoscopy
Electrolyte abnormality	Correct as appropriate (see *Endocrinology*, Sections 1.4.1 and 1.4.2)

DXT, deep X-ray therapy.

Recent government-sponsored initiatives in the UK may lead to increased availability of clinics to help people quit smoking. It is worth knowing what is available in your area so that you can readily advise. More often than not, nicotine-replacement therapies are available on NHS hospital formularies, so have an idea of what is available and encourage patients to see their GPs for further advice. Preparations include nicotine patches, gum, vaporiser (inhalator), sublingual tablets and nasal spray.

Encourage patients to quit, help them set a date on which to stop and refer them to a specialist smokers' clinic if appropriate. Record your advice in their notes and GP letter, and take the opportunity to ask how they are getting on if you see them again in clinic.

FURTHER READING

Brown JS and Spiro SG. Update on lung cancer and mesothelioma. *J. R. Coll. Physicians Lond.* 1999; 33: 506–12.

Fergusson RJ. Lung cancer. In: Seaton A, Seaton D and Leitch AG, eds. *Crofton and Douglas's Respiratory Disease*, 5th edn. Oxford: Blackwell Science, 1995: 1077–123.

Jett JR. Is there a role for adjuvant therapy for resected non-small cell lung cancer? *Thorax* 1999; 54: S37–S41.

McEwen A and West R. How to intervene against smoking. *J. R. Coll. Physicians Lond.* 1999; 33: 513–15.

Spiro SG. Bronchial tumours. In: Brewis RAL, Corrin B, Geddes DM and Gibson GJ, eds. *Respiratory Medicine*, 2nd edn. London: WB Saunders, 1995: 924–61.

2.9.2 Mesothelioma

Aetiology

Asbestos fibre has been used extensively for its fire-resistant properties in the building industry, in shipbuilding and for brake and clutch liners in cars. It was mined in countries as far apart as the former USSR, Canada and South Africa, and transported to countries such as the UK by boat. The crocidolite form of asbestos is now known to be particularly hazardous in causing the associated lung diseases.

Asbestos fibres are inhaled and become lodged in the alveoli where they are incompletely phagocytosed by macrophages. The resulting inflammatory reaction leads to local tissue damage and fibrosis, and is thought to increase susceptibility to malignant change.

Epidemiology

The effects of asbestos tend to occur 20–40 years after initial exposure. Therefore, as asbestos controls only became law in the late 1970s, it is predicted that we will continue seeing cases well into the twenty-first century.

Clinical presentation

- Shortness of breath.
- Weight loss.
- Chest wall pain.

Physical signs

Evidence of a pleural effusion and/or pleural thickening with:

- decreased expansion on the affected side;
- decreased breath sounds on the affected side.

A careful occupational history is required from anyone presenting in this way (see Section 1.1.7).

Investigations

Despite vigorous investigation it is sometimes not possible to obtain diagnostic histology confirming mesothelioma in life. Special stains can help and it may be worth discussing this with the pathologist (see Section 1.1.7):

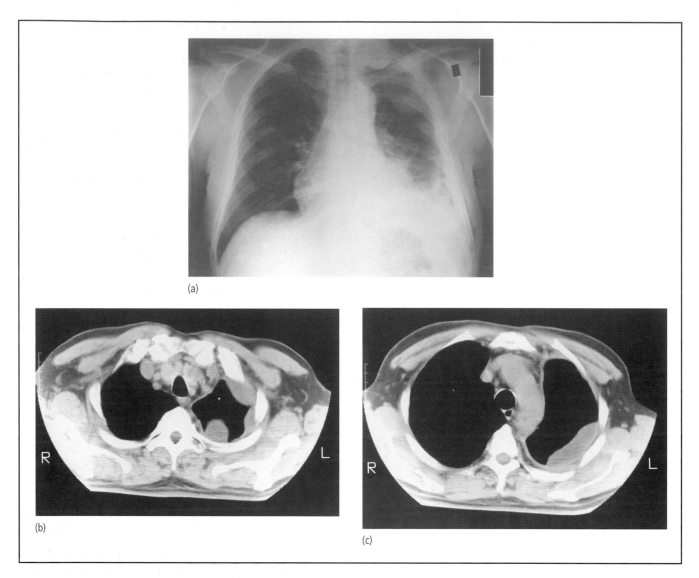

▲ **Fig. 32** (**a**) CXR of a man with left-sided mesothelioma. (**b**) A CT scan of the thorax shows extensive mesothelioma extending from apex and (**c**) from the pleura into the thoracic cavity at the level of the left upper lobe. (Courtesy of Dr J. Moore-Gillon.)

- pleural biopsy and aspiration;

- thoracoscopy and biopsy;

- CT scan of the chest (Fig. 32).

Differential diagnosis

- Lung cancer: there is a symbiotic relationship between asbestos and smoking, with lung cancer being five times more common in smokers exposed to asbestos than smokers who have no exposure.

- Sarcoma.

- Benign pleural thickening.

Treatment

Emergency

- Drain the associated pleural effusions if the patient is very short of breath.

- Only consider pleurodesis once you have a tissue diagnosis.

Short term

- Radical surgery, involving rib and lung resection, is attempted in a very few patients with limited disease.

- Pain can be a major problem and difficult to control, even with opiates; involve the experts, ie the palliative care (Macmillan) team early. Local radiotherapy (deep X-ray therapy) may sometimes help. Cervical cordotomy can help intractable unilateral pain.

- Surgical or medical pleurodesis can help prevent recurrent pleural effusions.

- Drain sites should be irradiated to prevent recurrence; mesothelioma is notorious for seeding along tracks.

Long term

As usual for diseases where the prognosis is poor and treatments ineffective, various trials are underway testing different treatment strategies. These include comparative chemotherapy trials, as well as a trial of tumour debulking plus chemotherapy versus chemotherapy alone.

Complications

- Repeated pleural effusions.

- Severe pain.

Prognosis

Poor, with limited response to therapy. Median survival is 12–18 months.

Prevention

There will continue to be a rise in the number of cases until at least 2015 as the rules controlling the use and handling of asbestos were only enforced in the late 1970s. The 20–40 year latency from exposure to symptoms means that patients who were youngsters then will continue to present for some time.

practice to record that you advised the patient of this point when you diagnose an asbestos-related condition.

Similar procedures for both state benefits and claims against employers may be followed for coal worker's pneumoconiosis, occupational asthma and a small number of other industrial lung diseases.

Disease associations

- Non-pleural mesotheliomas may occur as a primary disease on the pericardium, usually presenting as constrictive pericarditis. Diagnosis is normally made by pericardial biopsy.

- Peritoneal mesothelioma causes vague symptoms of tiredness, lethargy and loss of appetite, followed by abdominal distension caused by ascites. Diagnosis may be made by laparoscopic omental biopsy.

Compensation claims

Patients with mesothelioma, asbestosis, diffuse pleural thickening and lung cancer associated with asbestosis are entitled to state compensation and receive a disability pension. Patients may also be able to make a claim against previous employers for any asbestos-related condition, including pleural plaques, and may receive compensation if the employers have been negligent in exposing them to asbestos.

If patients wish to pursue this course of action, the law generally allows them only 3 years in which to commence legal action after the date on which they first knew they had an asbestos-related condition. It is good

FURTHER READING

Brown JS and Spiro SG. Update on lung cancer and mesothelioma. *J. R. Coll. Physicians Lond.* 1999; 33: 506–12.

- - - - - - - - - - - - - - - - - - -

Edge JR. Mesothelioma. *Br. J. Hosp. Med.* 1983; 29: 521–36.

- - - - - - - - - - - - - - - - - - -

Morgan WKC and Gee JBL. Asbestos-related disease. In: Morgan WKC and Seaton A, eds. *Occupational Lung Diseases*, 3rd edn. London: WB Saunders, 1995: 308–73.

- - - - - - - - - - - - - - - - - - -

Rudd RM. Asbestos-related disease. In: Brewis RAL, Corrin B, Geddes DM and Gibson GJ, eds. *Respiratory Medicine*, 2nd edn. London: WB Saunders, 1995: 545–69.

2.9.3 Mediastinal tumours

Aetiology

The mediastinum is the part of the thorax lying between the two pleural sacs and contains the heart and various other thoracic viscera. It is a site where masses of different pathology are not uncommon: they can occur at any age and may be solid or cystic.

Based on a lateral CXR, the mediastinum can be divided into three compartments (Fig. 33). Table 37 shows the normal constituents of the three compartments of the mediastinum as well as the tumours and cysts that may occur in each compartment.

Clinical presentation

Half of all mediastinal masses are asymptomatic and 90% of these are benign. The likelihood of malignancy is higher in infants and children than in adults. The signs and symptoms of mediastinal masses depend on the compression and invasion of nearby intrathoracic structures (Table 38). Mediastinal tumours may also be associated with various endocrine syndromes, myasthenia gravis with thymoma being particularly noteworthy (see *Neurology*, Section 2.2.5).

Investigations

The diagnostic approach to mediastinal masses can be divided into:

- imaging techniques;

- techniques for obtaining tissue samples.

Imaging techniques

Chest radiograph Most mediastinal tumours are discovered incidentally by posteroanterior or lateral CXRs.

CT This helps evaluate the origin of a mediastinal mass and can also

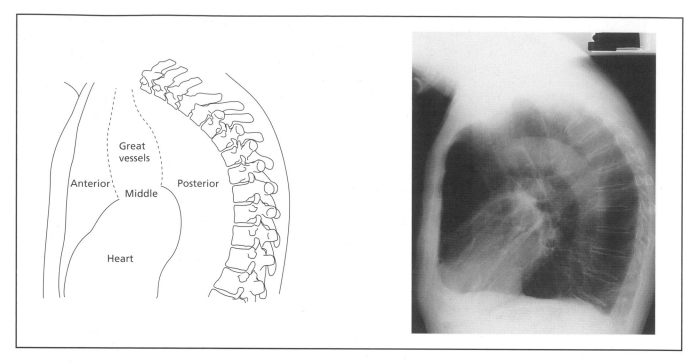

▲ **Fig. 33** Lateral CXR showing division of the mediastinum into anterior, middle and posterior compartments, the middle compartment containing the heart and great vessels

diagnose certain lesions confidently, eg teratoma.

MRI This can offer superior definition to CT scanning and may be preferred prior to surgery.

Radionuclide scanning These techniques can be used for specific lesions such as:

- radioiodine scanning for ectopic thyroid tissue;

- uptake of thallium (^{201}Tl) by Hodgkin's lymphoma;

- radioactive gold may be useful in localising extramedullary haematopoiesis.

Techniques for obtaining mediastinal tissue
Mediastinoscopy and mediastinotomy.

Treatment
The treatment of a mediastinal mass would depend on the nature and location of the lesion.

TABLE 37 NORMAL CONSTITUENTS OF THE MEDIASTINUM AND TUMOURS ARISING FROM THEM

Compartment	Location	Normal contents	Examples of mediastinal mass
Anterior	Superior and anterior to the heart shadow	Thymus gland (remnant), internal mammary artery and veins, lymph nodes, fat	Thymoma, lymphoma, retrosternal thyroid and parathyroid mass, fibroma, lipoma, teratoma, seminoma, choriocarcinoma
Middle	Posterior and inferior to the anterior compartment	Heart, pericardium, great vessels, trachea, major bronchi, phrenic nerves	Aortic arch aneurysm, pericardial cysts, left ventricular aneurysm, vascular lesions
Posterior	Lies within the margins of the thoracic vertebrae	Oesophagus, thoracic duct, descending thoracic aorta, azygos and hemiazygos veins, sympathetic chain	Oesophageal tumours, neurogenic tumours (neurofibroma, neurilemoma, neurosarcoma, ganglioneuroma, neuroblastoma, chemodectoma, phaeochromocytoma), diaphragmatic hernia, rare tumours (Adkin's tumour, descending aortic aneurysm chordoma, mediastinal sarcoma)

TABLE 38 CLINICAL PRESENTATION OF MEDIASTINAL TUMOURS

Structure involved	Signs and symptoms
Trachea and main bronchus	Stridor, cough, dyspnoea and recurrent chest infections
Phrenic nerve	Diaphragmatic paralysis
Oesophagus	Dysphagia
Sympathetic trunk	Horner's syndrome
Superior vena cava	Non-pulsatile distension of neck veins, cyanosis and swelling of the face, neck and upper arm, and dilated veins on chest wall
Pericardium	Pericardial effusion and pericarditis
Left recurrent laryngeal nerve	Left vocal cord palsy with hoarse voice

FURTHER READING

Benjamin SP, McCormack LJ, Effler DB, *et al*. Primary tumours of the mediastinum. *Chest* 1972; 62: 297–303.

Pierson DJ. Disorders of the pleura, mediastinum and diaphragm. In: Wilson JD, Braunwald E, Isselbacher KJ, *et al. Harrison's Principles of Internal Medicine*, 12th edn. New York: McGraw-Hill, 1991: 1111–16.

Pierson DJ. Tumours and cysts of the mediastinum. In: Murray JF and Nadel JA, eds. *Textbook of Respiratory Medicine*, 2nd edn. Philadelphia: WB Saunders, 1994: 2278–90.

Treatment

The treatment of a mediastinal mass would depend on the nature and location of the lesion.

2.10 Disorders of the chest wall and diaphragm

A variety of chest wall and diaphragmatic disorders can lead to nocturnal hypoventilation and chronic respiratory failure, which occurs when the load placed on the respiratory muscle pump exceeds the pump's capacity. Abnormalities are initially present at night when the patient is supine, which increases the load, and drive is physiologically reduced.

Aetiology

Chest wall disorder

The commonest chest wall disorder causing chronic respiratory problems is kyphoscoliosis, which is often idiopathic (cause unknown), but can be caused by/associated with:

- Neuromuscular disease – muscular dystrophy, poliomyelitis, cerebral palsy and Friedreich's ataxia.

- Vertebral disease – osteoporosis, osteomalacia, tuberculous spondylitis, neurofibromatosis and vitamin D resistant rickets.

- Disorders of connective tissue – Ehlers–Danlos syndrome and Marfan's syndrome

- Thoracic cage abnormality – thoracoplasty, empyema.

Other causes of significant chronic chest wall disorder include fibrothorax (following pleural disease such as caused by haemothorax, tuberculous empyema or asbestos exposure) and ankylosing spondylitis (usually in association with additional lung disease).

Diaphragmatic paralysis

Paralysis of one or both hemidiaphragms, often called eventration of the diaphragm, is a common clinical finding. A leading cause of unilateral phrenic palsy is open-heart surgery, with an incidence of 2–20%: the left side is most commonly affected, but right and bilateral involvement are not uncommon. Thoracotomy, pleurectomy and pneumonectomy are generally not accompanied by the risk of phrenic nerve injury, unlike mediastinal and oesophageal procedures. Other causes of phrenic nerve palsy/diaphragmatic paralysis are shown in Table 39.

Clinical presentation

Chest wall disorder

Common – dyspnoea on exertion, orthopnoea and symptoms of

TABLE 39 CAUSES OF PHRENIC NERVE PALSY/ DIAPHRAGMATIC PARALYSIS

Traumatic	Compression	Inflammatory	Others
Cervical spine	Bronchogenic	Pleurisy	Peripheral neuropathy
Birth trauma	carcinoma	Pneumonia	Anterior horn cell disease
Iatrogenic (during	Mediastinal masses	Herpes zoster	Myopathies
subclavian and jugular	Aortic aneurysms	Vasculitis	Multiple sclerosis
catheterisation)	Substernal thyroid		Neuralgic amyotrophy
			Acid maltase deficiency
			Idiopathic

nocturnal hypoventilation (morning headache, daytime somnolence and mood or personality change due to associated sleep disturbance). Less common – acute respiratory failure and cor pulmonale.

Diaphragmatic paralysis

The clinical manifestations of diaphragmatic paresis depend on the severity of the weakness, whether it is unilateral or bilateral, the rapidity of onset and the presence or absence of any underlying respiratory illness.

- Unilateral Paralysis: 50% of patients may be asymptomatic. Others complain of dyspnoea at rest or exertion, cough, fatigue and chest wall discomfort; some may complain of dyspnoea on lying with the paralysed side down.

- Bilateral paralysis: this is almost always associated with severe symptoms, particularly severe exertional dyspnoea and orthopnoea. Ventilatory failure, cor pulmonale, atelectasis and pneumonia are frequent. Due to the respiratory dysfunction in the supine position, sleep disturbances are common; and during rapid eye movement (REM) sleep, when generalised hypotonia is present, ventilatory function is seriously compromised with nocturnal hypoxia and hypercapnia leading to daytime somnolence, morning headaches and anxiety.

Physical signs

Look in particular for evidence of:

- Respiratory failure – cyanosis, carbon dioxide retention (flap and dilated veins) and cor pulmonale.

- Skeletal/rib cage deformity, including surgical scars (phrenic nerve crush).

- Diaphragmatic movement – with the patient lying down, does their abdomen move out (normal) or in (abnormal) when they breath in or sniff?

Investigations

- FBC – polycythaemia due to hypoxia.

- Arterial blood gases (ABG) – daytime hypercapnia. Early morning ABG (7am) reflects nocturnal gas exchange and may reveal hypercapnia with acute respiratory acidosis (pH < 7.35).

- ECG – Signs of right ventricular hypertrophy.

- Pulmonary function – may show a restrictive pattern.

- CXR – may be impossible to interpret in severe scoliosis. Spinal radiographs can be examined to determine the Cobb angle (Fig. 34), an angle of less than 70° seldom being associated with respiratory failure unless there is another pathology.

- Overnight pulse oximetry – may reveal severe nocturnal hypoxia.

- Sleep study – may reveal hypoxias occurring during REM sleep. May reveal the presence of obstructive sleep apnoea syndrome in obese patients.

- Thoracic ultrasound – can be very useful to assess diaphragmatic paralysis. Normally on sniffing the diaphragm moves downwards, but a paralysed diaphragm or hemidiaphragm moves upwards.

Treatment

General measures

Avoid smoking; treat any underlying obstructive airway disease; pulmonary rehabilitation; chest physiotherapy; and immunisation in patients with recurrent chest infections. In cases of obesity – weight reduction, and treat the underlying obstructive sleep apnoea with nasal continuous positive airway pressure or dental devices. For more details on the treatment of respiratory failure, see Section 2.12.

Chest wall disorder

Surgical correction of thoracic cage deformity does not seem to be of much benefit, excepting to prevent worsening of curvature in children who are still growing by spinal stabilisation.

Diaphragmatic paralysis

Unilateral paralysis does not require any treatment as the symptoms are usually mild. In bilateral paralysis most patients will require some form of ventilatory support. Diaphragmatic pacing may be an option in those with an intact phrenic nerve and diaphragm muscle.

Complications

Atelectasis; frequent chest infections; type I respiratory failure; type II respiratory failure; pulmonary hypertension; and cor pulmonale.

2.11 Complications of respiratory disease

2.11.1 Chronic respiratory failure

Aetiology

In health, the arterial partial pressure of carbon dioxide (Paco$_2$) is maintained within a narrow range by adjusting alveolar ventilation to match the fluctuating rate of carbon dioxide production. Respiratory failure results from a disorder in which lung function is inadequate for the metabolic requirements of the individual. It can be classified into two types.

- Type I respiratory failure: this is characterised by a low Pao_2 (<8 kPa) and normal or low $Paco_2$. It is mainly due to diseases that affect lung parenchyma with hypoxaemia due to right-to-left shunts or ventilation–perfusion mismatch. Such conditions include pneumonia, pulmonary oedema, acute respiratory distress syndrome, fibrosing alveolitis and pulmonary embolism.

- Type II respiratory failure: also called ventilatory failure, it is characterised by a low Pao_2 and a high $Paco_2$. This occurs when alveolar ventilation is insufficient to excrete the carbon dioxide produced by tissue metabolism. The most common conditions include chronic obstructive pulmonary disease (COPD), obesity, chest wall disorders, respiratory muscle weakness and depression of the respiratory centre.

Both types of respiratory failure may be acute or chronic depending on the speed of their development.

Inadequate ventilation occurring acutely will result in a low Pao_2 and a rising $Paco_2$, which will result in the lowering of blood pH (respiratory acidosis). A chronically raised $Paco_2$ is compensated for by the renal retention of bicarbonate and, as a result, the pH returns towards normal (compensated type II failure). This can be called chronic respiratory failure (chronic respiratory failure).

Chronic respiratory failure can be due to:

- COPD (see Section 2.3);

- chest wall disorders (see Section 2.10);

- disorders of the diaphragm (see Section 2.10);

- obstructive sleep apnoea (see Section 2.1.1);

- obesity hypoventilation syndrome (see Section 2.10);

- disorders of respiratory muscles (see Section 2.10);

- respiratory centre inhibition (drugs, stroke, etc.);

- diffuse parenchymal lung diseases (see Section 2.7);

- chronic lung diseases such as bronchiectasis (see Section 2.4), cystic fibrosis (see Section 2.5) and sarcoidosis (see Section 2.8.2);

- occupational lung disease (see Section 2.6).

In fact chronic respiratory failure can be the end result of any chronic lung disease.

Assessment of patients with chronic respiratory failure

Patients with chronic respiratory failure may have one or more of the following features:

- use of accessory muscles of respiration;

- tachypnoea;

- tachycardia;

- sweating;

- pulsus paradoxus;

- inability to speak;

- signs of carbon dioxide retention (bounding pulse, headaches, peripheral vasodilatation, flapping tremor of the outstretched hands, confusion, drowsiness and papilloedema).

Investigations

Diagnosis of chronic respiratory failure is simple. An arterial blood gas measurement will establish the diagnosis. However it is essential to arrange other tests to find an underlying cause:

- CXR;

- lung function test;

- ultrasound of the diaphragm;

- high-resolution CT scan.

Treatment

- Treat underlying disorder.

- Controlled oxygen therapy (see Section 2.12.1).

- Non-invasive ventilation (see Section 2.12.3).

2.11.2 Cor pulmonale

This is defined as enlargement of the right ventricle (dilatation and/or hypertrophy) due to increased right ventricular afterload caused by diseases of the lungs, chest wall or ventilation control centre. Primary diseases of the pulmonary circulation (eg chronic pulmonary thromboembolism, vasculitis and idiopathic pulmonary arterial hypertension) are included by some, but in this module are dealt with in *Cardiology*, Sections 2.12 and 2.18.1). Right ventricular failure is not necessary for a diagnosis of cor pulmonale.

Physiology

- The pulmonary circulation lies between the right ventricle and the left side of the heart.

- It carries deoxygenated blood, which takes part in gas exchange in the lungs.

- Blood flow through the pulmonary circulation depends on the left ventricle and respiratory movements (negative intrathoracic pressure during inspiration sucks blood into the pulmonary circulation, while positive pressure on expiration pushes it forwards).

- The right ventricle acts as a pump only when there is obstruction to the pulmonary blood flow.

- Cor pulmonale is due to an increase in right ventricular afterload. This occurs secondary to an increase in pulmonary artery pressure (pulmonary arterial hypertension).

Pathophysiology

Hypoxic vasoconstriction is the most common cause of pulmonary arterial hypertension (PAH). Hypoxia may be episodic as seen in obstructive sleep apnoea (see Section 2.1.1) or chronic as seen in any other chronic lung condition. Once PAH is present, there is an increase in right ventricular workload to maintain an adequate cardiac output. PAH may be worsened by the increase in blood viscosity that accompanies polycythaemia, which in turn is due to hypoxaemia. It may also occur in some people who live at high altitudes and is known as chronic mountain sickness or Monge's disease.

Clinical presentation

The symptoms of PAH are non-specific in the early stages of the disease and may not be apparent for months or even years. As the disease progresses, symptoms become more noticeable and include:

- dyspnoea (exertional initially);

- fatigue;

- presyncope or syncope on exertion due to inability to increase cardiac output during exercise;

- chest pain (may be due to ventricular ischaemia);

- leg swelling;

- palpitations;

- cough;

- haemoptysis;

- in rare cases there is hoarseness of the voice due to compression of the left recurrent laryngeal nerve by the dilated pulmonary artery;

- in advanced cases, passive hepatic congestion may cause right upper quadrant abdominal pain and jaundice.

Examination

Check for:

- features of underlying conditions;

- oedema;

- cyanosis (central and peripheral);

- tachypnoea;

- left parasternal heave (due to right ventricular hypertrophy);

- pulsatile hepatomegaly;

- splitting of second heart sound with accentuation of the pulmonary component;

- ejection systolic murmur over the pulmonary area;

- distended neck veins (with a prominent v wave and a pansystolic murmur at the left sternal edge due to tricuspid regurgitation) occur in right ventricular failure;

- pleural effusions are very rarely a feature of cor pulmonale (eg when associated with the underlying cause).

Diagnosis

Perform the following to establish a case of cor pulmonale:

- FBC;

- ECG may show right-axis deviation, P pulmonale, rhythm disturbances and right bundle branch block;

- arterial blood gases;

- CXR;

- lung function tests;

- high-resolution CT scan;

- CT pulmonary angiography if recurrent pulmonary embolism is suspected;

- overnight pulse oximetry may demonstrate nocturnal hypoxaemia;

- polysomnography if obstructive sleep apnoea is suspected (see Section 2.1.1).

Treatment

- Treat the underlying condition (eg chronic obstructive pulmonary disease, diffuse parenchymal lung disease).

- Maximise oxygenation.

- Diuresis.

- Consider preventive anticoagulation, even if PAH is not caused by thromboembolism.

2.12 Treatments in respiratory disease

2.12.1 Domiciliary oxygen therapy

Blood returning to the heart from the tissues has a low Po_2 and travels to the lungs via the pulmonary arteries. The pulmonary arteries form pulmonary capillaries, which surround alveoli. Oxygen diffuses from the high pressure in the alveoli to the lower pressure of the blood in the pulmonary capillaries. After oxygenation blood moves into the pulmonary veins and is returned to the left side of the heart to be pumped to the systemic tissues. In a 'perfect lung' the Po_2 of pulmonary venous blood would be equal to the Po_2 in the alveolus. Three factors may cause the Po_2 in the pulmonary veins to be less than the alveolar Po_2.

- Ventilation–perfusion mismatch: in a 'perfect lung' all alveoli would receive an equal share of alveolar ventilation and the pulmonary capillaries that surround different alveoli would receive an equal share of cardiac output (ventilation and perfusion would be perfectly matched). Diseased lungs may have a marked mismatch between ventilation and perfusion. Some alveoli are relatively over-ventilated while others are relatively over-perfused (the most extreme form of this is a shunt).

- Shunt: occurs when deoxygenated venous blood from the body passes unventilated alveoli to enter the pulmonary veins and the systemic arterial system with an unchanged Po_2.

- Slow diffusion: in the normal lung, the diffusion of oxygen into the blood is very rapid and is complete, even if the cardiac output is increased (exercise) and the blood spends less time in contact with the alveolus. This may not happen when the alveolar capillary network is abnormal (if there is lung fibrosis and emphysema).

Domiciliary oxygen therapy is the domiciliary administration of oxygen to patients with lung disorders with the aim of correcting hypoxia while maintaining $Paco_2$ and subsequently pH within an acceptable range. The advantages of domiciliary oxygen therapy include the following.

- Increased survival: two studies have established a place for prolonged oxygen treatment in the management of chronic obstructive pulmonary disease (COPD): the British Medical Research Council trial, which evaluated oxygen for 15 hours daily versus no oxygen, and the National Institutes of Health Nocturnal Oxygen Therapy Trial (NIH NOT Trial), which compared 12 versus 24 hours of oxygen daily. Both studies showed a survival benefit in selected patients with cor pulmonale. In addition, the NIH NOT Trial showed better survival in patients with continuous oxygen therapy compared with nocturnal oxygen therapy only.

- Reduction in haematocrit: this leads to improved pulmonary and systemic blood flow.

- Neuropsychological improvement.

Indications for long-term oxygen therapy

- Chronic hypoxaemia due to COPD, chronic asthma, diffuse parenchymal lung disease, bronchiectasis, pulmonary vascular disease, cystic fibrosis, idiopathic pulmonary arterial hypertension, pulmonary malignancy and heart failure.

- Nocturnal hypoventilation due to obesity, neuromuscular disease, chest wall disorders and obstructive sleep apnoea.

- Palliative use.

Patient selection

The need for oxygen therapy should be assessed in:

- all patients with cyanosis;

- patients with polycythaemia;

- patients with cor pulmonale (oedema);

- in COPD, patients with a forced expiratory volume in 1 second <30% of predicted.

All patients should be on optimum treatment prior to assessment for long-term oxygen therapy (LTOT).

LTOT is indicated in patients with:

- daytime Pao_2 <7.3 kPa on two occasions, 3 weeks apart during a period of clinical stability;

- daytime Pao_2 7.3–8.0 kPa, in the presence of cor pulmonale (oedema), polycythaemia or nocturnal hypoxaemia (Sao_2 <90% for more than 30% of the time).

Once a patient fulfils the criteria for LTOT, the appropriate flow rate that can achieve a Pao_2 >7.3 kPa, should be determined by checking the arterial blood gases on oxygen. In the NIH NOT Trial, the majority of patients needed 1–2 L/min of oxygen delivered by nasal cannulae. Patients will need an additional 1 L of oxygen during exercise and while sleeping.

Ambulatory oxygen

All patients with chronic lung disorders should be assessed for ambulatory oxygen requirements. The 6-minute walk test is a simple and widely used stress test that makes it possible to evaluate the functional status of patients with lung disorders and their ability to carry out activities of daily living. The test measures the distance walked on a flat surface in 6 minutes and requires a constant level of effort similar to that needed by the patient to carry out activities of daily living. The test has also been used to assess exercise-induced desaturation.

The American Thoracic Society guidelines for domiciliary oxygen state that 'ambulatory O_2 should be prescribed to patients normoxaemic at rest with evidence of exertional desaturation to 88% or less'. Short-term ambulatory oxygen is associated with significant improvements in health-related quality of life. Ambulatory oxygen can be prescribed in three groups of patients:

1. patients on LTOT who are mobile and need to leave the home on a regular basis;

2. patients on LTOT who are housebound and unable to leave the home unaided, but may use ambulatory oxygen for short, intermittent periods only;

3. patients without chronic hypoxaemia but who show evidence of arterial oxygen desaturation on exercise.

Short-burst oxygen therapy

- Short-burst oxygen therapy (SBOT) is commonly prescribed for patients who do not fit the criteria for LTOT but remain breathless after minimal exertion. It is usually provided from cylinders.

- SBOT either before or after exercise probably does not benefit the majority of patients with moderately severe COPD who exercise for more than a very short period of time.

Modes of administration of oxygen

- Oxygen cylinders.

- Oxygen concentrator.

- Portable small lightweight cylinders for ambulatory oxygen delivering liquid oxygen.

2.12.2 Continuous positive airways pressure

Continuous positive airways pressure (CPAP) is a system that delivers a constant pressure to the airway, via a tube and a mask, thus acting as a pneumatic splint preventing upper airway collapse. Colin Sullivan introduced it in the early 1980s for the treatment of obstructive sleep apnoea (OSA). Prior to this, the treatment of choice for OSA was tracheostomy. The pressure delivered can be titrated to achieve adequate upper airway patency. The interface delivering the pressure can be nasal, full face or nasal pillows. The advantage of the nasal pillow is that no headgear is required to keep it in place. If needed, oxygen can be delivered via the CPAP.

Indications

- OSA: the treatment of choice for this is nasal CPAP. This prevents the nocturnal collapse of the upper airway (causing apnoea and hypopnoea), thus preventing sleep fragmentation and daytime somnolence. The pressure needed to achieve this can be titrated by repeating sleep studies on CPAP. However, autotitrating machines are now available, thus avoiding repeated sleep studies.

- Neuromuscular diseases: inspiratory upper airway collapse can complicate neuromuscular diseases affecting the chest wall, but CPAP can prevent these episodes. CPAP also prevents atelectasis in neuromuscular and chest wall diseases. Thus in such patients with type I respiratory failure, nasal CPAP should be considered.

- Paralysed hemidiaphragm: CPAP can prevent the flail action of a paralysed hemidiaphragm and

thus improve the efficiency of inspiration.

- CPAP may be indicated in any pulmonary disorder that results in severe oxygenation abnormalities (F_{IO_2} >0.6 is needed to maintain P_{aO_2} >8 kPa) in the presence of a normal P_{aCO_2}.

- Pulmonary oedema: CPAP in patients with severe cardiogenic pulmonary oedema can result in early physiological improvement and reduce the need for intubation and mechanical ventilation.

- Central sleep apnoea (CSA): up to 50% of patients with severe heart failure (ejection fraction <45%) suffer from nocturnal CSA, presenting with daytime somnolence and paroxysmal nocturnal dyspnoea. These patients have increased morbidity in comparison with patients who have congestive cardiac failure without CSA. CPAP can help relieve their daytime symptoms.

Complications

- Dry nose, nose-bleeds and sore throat.

- Nasal congestion, runny nose and sneezing.

- Irritation of the eyes and the skin on the face.

- Abdominal bloating.

- Headaches.

- Leaks around the mask because it does not fit properly.

2.12.3 Non-invasive ventilation

Respiratory failure results from an imbalance between the capacity of the 'ventilatory apparatus' (including respiratory centre, spinal cord, intercostal nerves, chest wall, bronchi and lungs) and the load placed upon it. This imbalance can be acute or chronic. In acute respiratory failure leading to respiratory acidosis, some form of transient ventilatory support is needed, while medical therapy corrects the insult.

Non-invasive ventilation (NIV) is the delivery of ventilatory support without the need for an invasive artificial airway. It has a role in the management of acute or chronic respiratory failure in many patients, and may have a role for some patients with heart failure. NIV can often eliminate the need for intubation or tracheostomy, and preserve normal swallowing and speech and cough mechanisms. There are two types of NIV.

Non-invasive positive-pressure ventilation

Non-invasive positive-pressure ventilation (NIPPV) is usually delivered nasally or via a face mask, therefore eliminating the need for intubation or tracheostomy. It can be administered in a volume-controlled or pressure-controlled manner. A bi-level positive airway pressure device is used, which delivers different pressures during inspiration (inspiratory positive airway pressure, IPAP) and expiration (expiratory positive airway pressure, EPAP). Volume ventilators are often not tolerated because they generate high inspiratory pressures that result in discomfort and mouth leaks. Although positive-pressure support is usually well tolerated by patients, mouth leaks or other difficulties are sometimes encountered. Supplementary oxygen can be given via the mask.

Negative-pressure ventilation

Negative-pressure ventilation involves devices such as the iron lung, tortoise shell or cuirass. The concept of mechanical ventilation first evolved with negative-pressure ventilation. In the late 1920s, Philip Drinker introduced negative-pressure ventilation and popularised the iron lung. He maintained an 8-year-old girl with acute poliomyelitis on artificial respiration continuously for 122 hours. The polio epidemics of the 1930s, 1940s and 1950s led to the development of pulmonary medicine as a specialty and the iron lung as a workhorse. Ventilators delivering negative-pressure ventilation fell out of favour as the use of NIPPV increased during the 1960s. This was primarily due to an improvement in anaesthetic procedures. Negative-pressure ventilators support ventilation by lowering the pressure surrounding the chest wall during inspiration and reversing the pressure to atmospheric level during expiration. These devices augment tidal volume by generating negative extrathoracic pressure. Several of these devices, such as body ventilators and iron lungs, are available and either cover the whole body below the neck or apply negative pressure to the thorax and abdomen. Although studies of body ventilators have shown benefit in patients with chronic obstructive pulmonary disease (COPD), neuromuscular disease and chest wall deformities who develop acute respiratory failure, prospective and controlled studies are lacking. Several uncontrolled studies have reported benefits of intermittent negative-pressure ventilation in patients with chronic respiratory failure resulting from chest wall, neuromuscular or central hypoventilation. However, no benefit has been demonstrated in patients with stable but severe COPD.

Because of their awkward size and their tendency to cause upper airway obstructions in some patients, negative-pressure ventilators are not readily acceptable and NIPPV is the modality of choice for NIV.

Mechanism of action

- NIPPV decreases the work of breathing and the IPAP improves alveolar ventilation while simultaneously resting the respiratory musculature. This helps in blowing off carbon dioxide.

- The IPAP prevents any atelectasis and hence recruits alveoli in gas exchange.

- Externally applied EPAP decreases the work of breathing by partially overcoming the auto-positive end-expiratory pressure, which is frequently present in these patients. The patient generates a less negative inspiratory force to initiate a breathing cycle.

Indications

- Acute respiratory failure leading to respiratory acidosis: this may be due to exacerbation of COPD, cystic fibrosis or bronchiectasis, or pulmonary oedema or pneumonia. Patients with one of the above conditions may develop acute respiratory failure and respiratory acidosis (pH <7.35 with raised Paco$_2$).

- Chronic respiratory failure: patients with neuromuscular and chest wall diseases, obesity hypoventilation syndrome, obstructive sleep apnoea with hypoventilation, COPD with hypoventilation and, in fact, any respiratory disorder with hypoventilation may not be able to breathe out carbon dioxide, causing respiratory acidosis. Initially this occurs during the night and can be detected by overnight monitoring of transcutaneous carbon dioxide. Measurement of arterial blood gases at 7 a.m. is also helpful as it reflects nocturnal gas exchange. Such patients may also complain of morning headaches due to raised $Paco_2$. Nocturnal NIPPV can improve their gas exchange and symptoms. With disease progression, their need for NIPPV will increase.

Contraindications

- Respiratory arrest.

- Inability to use a mask because of trauma or surgery.

- Excessive secretions.

- Haemodynamic instability or life-threatening arrhythmia.

- High risk of aspiration.

- Impaired mental status.

- An uncooperative or agitated patient.

- Life-threatening refractory hypoxaemia.

Complications

- Ulceration of the nasal bridge due to a tight mask: this can be avoided by choosing the correct size mask and applying gel foam at pressure points.

- Gastric distension.

- Hypotension.

- Barotrauma.

Practical details

- If NIPPV is indicated, it should be started as soon as possible.

Delays due to non-availability of a bed are unacceptable, as respiratory acidosis worsens with time.

- Before starting NIPPV in a patient with acute respiratory failure, decide whether the patient will be a candidate for intubation and mechanical ventilation should NIPPV fail. If so, the intensive care unit (ICU) team should be informed as early as possible.

- The initial IPAP and EPAP should be set up as per the hospital guidelines.

- Once NIPPV is started, measurement of arterial blood gases should be repeated in approximately 1 hour (earlier if there is clinical deterioration). If there is an improvement, treatment should continue on the same inspiratory and expiratory pressures. If $Paco_2$ is increasing, IPAP can be increased to help blow it off.

- If arterial blood gases are improving, they should be checked at increasing intervals. Once the acidosis is corrected, NIPPV can be stopped. However, if this occurs in late evening, it will be prudent to continue NIPPV overnight and stop it next morning.

- Always remember to optimise medical treatment for the underlying condition.

- Though NIPPV may be effective in respiratory acidosis due to exacerbation of asthma, such patients should be managed in an ICU with access to immediate intubation.

2.13 Lung transplantation

General guidelines

Any patient less than 65 years old with end-stage pulmonary disease in the absence of other significant organ dysfunction should be considered for referral for lung transplant assessment. Other criteria include the following:

- medical therapy is ineffective or unavailable;

- the patient is experiencing substantially limited daily activity;

- the patient has a limited life expectancy, usually less than 2 or 3 years, without transplantation;

- the patient is ambulatory with rehabilitation potential;

- the patient's nutritional status is acceptable (usually 80–120% of ideal body weight);

- the patient has a satisfactory psychosocial profile and support system;

- the patient has normal left ventricular function;

- the patient has a creatinine clearance >50 mL/min;

- the patient is seronegative for hepatitis B and C, and HIV;

- the patient is not osteoporotic;

- the patient has been free from malignancy for over 5 years.

- the patient has been a non-smoker for 6 months.

Indications

Common

- Chronic obstructive pulmonary disease.

- Emphysema due to α_1-antitrypsin deficiency.

- Cystic fibrosis.

- Idiopathic pulmonary arterial hypertension.

- Eisenmenger's syndrome.

Less common

- Bronchiectasis.

- Sarcoidosis.

- Lymphangioleiomyomatosis.

- Pulmonary Langerhans' cell histiocytosis.

Note that where there is concurrent cardiac disease, as there is in many of these patients at this stage, heart–lung transplantation is necessary.

Contraindications

- Acutely ill or unstable clinical status.

- Uncontrolled or untreatable pulmonary or extrapulmonary infection: this does not disqualify patients with airway colonisation.

- Uncured malignancy.

- Significant dysfunction of other vital organs.

- Significant coronary disease or left ventricular dysfunction (unless heart–lung transplantation is considered).

- Active cigarette smoking.

- Drug or alcohol dependency.

- Unresolved psychological problems or non-compliance with medical management.

- HIV infection.

- Hepatitis B antigenaemia or hepatitis C infection with histopathological evidence of liver disease.

Types of transplant procedure and age limits

While strictly speaking there are no age-based cut-offs for transplantation, organs are of course severely limited and hence priority is always given to those recipients most likely to enjoy sustained benefit.

- Single lung transplantation: 65 years.

- Bilateral lung transplantation: 60 years.

- Heart–lung transplantation: 55 years.

- Transplantation of lobes from living related donors.

Practical details

Preoperative

Ideally the patient should be on as low a dose of corticosteroids as possible. Bridging strategies such as target therapies for pulmonary arterial hypertension (see *Cardiology*, Section 2.12) and non-invasive ventilation are of value. Ventilator-dependent patients have a much higher mortality rate after transplantation.

Operative

Surgical details are beyond the scope of a medical text, but it should be noted that organ retrieval, preservation and assessment are crucial. Previous cardiac surgery, pleurectomy or pleurodesis increases operative difficulty and risk.

Postoperative

Regular follow-up of the patient with careful monitoring (CXR, spirometry, bronchoscopy and blood tests to control immunosuppressive therapy) must continue for the lifetime of the patient in order to prevent complications and detect them as soon as possible. A sustained decline of 10–15% or more in forced vital capacity or forced expiratory volume in 1 second (FEV_1) suggests a potentially significant problem.

Complications

- Acute rejection: most common in the first 6 months (fever, chills, malaise, increasing tightness in the chest, cough and worsening dyspnoea); complicates up to 10% of transplant procedures and accounts for more than 40% of 30-day mortality. The gold standard for diagnosis of acute rejection is tissue confirmation; the sensitivity of transbronchial lung biopsy for detecting acute rejection varies between 72 and 94%.

- Chronic rejection (bronchiolitis obliterans): most common between the first and fifth postoperative years (dyspnoea on exertion associated with a decline in FEV_1) (see Section 2.7.3).

- Infection: the main cause of early postoperative death due to typical pneumonia organisms, with high incidence of Gram-negative rods (*Pseudomonas* spp.), cytomegalovirus, herpesviruses, *Pneumocystis carinii*, *Candida* spp. and *Aspergillus* spp.

- Other complications affecting intermediate and long-term survival include drug-induced renal failure (virtually all patients), osteoporosis (in 73%), hypertension (in 66%), neurological problems (in 25%), gastrointestinal problems (in 20%), non-lymphoproliferative malignancies and disease recurrence.

Retransplantation

This is rarely performed (4% of lung and heart–lung procedures) due to donor shortage and the poor medical condition of potential candidates because of other medical problems or complications related to the first transplant.

FURTHER READING

American Society for Transplant Physicians (ASTP), American Thoracic Society (ATS), European Respiratory Society (ERS) and International Society for Heart and Lung Transplantation (ISHLT). International guidelines for the selection of lung transplant candidates. *Am. J. Respir. Crit. Care Med.* 1998; 158: 335–9.

- - - - - - - - - - - - - - - - -

Nathan, SD. Lung transplantation: disease-specific considerations for referral. *Chest* 2005; 127:1006–16.

3.1 Arterial blood gas sampling

Principle
To measure the oxygen and carbon dioxide tensions and acid–base status of arterial blood.

Indications
Arterial blood gas sampling was a research procedure until the mid-1960s but is now widely performed, either by direct arterial puncture or from indwelling arterial lines. Indications include:

- respiratory failure (type I or II);
- renal failure;
- hepatic failure;
- cardiac failure;
- drug intoxication (aspirin and narcotics);
- endogenous acid overproduction (ketoacidosis or lactic acidosis);
- severe illness, cause unknown.

For interpretation of data, see Section 3.6.1.

Contraindications
Care should be taken in the presence of bleeding disorders. Renal physicians will be appropriately unimpressed if an arterial blood gas sample is taken from an arteriovenous fistula.

Important information for patients
The procedure should be explained to the patient. The possibility of requiring more than one attempt should be mentioned.

Practical details

Before investigation
The patient should be lying or sitting comfortably and an appropriate site selected. The radial artery of the non-dominant arm is most commonly used, but the brachial or femoral arteries can be used. Make sure you have enough sterile gauze to apply immediate pressure after the procedure.

The investigation

- Clean the skin over the wrist with antiseptic solution. Palpate the artery between the tips of the forefinger and the middle finger of one hand.

- Holding it between your fingers, introduce the needle (with heparinised syringe attached) at an angle of 45° and slowly advance the needle along the line of the artery. On puncturing the artery, a small spurt of blood will be seen entering the syringe.

- Withdraw 3–4 mL of blood and press a sterile dressing over the site of puncture.

- Expel any air bubbles and cap the syringe. The syringe should be labelled and sent to the laboratory immediately on ice if a blood gas machine is not available at the bedside.

- The role of local anaesthesia remains controversial. Although used by some, especially in paediatric practice, skilled operators maintain that it adds unnecessary complexity to the procedure.

After investigation
It would be best if an assistant or the patient could apply direct pressure for the required minimum 5 minutes.

Complications
In practice, complications are rare:

- haematoma;
- arterial spasm leading to distal ischaemia;
- femoral nerve lies lateral to the femoral artery and can be injured if femoral artery is the chosen site;
- median nerve lies medial to the brachial artery and can be injured.

FURTHER READING
Lightowler JV and Elliott MW. Local anaesthetic infiltration prior to arterial puncture for blood gas analysis: a survey of current practice and a randomised double blind placebo controlled trial. *J. R. Coll. Physicians Lond.* 1997; 31: 645–6.

3.2 Aspiration of pleural effusion or pneumothorax

Principle

To aspirate fluid from a pleural effusion or air from a pneumothorax. This can be carried out using a syringe and a cannula, which is less traumatic than a chest drain (see Section 3.4) and should be considered before chest drain insertion in most cases.

Indications

- Pleural effusion: aspiration is preferred where the aim is to collect a diagnostic sample (a few millilitres) or if the aim is simply to palliate symptoms by removing fluid where the cause is known. The British Thoracic Society guidelines for investigation of a pleural effusion are shown in Fig. 34.

- Pneumothorax: aspiration is preferred unless there is respiratory embarrassment or bilateral pneumothoraces

Contraindications

Gross abnormalities of coagulation require correction.

Important information for patients

The procedure should be explained to the patient and the possibility of developing a pneumothorax should be mentioned.

Practical details

Before procedure

A simple aspiration may be performed with or without local anaesthesia depending on patient/operator preferences. If required, lidocaine should be infiltrated into the skin and the parietal pleura. Except in the case of a diagnostic aspiration of fluid (when a 20-mL syringe and green needle suffice), the equipment required includes:

- wide-bore (grey) venflon;

- three-way tap;

- 50-mL Luer lock syringe.

In the case of an effusion, a jug and a giving set with fluid chamber cut off will also be required.

Pleural effusion technique

- The patient should be seated comfortably, either on the edge of a bed resting forward onto one or more pillows on a bedside table, or 'cowboy style' on a chair (back-to-front, facing the chair back, with arms resting on the chair back).

- The area of stony dullness corresponding to the radiograph should be identified and one interspace below this marked with a biro, usually in the line of the scapula.

- Having cleaned the skin, the venflon is inserted while aspirating with a syringe. Remember to enter the pleural cavity just above the rib to avoid injury to the neurovascular bundle.

- When fluid is obtained, advance the cannula while removing the stylet and connect the three-way tap with the 50-mL syringe and giving set attached.

- The effusion is removed by aspirating and then expelling into the jug. The purpose of the giving set is to avoid air inadvertently entering the pleural space.

- Not more than 1500 mL of fluid should be aspirated in a single session as re-expansion pulmonary oedema may occur. Discontinue aspiration if the patient experiences persistent cough, dyspnoea or faintness (signs of rapid mediastinal shift).

Pneumothorax technique

With the patient in the supine position, aspirate the air from the second intercostal space in the mid-clavicular line. Discontinue the procedure if more than 1.5 L are aspirated (a large leak will need a chest drain), if resistance is felt or if the patient experiences persistent cough, dyspnoea or faintness.

After procedure

Apply a dressing and request a CXR.

Complications

- Entry into the pleural cavity may precipitate vasovagal syncope (give intravenous atropine).

- Rapid aspiration can lead to re-expansion pulmonary oedema.

- Pneumothorax.

- Haemothorax.

FURTHER READING

Davies G. Pleural procedures. *Medicine* 2004; 32; 164–6.

3.3 Pleural biopsy

Principle

Pleural biopsy is used to obtain a sample of the parietal pleura for histological and microbiological examination.

Indications

All cases of exudative pleural effusion of undetermined cause. Discrete pleural lesions are best biopsied under radiological control because of the difficulty matching

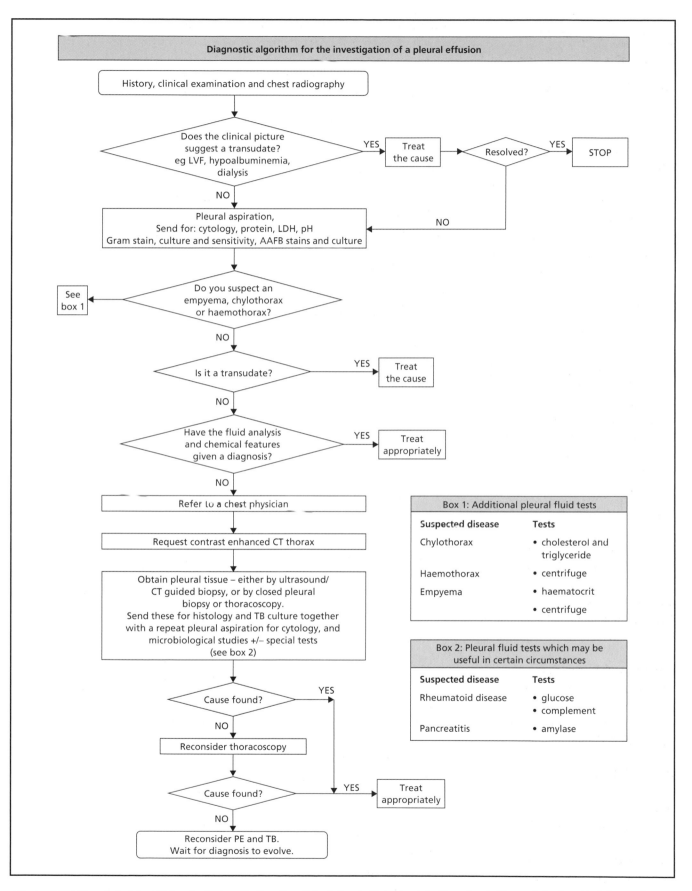

Diagnostic algorithm for the investigation of a pleural effusion

History, clinical examination and chest radiography

Does the clinical picture suggest a transudate? eg LVF, hypoalbuminemia, dialysis — YES → Treat the cause → Resolved? — YES → STOP

NO ↓

Resolved? — NO →

Pleural aspiration, Send for: cytology, protein, LDH, pH Gram stain, culture and sensitivity, AAFB stains and culture

Do you suspect an empyema, chylothorax or haemothorax? — (YES) → See box 1

NO ↓

Is it a transudate? — YES → Treat the cause

NO ↓

Have the fluid analysis and chemical features given a diagnosis? — YES → Treat appropriately

NO ↓

Refer to a chest physician

Request contrast enhanced CT thorax

Obtain pleural tissue – either by ultrasound/ CT guided biopsy, or by closed pleural biopsy or thoracoscopy. Send these for histology and TB culture together with a repeat pleural aspiration for cytology, and microbiological studies +/– special tests (see box 2)

Cause found? — YES →

NO ↓

Reconsider thoracoscopy

Cause found? — YES → Treat appropriately

NO ↓

Reconsider PE and TB. Wait for diagnosis to evolve.

Box 1: Additional pleural fluid tests

Suspected disease	Tests
Chylothorax	• cholesterol and triglyceride
Haemothorax	• centrifuge
Empyema	• haematocrit
	• centrifuge

Box 2: Pleural fluid tests which may be useful in certain circumstances

Suspected disease	Tests
Rheumatoid disease	• glucose
	• complement
Pancreatitis	• amylase

▲ **Fig. 34** British Thoracic Society guidelines for the investigation of a unilateral pleural effusion in adults. (Reproduced with permission from Maskell NA and Butland RJA. *Thorax* 2003; 58(Suppl. 2): ii8–ii17.)

the surface landmarks to radiological anatomy.

Contraindications

- Absence of adequate pleural fluid.

- Borderline respiratory function: production of a pneumothorax can precipitate respiratory failure.

- Empyema: risk of development of multiple subcutaneous abscesses.

- Presence of a bleeding diathesis.

- Thrombocytopenia: if platelets $<50 \times 10^9$/L, platelets should be transfused before the procedure.

Important information for patients

The procedure should be explained to the patient and the possibility of developing a pneumothorax should be mentioned.

Practical details

Before procedure

Premedication with an opiate or midazolam will help to reduce pain and anxiety.

The patient should be comfortable during the procedure and this is best achieved by having him or her sitting on the edge of the bed or on a stool with arms and head resting on one or more pillows on a bedside table. The operator stands behind the patient.

The site for the biopsy should be selected with care on the basis of a recent CXR and clinical presentation. The best site is in the intercostal space below the spot where the tactile fremitus is lost and the percussion note becomes dull, just superior to the rib below and hence avoiding the neurovascular bundle.

The procedure

The procedure can be performed using either Abrams' needle or Cope's needle. The Abrams' needle technique is more common and hence is described here.

- After positioning the patient and cleaning the skin with sterile solution, the skin and underlying tissues are infiltrated with 1% lidocaine. It is essential to anaesthetise the parietal pleura, which is rich in pain receptors. Do this as follows: once you have entered the pleural cavity and are aspirating pleural fluid, withdraw the needle slightly until nothing appears on aspiration. At this stage the needle is in contact with the parietal pleura: infiltrate with lidocaine, and allow 5 minutes for it to act.

- Prepare for the biopsy by using a scalpel to make a small incision (0.5 cm) in the skin and the tissues, dissecting if necessary with forceps.

- Introduce the Abrams' needle into the pleural space using constant and firm pressure. Using a twisting motion will reduce the amount of forward pressure required, and hence the chances of damaging the visceral pleura. Then remove the stylet and, with the inner cannula in the closed position, attach a syringe to the inner cannula.

- Rotate the inner cannula anticlockwise in the outer cannula to open the distal notch.

- Aspirate pleural fluid and withdraw the needle slowly until it hooks onto the pleura.

- Rotate the inner cannula into the closed position and remove the whole needle.

- A specimen of the pleura should be found in the tip of the needle. Three specimens are normally obtained at the 3 o'clock, 6 o'clock and 9 o'clock positions.

- Do not forget to send a sample in saline (*not formalin*) to microbiology for mycobacterial microscopy and culture.

After procedure

A dressing at the site should be applied and a CXR should be requested.

Complications

Although many complications are possible, these are not common in practice:

- vasovagal syncope (give intravenous atropine);

- pneumothorax/ haemopneumothorax;

- bronchopleural fistula if visceral pleura is damaged;

- bleeding because of damage to the intercostal artery or vein;

- visceral damage (spleen, liver or kidney).

3.4 Intercostal tube insertion

Principle

Intercostal tube insertion enables drainage of fluid, air, blood or pus from the pleural cavity. It can be life-saving, and may have to be performed rapidly and in unusual places. All doctors should be able to perform it.

Indications

- Tension pneumothorax.

- Bilateral pneumothorax.

- Empyema (use a large-diameter tube 28–32F).

- Any patient with pneumothorax who is to be ventilated.

- Haemothorax.

- Any pleural effusion adversely affecting the patient's breathing (and not relieved by aspiration).

- To drain the pleural cavity dry prior to pleurodesis.

Contraindications

There are no absolute contraindications. However, note the following:

- bleeding diatheses should be corrected before chest drain insertion when possible;

- it can be difficult to insert a drain if the pleura is thickened.

 Patients with chronic obstructive pulmonary disease may have large bullae that resemble pneumothoraces. Inserting a chest drain into a bulla may lead to development of a bronchopleural fistula and have life-threatening long-term sequelae.

Important information for patients

The procedure should be explained to the patient and the possibility of developing a haemothorax should be mentioned. Verbal consent should be obtained and documented in the notes.

Practical details

Before procedure

Premedication with an opiate or midazolam will reduce pain and anxiety; however, bear in mind the respiratory depression that can occur as a result of these drugs.

The patient should be lying supine with the head end of the bed elevated 30–45° and the arm held behind the head. A recent CXR should be reviewed and the site of insertion should be marked. The drain should be inserted in the triangle of safety:

- between the anterior and posterior axillary lines, preferably anterior to the mid-axillary line;

- below the axillary vessels;

- in the level of or above the nipple (ie fifth intercostal space);

- above the rib avoiding the neurovascular bundle.

The procedure

- Infiltrate the clean skin and parietal pleura with 1% lidocaine.

- Incise the skin in the line of the ribs (2 cm) and dissect soft tissue with artery forceps.

- Insert two strong non-absorbable sutures: one simple suture to secure the drain and one vertical mattress suture to close the wound after removal of the drain. A pursestring suture results in a circular wound, which heals with a scar and so should not be used.

- When the pleura is breached, insert the drain with the trocar retracted so that it acts as a rigid directional guide only. Do not use excessive force as you may damage the underlying viscera.

- In the case of a pneumothorax, aim the drain towards the apex. In the case of an effusion, aim the drain inferiorly.

- Once the drain is inserted, remove the trocar slowly and connect the tube to the underwater seal system.

- Secure the drain and apply sterile dressing.

After procedure

- Obtain a CXR to check position of the drain.

- Always maintain the level of water above the bottom of the tube in the underwater seal system.

- The bottle should be kept below chest level.

- Never clamp the chest drain in a case of pneumothorax (risk of developing a tension pneumothorax).

- Check daily if it is draining, bubbling or swinging.

Removal of chest drain

- In the case of a pneumothorax, it can be removed once there is no bubbling, minimal swinging with respiration and a CXR shows a fully expanded lung.

- In the case of a pleural effusion, it can be removed once it is draining less than 30 mL of fluid in 24 hours.

The drain should be removed with the patient performing a Valsalva manoeuvre. A CXR should be performed afterwards to check for pneumothorax.

Complications

These can include:

- bronchopleural fistula caused by injury to the lung;

- visceral injury (liver, heart, diaphragm, spleen and stomach);

- thoracic duct injury causing chylothorax;

- long thoracic nerve damage causing winging of the scapula;

- haemothorax.

FURTHER READING

Light RW. *Pleural diseases*, 2nd edn. Philadelphia: Lea and Febiger, 1990: 311–20.

– – – – – – – – – – – – – – – – –

Laws D, Neville E and Duffy J. BTS guidelines for the insertion of a chest drain. *Thorax* 2003; 58(Suppl. 2): ii53–ii59.

3.5 Fibreoptic bronchoscopy and transbronchial biopsy

3.5.1 Fibreoptic bronchoscopy

Principle
Fibreoptic bronchoscopy allows inspection of the bronchial tree and the biopsy of abnormal lesions. It should be performed only by trained respiratory physicians.

Indications
- Diagnostic.
- Therapeutic.

Diagnostic
- Evaluate lung lesions that appear on the CXR.
- Assess airway patency.
- Investigate unexplained haemoptysis.
- Search for the origin of suspicious or positive sputum cytology.
- Obtain specimen for microbiological examination in suspected infections.
- Investigate cause of superior vena cava obstruction, vocal cord palsy, unexplained pleural effusion and paralysis of hemidiaphragm.
- Evaluate a suspected tracheo-oesophageal fistula.
- Evaluate the airways for a suspected bronchial tear after thoracic trauma.
- Determine the extent of respiratory injury after inhalation of noxious fumes or aspiration of gastric juice.

Therapeutic
These are often performed via an endotracheal tube:

- removal of foreign bodies;
- removal of secretions or mucous plugs;
- difficult intubations.

3.5.2 Transbronchial biopsy

Principle
To obtain diagnostic tissue, usually in cases of suspected diffuse parenchymal lung disease.

Indications
Although the samples obtained are small and sometimes crushed, transbronchial biopsy achieves a high diagnostic yield in diffuse parenchymal lung diseases that have centrilobular accentuation, such as granulomatous and metastatic diseases. These include:

- sarcoidosis (75–89% diagnostic yield);
- carcinoma (64–68% diagnostic yield);
- infection;
- eosinophilic pneumonia;
- alveolar proteinosis.

Complications
The risk of developing a pneumothorax is 10%; however, this can be reduced by avoiding the middle lobe and the lingula and possibly with the use of fluoroscopy.

FURTHER READING

British Thoracic Society. The diagnosis, assessment and treatment of diffuse parenchymal lung disease in adults. *Thorax* 1999; 54: S1–S14.

— — — — — — — — — — — —

Sokolowski RW, Burgher LW, Jones FL, *et al*. Guidelines for fibreoptic bronchoscopy in adults. American Thoracic Society. Medical Section of the American Lung Association. *Am. Rev. Respir. Dis.* 1987; 136: 1066.

3.6 Interpretation of clinical data

3.6.1 Arterial blood gases

What is measured

> Whenever you take a set of blood gases, make sure that you clearly record the date, time, patient's name and inspired concentration of oxygen. This is crucial for interpretation and comparison with other results: a Po_2 of 12 kPa is normal if the patient is breathing air but grossly abnormal if they are on 60% oxygen!

Blood gas machines record various data (Table 40), and many also give a value for base excess/deficit. Calculation of base excess/deficit is designed to make it easy to separate metabolic from respiratory causes of pH disturbance. Various algorithms are used in these calculations, the principles being as follows.

- Predict the pH that would arise in normal blood in the presence of the Pco_2 actually measured. If Pco_2 is high, then the predicted pH is low; if Pco_2 is low, then the predicted pH is high.

- Calculate the amount of acid or base that would have to be added to the blood to change the predicted pH into the pH actually measured. This is the base deficit/excess (in mmol/L) and is a measure of the degree of 'metabolic', as opposed to 'respiratory', disturbance. A normal value is between −2 and +2.

If the blood gas machine that you have used does not provide base deficit/excess, then a useful

TABLE 40 MEASUREMENTS MADE BY BLOOD GAS MACHINES

	Normal range	Notes
pH	pH 7.35–7.45	
H$^+$	37–43 nmol/L	
Po_2	>10.6 kPa (breathing air)	Respiratory failure: Type I: Po_2 <8 kPa, Pco_2 <6.5 kPa Type II: Pco_2 >6.5 kPa
Pco_2	4.7–6.0 kPa	
HCO$_3^-$	22–28 mmol/L	In dealing with problems of respiratory failure or acid–base disturbance, measurement of plasma bicarbonate is often helpful

rule of thumb is as follows: in uncompensated metabolic disorders, the steady-state Pco_2 (measured in mmHg, where 1 kPa = 7.6 mmHg) should be numerically equal to the last two digits of the pH. For example, a normal Pco_2 is 5.3 kPa or 40 mmHg, and a normal pH is 7.40.

If this picture is not observed, then either:

- the problem is not simply metabolic – there is a primary respiratory element to the acid–base disorder;

- the metabolic change is very acute and respiratory compensation has not had time to develop (unlikely, because respiratory compensation is very rapid).

Interpreting results

Low Po_2
See Section 1.4.2.

Because it is not possible to specify the precise concentration of oxygen that a patient receives, unless he or she is intubated and ventilated, normal values for Po_2 cannot be quoted for those breathing on 24%, 28% or other oxygen masks. As a very rough guide, the 'hypoxaemia score' can be calculated as follows:

Hypoxaemia score = Po_2/Fio_2

where Po_2 is measured in mmHg (1 kPa = 7.6 mmHg) and Fio_2 is fraction of oxygen inspired (in air 0.21).

If the patient were breathing air, then applying the lower limit of normal Po_2 (10.6 kPa) would give a score of 384; and the value of Po_2 taken conventionally to define hypoxia (8 kPa) would score 290. In assessing a patient breathing supplementary oxygen, a value of <300 is usually taken as indicating significant compromise.

High Po_2
Air has a Po_2 of 21 kPa. Allowing for the Pco_2, the highest Po_2 that can be achieved breathing air is around 15 kPa. If a value higher than this is obtained, then the patient must have been breathing supplementary oxygen.

Low Pco_2
Hyperventilation may be:

- primary (most commonly caused by anxiety);

- secondary – to metabolic acidosis (respiratory compensation) or when attempting to maintain normoxia (eg in pulmonary embolus, acute severe asthma, pneumonia).

How can you tell if the patient has a metabolic acidosis? Look for

reduction in pH and increased 'negative base excess', ie a base excess more negative than –2. For the clinical approach to metabolic acidosis, see *Acute Medicine*, Sections 1.2.20 and 1.2.31.

High Pco_2
Hypoventilation may be caused by problems with the respiratory (airway, lungs, respiratory muscles and chest wall) or neurological (central and neuropathic) components of respiration.

How can you tell if this is acute or chronic? In chronic carbon dioxide retention the bicarbonate rises (secondary metabolic alkalosis) and the chloride falls.

Much more rarely a high Pco_2 is secondary to metabolic alkalosis, which would be known as respiratory compensation. How can you tell if the patient has a metabolic alkalosis? Look for elevation in pH and increased 'base excess', ie a base excess more positive than +2.

pH or H$^{+?}$
Alterations in acid–base status can result from changes in Pco_2, bicarbonate concentration or both.

- If the primary process affects Pco_2, then the alteration is described as a respiratory acidosis/alkalosis.

- If the primary process affects bicarbonate, then the terms metabolic acidosis/alkalosis are used.

- 'Mixed' disorders are those that arise as a result of more than one 'primary' process.

Whatever the primary process, it will usually be accompanied by secondary change in either Pco_2 or bicarbonate concentration, such that change in blood pH is minimised.

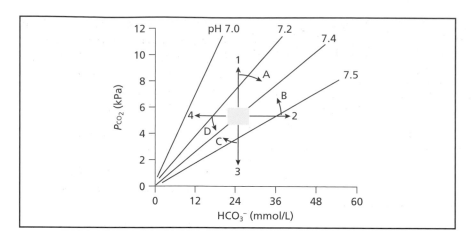

▲ **Fig. 35** Nomogram showing relationships between P_{CO_2}, pH and bicarbonate. Shaded area depicts normal range. Perturbations: (**1**) respiratory acidosis with (**A**) secondary metabolic alkalosis; (**2**) metabolic alkalosis with (**B**) secondary respiratory acidosis; (**3**) respiratory alkalosis with (**C**) secondary metabolic acidosis; and (**4**) metabolic acidosis with (**D**) secondary respiratory alkalosis.

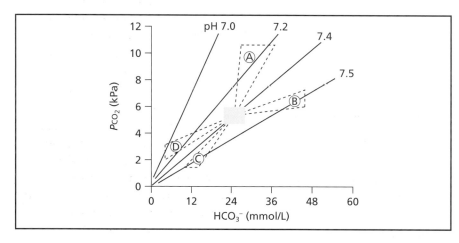

▲ **Fig. 36** Relationships between P_{CO_2}, pH and bicarbonate seen clinically in the four simple types of acid–base disturbance. Shaded area depicts normal range. Perturbations: (**A**) respiratory acidosis; (**B**) metabolic alkalosis; (**C**) respiratory alkalosis; (**D**) metabolic acidosis.

Plotting the values for P_{CO_2}, pH and bicarbonate for any particular patient on the nomograms shown in Figs 35 and 36 will define the type of acid–base disturbance, as is done by calculation of the base deficit/excess shown above.

Once the type of acid–base disturbance is known, consideration must be directed towards specific causes.

- Respiratory acidosis: see Sections 1.8 and 1.15.
- Respiratory alkalosis: see *Acute Medicine*, Section 3.6.2.
- Metabolic acidosis: see *Acute Medicine*, Section 3.6.2.

3.6.2 Lung function tests
See Table 41.

Peak flow
This is a valuable guide to airway obstruction, but is also influenced by patient aptitude and lung volume amongst other factors.

Spirometry
There are portable spirometers that can be transported to the wards. The vital capacity may be reduced by many disorders, but the FEV_1 is disproportionately reduced in obstructive conditions. This may be quantified from the FEV_1/FVC ratio (Table 42 and Fig. 37). This ratio is normally 80% (range 70–85%), although the 'normal ratio' tends to decline with age.

- A decreased ratio indicates an obstructive lung defect.

Abbreviation	Meaning (units)	Description
	TABLE 41 DEFINITIONS OF LUNG FUNCTION	
PEF	Peak expiratory flow (L/s)	Maximum rate of expiratory airflow during maximum forced expiration
FEV_1	Forced expiratory volume in 1 second (L)	Volume of air expired during first second of a forced expiration
FVC	Forced vital capacity (L)	Volume of air expired by a forceful expiration after taking a full inflation
FEV_1/FVC	Ratio (%)	
TLC	Total lung capacity (L)	Total volume of air in the lungs after maximum inspiration
RV	Residual volume (L)	Volume of air remaining in the lung after a maximum expiration
FRC	Functional residual capacity (L)	Volume of air remaining in the lungs at the end of normal expiration without any muscle activity. The 'neutral point' of the respiratory system

TABLE 42 CAUSES OF RESTRICTIVE AND OBSTRUCTIVE LUNG DEFECTS

Type of defect	Spirometric pattern	Examples
Restrictive	Increased FEV$_1$/FVC ratio	Pulmonary fibrosis, respiratory muscle weakness, obesity, pleural disease, chest wall and skeletal disorders
Obstructive	Decreased FEV$_1$/FVC ratio	COPD and asthma

COPD, chronic obstructive pulmonary disease.

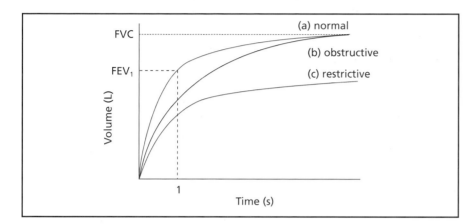

▲ **Fig. 37** Spirometry curves for (**a**) a normal patient, (**b**) a patient with a obstructive lung defect and (**c**) a patient with a restrictive lung defect.

- A raised ratio is suggestive of a restrictive defect.

This distinction can only be made absolutely by measurement of TLC (see *Scientific Background to Medicine 1*, Respiratory System).

Laboratory lung function

This needs the patient to be relatively well: it is not possible for really sick patients. It records lung volumes (TLC and RV), flow–volume loops and estimates the efficiency of gas transfer into the lung using carbon monoxide (TLCO, KCO).

Lung volumes

After looking at the FEV$_1$ and FVC, lung volumes are helpful in further interpretation of the underlying pathology.

Gas transfer

TLCO and KCO are measurements of gas diffusion across the alveolar membrane. KCO is corrected for lung volume as KCO = TLCO/Va, where Va is the alveolar volume available for gas exchange. In the laboratory, carbon monoxide is used to calculate this diffusion capacity, hence the 'CO' after the terms.

If you imagine the alveolar membrane in its healthy state as being thin and permeable, say like a sheet of tissue paper, any pathological process that causes it to become thickened and coarse will slow down the movement of carbon monoxide (or oxygen) from the lung into the bloodstream. Conversely, increased levels of blood and therefore haemoglobin, either in the bloodstream or in the alveoli, will cause an increase in the uptake of oxygen (Table 43).

Flow–volume loops

These measure the expiratory and inspiratory flow of air (L/s) against actual volume exhaled or inhaled. The upper, expiratory curve starts with the patient at maximum/forced inhalation (TLC) and ends at total/forced expiration (RV).

The curves have characteristic shapes according to the underlying disease process and whether the pathology is causing intrathoracic or extrathoracic obstruction to airflow, thus distorting the shape of the curve from normal. The most important patterns are those of expiratory flow limitation (Fig. 38).

TABLE 43 CAUSES OF INCREASED AND DECREASED KCO

Change in KCO	Mechanism	Examples
Increased	Reduced alveolar volume	Skeletal deformity, pleural disease, respiratory muscle weakness
	Increased capillary blood volume	Left-to-right shunt, lung haemorrhage, polycythaemia
Reduced	Destruction of lung tissue	Emphysema
	Impairment to diffusion by disease	Fibrosing alveolitis
	Reduced blood flow to pulmonary capillaries	Pulmonary vascular disease or hypertension, right-to-left shunt
	Reduced uptake by blood	Anaemia

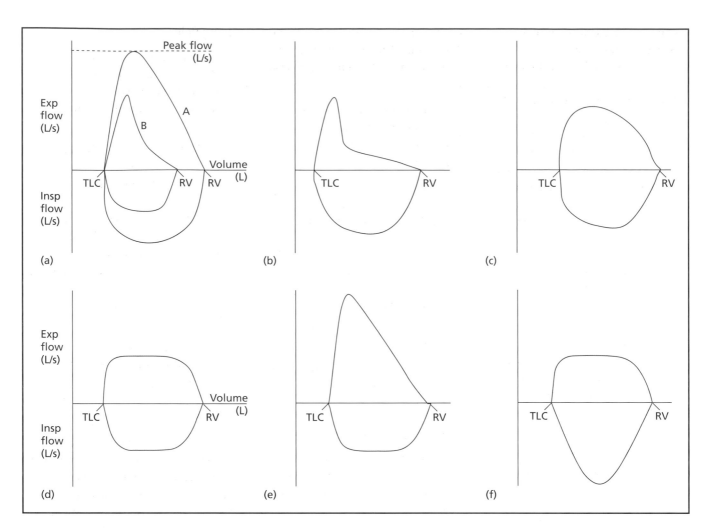

▲**Fig. 38** Flow–volume loops: (**a**) normal patient (**A**) and obstructive lung disease (**B**), eg asthma or chronic obstructive pulmonary disease; (**b**) emphysema; (**c**) restrictive lung defect, eg pulmonary fibrosis; (**d**) fixed intrathoracic or extrathoracic obstruction, eg tracheal tumour; (**e**) variable extrathoracic obstruction, eg tracheal stenosis outside the thoracic cavity, works like a one-way valve, opening on expiration while collapsing on inspiration; (**f**) variable intrathoracic obstruction.

3.6.3 Overnight oximetry

This relatively cheap and easy test can be used as a baseline investigation to screen for possible sleep apnoea in patients who report disturbed sleep and/or daytime somnolence. The patient's Sao_2 is continuously recorded via a finger probe while resting.

Analysis of the results looks for reductions in Sao_2 and the frequency of these events, which may represent episodes of apnoea (see Section 2.1.1). Patients with recurrent hypoxic episodes and/or large dips in their Sao_2 should be referred for formal assessment by a physician interested in sleep disorders.

3.6.4 Chest radiograph

Before interpreting a CXR, check the name, date, side label and projection, usually PA (posteroanterior) or AP (anteroposterior). Then stand back and take a long hard look. Does anything strike you straight away? If so, fine, but do not ignore the rest. Always examine the various parts of a CXR in a systematic manner. The following routine is suggested.

Always check for patient rotation: this causes asymmetry of the soft-tissue shadows and may produce apparent increased density in one lung or simulate mediastinal shift.

Tracheobronchial tree

- Follow the trachea and main bronchi (study for displacement, narrowing or intraluminal masses). If the trachea is not central, it may be pushed across by superior mediastinal mass (eg retrosternal goitre) or pulled over to the side of the lesion by fibrosis or collapsed lung.

- Assess the mediastinal contour. Are there any abnormal shadows (tumour, goitre or paratracheal lymphadenopathy)?

- Look at the position, outline and density of the hilar shadow. Displacement of the hila is common in collapse, fibrosis or resection of the lung. Enlarged and lobulated hila are characteristic of hilar adenopathy. Enlarged but otherwise normal hila occur with dilatation of the pulmonary arteries. Unilateral enlargement of a pulmonary artery (distended by a thrombus) may be seen in massive embolism. Perihilar haze is an early sign of pulmonary oedema. Check whether both hilar shadows are of equal density; increased density of the hilum is the most common manifestation of a hilar mass. Do not miss it!

Cardiac shadow

Is the heart size normal, enlarged or narrow (chronic obstructive pulmonary disease – COPD)? Estimate the cardiothoracic ratio; the heart should fill less than half the thoracic width.

Follow the contours of the heart. Are all heart borders well defined?

- Right middle lobe collapse: hazy (blurred) right heart border.

- Lingular collapse: hazy left heart border.

- Right lower lobe collapse: heart border is preserved, and there is an additional wedge-shaped density and a blurred medial diaphragm.

- Left lower lobe collapse: there is a wedge-shape density behind the heart ('sail sign', or an apparent double heart border) that obscures the medial diaphragm, which is elevated.

Check the areas behind the heart. Do not miss hiatus hernia, tumour of the oesophagus or lung collapse.

Diaphragm

In full inspiration the mid-point of the right diaphragm lies at the level of the anterior end of the sixth rib. The dome of the right diaphragm is normally up to 1 cm higher than the left.

- Is the diaphragm elevated? This suggests paralysis, eventration or infrapulmonary effusion.

- Are both diaphragms, the costophrenic angles and the cardiophrenic angles well defined? A blurring of the diaphragm indicates either pleural fluid or disease in the adjacent lung field. A minimal pleural effusion or pleural thickening obliterates the costophrenic angle.

- Is there any calcification over the diaphragm? This would indicate asbestos plaques.

Soft tissues and bones

The soft tissues and bones may give a false impression of pulmonary disease and should be examined before analysing the lung fields.

- Look at the breast shadow: mastectomy produces ipsilateral hyperlucency (a 'blacker' lung).

- Examine the clavicles, ribs and scapula for evidence of metastasis (indicates lytic or sclerotic lesions) and for evidence of old or new fractures (ie pathological). Turning the CXR on its side and studying the ribs helps distract your attention from everything else.

- Look for subcutaneous emphysema.

Lung parenchyma

First, ignore the lung fields and take a good look around the edge of the lung at the pleura. Is it thickened (pleural plaques) or calcified? Do not miss a small pneumothorax (especially apical).

Lung fields

- Assess the size of the lungs: if they are small, the problem could be poor inspiration or fibrosis, whereas if they are large then this suggests COPD.

- Is the transradiancy of each zone equal? Compare the relative parts of the opposite lung in order to detect more subtle parenchymal changes. If there is any abnormally increased or decreased density, describe its location, size (localised or diffuse), shape (irregular, round, wedge-shaped or linear) and texture (reticulonodular or solid).

- Are all the pulmonary lobes and fissures intact or are they distorted? See Fig. 39.

If any abnormality is identified, compare its radiological appearance with the previous films, as the sequence and pattern of abnormalities may give you an important clue as to the most likely cause and may influence your management (eg long-standing changes often prevent unnecessary investigations). If in doubt, ask a radiologist!

FURTHER READING

Gurney JW and Winer-Muram HT. *Pocket Radiologist Chest: Top 100 Diagnoses.* Philadelphia: WB Saunders, 2003.

3.6.5 Computed tomography scan of the thorax

There are a number of indications for CT scans of the thorax and, as with all investigations, you need to give detailed reasons for the test on the request form in order for the radiologists to give you the best possible service. A variety of techniques are used.

Figure 40 shows the principal mediastinal structures seen on CT scanning of the thorax.

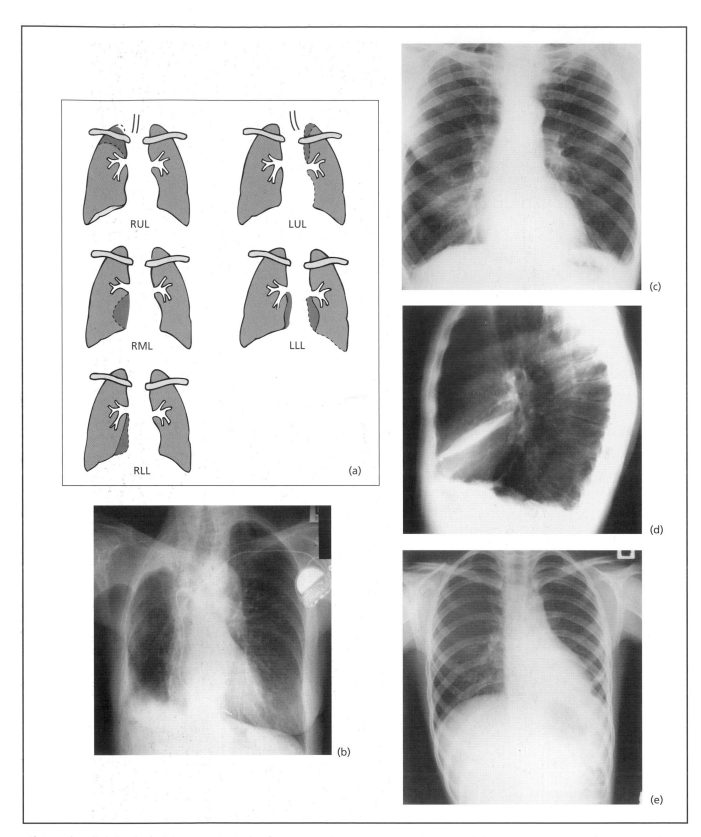

▲ **Fig. 39** Radiological signs of lobar collapses: (**a**) diagrammatic representation of the radiographic patterns of lobar collapse – right upper lobe (RUL), left upper lobe (LUL), right middle lobe (RML), left lower lobe (LLL) and right lower lobe (RLL); (**b**) RUL collapse secondary to tuberculosis infection (also pacemaker); (**c**) RML collapse, which can be difficult to diagnose; (**d**) RML collapse, which is clearly demonstrated on a lateral chest radiograph; and (**e**) LLL collapse, with the 'sail sign' where the collapse lobe lies behind the heart and the mediastrinum is shifted to the left, straightening the right heart border.

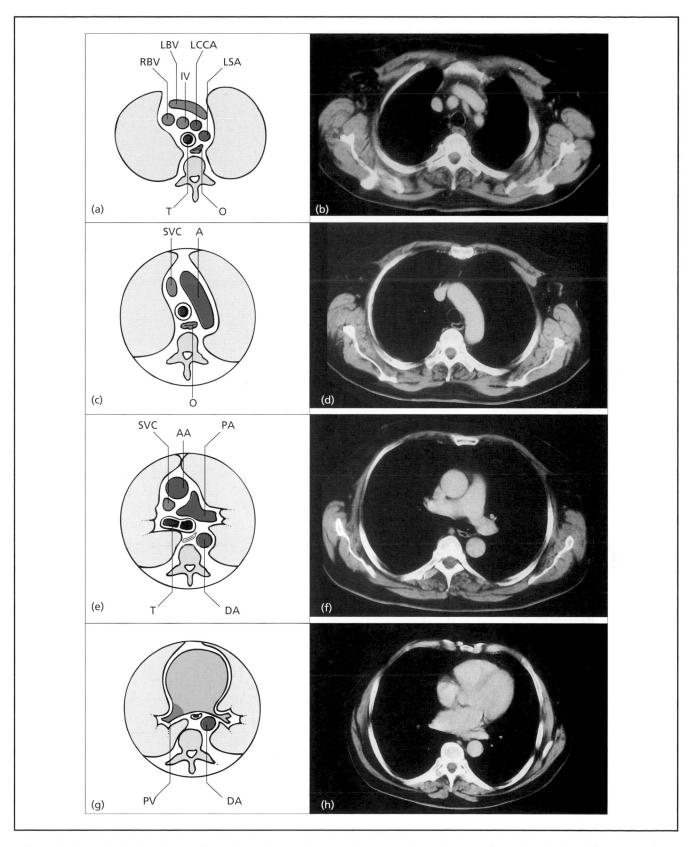

▲**Fig.40** Principal mediastinal structures on CT scanning of the thorax. Remember that you are viewing the sections from below, ie the left of the thorax is on the right of the figure. (**a, b**) Section above the aortic arch. The trachea (T), oesophagus (O), right brachiocephalic vein (RBV), left brachiocephalic vein (LBV), innominate vein (IV), left common carotid artery (LCCA) and left subclavian artery (LSA) are visible. (**c, d**) Section at the level of the aortic arch (A). The superior vena cava (SVC) is visible. (**e, f**) Section below aortic arch. Both ascending (AA) and descending (DA) aortas are visible. The trachea (T) is bifurcated and pulmonary arteries (PA) are seen. Note in (**f**) that the bifurcation of the trachea is present behind the pulmonary arteries but is difficult to see in cross-section. (**g, h**) Section at the level of the pulmonary veins (PV). Lower lobe intrapulmonary arteries and bronchi are not shown in the diagram. DA, descending aorta. (CT scans courtesy of Dr I. Vlahos.)

TABLE 44 TYPICAL HIGH-RESOLUTION CT APPEARANCES OF SOME DIFFUSE PARENCHYMAL LUNG DISEASES

Disorder	High-resolution CT appearances
Usual interstitial pneumonia (UIP)	Patchy abnormalities that are mainly peripheral and basal. Also look for reticular and honeycomb changes with ground-glass opacification and traction bronchiectasis
Asbestosis	Similar to UIP. Reticular nodular opacities and thickened interlobular septa. Pleural plaques are often present
Sarcoidosis	Lymph node enlargement, and micronodules with bronchovascular and subpleural distribution. Abnormalities mainly in the upper and mid zones
Lymphangitis carcinomatosa	Irregular thickening of the interlobular septa, peribronchial cuffing and thickening of fissures. No architectural distortion
Extrinsic allergic alveolitis	Ground-glass opacification and poorly defined centrilobular micronodules. Air trapping on expiratory scans
Langerhans' cell histiocytosis	Cysts of bizarre shape associated with nodules. Lung bases usually not affected
Lymphangioleiomyomatosis	Thin-walled cysts surrounded by normal lung

Types of scan

The images produced by CT scanning depend on the thickness of the cuts taken, and the distance between successive cuts. For example by taking 10-mm cuts at 10-mm intervals the whole lung can be imaged, but each individual cut will not show fine parenchymal detail, as effectively data from a thick slice of lung have been compressed onto a single two-dimensional plane. This would be appropriate when one is looking for lung cancer for example. On the other hand, taking 1-mm slices at 10-mm intervals will give much greater fine detail (and for a smaller total radiation dose), but 90% of the area included in the scan would not be visualised, and in theory a nodule under 1 cm in size could be missed. In reality, modern 'multislice' scanners are capable of scanning the whole lung and then using computer software to retrospectively reconstruct thin cuts.

High-resolution scans

Here the lung is imaged by taking thin cuts at regular intervals. These are often invaluable in the diagnosis of parenchymal lung disease and can be diagnostic of certain conditions, thus avoiding further more invasive investigations, eg sarcoidosis or usual interstitial pneumonia (Table 44).

If the changes are subtle, the radiologist may perform prone and supine films, ie scan the patient lying on both back and front. This is to ensure that pulmonary interstitial fluid is not mimicking the changes of fibrosis: fluid will move downwards, while fibrosis remains in the same area of the lung on both views (Fig. 41).

Conventional scans

Staging scans for suspected lung cancer (or other discrete lesions like abcesses) involve the scanner taking thick slices in order to cover the whole lung field. The images are reproduced in two settings.

- Bone or soft-tissue windows: these highlight lymph node enlargement, soft-tissue involvement and bony lesions.

- Lung windows: these concentrate on the lung parenchyma, producing images of the tumour as well as the condition of the surrounding lung, ie coexisting emphysema, bullae or fibrosis.

Helical scans

Spiral CT is the latest technological improvement in this form of scanning. It is fast and a complete scan can be completed in one breath-hold. They are increasingly useful in the diagnosis of pulmonary emboli when contrast media is used to create a pulmonary angiogram.

Reading a scan

When you assess a CT scan, remember that you are viewing it as though you are standing at the patient's feet looking upwards, so for example the patient's liver is on the left of the picture and the spleen on the right. Like the CXR, try to follow a system through the scans.

- Follow the main vessels such as the descending and ascending aorta and its arch.

- Look carefully for enlargement of the hilar and paratracheal lymph nodes and any other soft-tissue changes (Fig. 42).

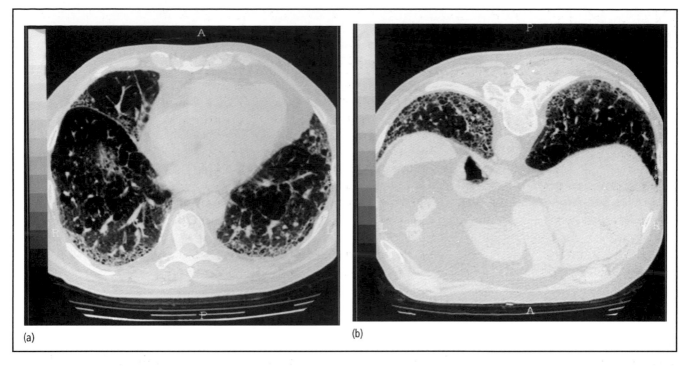

(a)   (b)

▲ **Fig. 41** CT scan of the thorax of a man with pulmonary fibrosis in (**a**) supine and (**b**) prone positions. Note the different positioning of the patient on the scanning table (at the bottom of both films). The honeycomb appearance of the lungs remains posterior in both views.

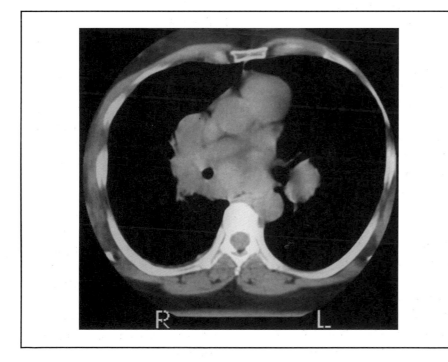

▲ **Fig. 42** CT of the thorax: note the mass of lymph nodes distorting the normal architecture of the mediastinum. This patient was subsequently diagnosed as having sarcoidosis.

- Look at the lung windows: study the lung parenchyma and run your eye carefully around the pleura looking for any thickening, plaques and/or adjacent fibrosis.

- Finally, for your education, ask a radiologist to talk you through the scan.

FURTHER READING

Hughes JMB and Pride NB. *Lung Function Tests, Physiological Principles and Clinical Applications.* London: WB Saunders, 1999.

4.1 Self-assessment questions

Question 1

Clinical scenario

A 72-year-old man with emphysema, an ex-smoker for 4 years, continues to be symptomatic on minimal exertion despite maximal medical therapy, including long-term oxygen treatment. A 6-week pulmonary rehabilitation programme has also failed to palliate his symptoms. His forced expiratory volume in 1 second is 0.6 L (28% of predicted) and his gas transfer is 45%. His CT chest scan shows severe heterogeneous emphysema with almost completely destroyed upper lobes.

Question

Which one of the following treatment options would you consider?

Answers

A Single lung transplantation
B Bilateral lung transplantation
C Heart–lung transplantation
D Lung volume reduction surgery
E Nebulised morphine.

Question 2

Clinical scenario

A 40-year-old man, a lifelong non-smoker, presents with a 6-month history of exertional shortness of breath. His CXR is shown in Fig. 43.

Question

What is the most likely diagnosis?

Answers

A Asthma
B Extrinsic allergic alveolitis
C Usual interstitial pneumonia
D Asbestosis
E Emphysema secondary to α_1-antitrypsin deficiency

Question 3

Clinical scenario

A 62-year-old woman with chronic obstructive pulmonary disease continues to complain of shortness of breath on exertion and presents with frequent lower respiratory tract infections requiring antibiotics and oral steroid treatment. Her medication consists of an inhaled short-acting anticholinergic and aminophylline tablets. She has been unable to tolerate inhaled long-acting β_2 agonists because of tremor. A trial of long-acting anticholinergic has proved unhelpful. Her forced expiratory volume in 1 second is 0.8 L (38% of predicted) and her Sao_2 is 95%.

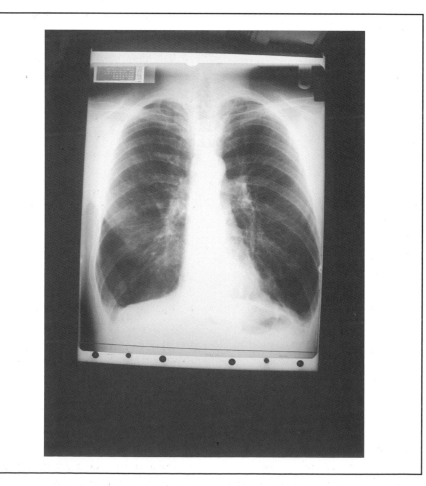

▲**Fig. 43** Question 2.

Question

What treatment would you recommend?

Answers

A Long-term oral corticosteroid treatment
B Nebulised bronchodilators
C Leukotriene receptor antagonist
D Prophylactic antibiotic treatment
E Inhaled corticosteroid treatment

Question 4

Clinical scenario

A 52-year-old married heathcare assistant gives a 6-week history of a dry hacking cough and progressive shortness of breath, which has failed to respond to two courses of antibiotics (penicillin and macrolide). Her CXR is reported as showing bilateral patchy consolidation, predominantly in the lower lobes. Routine blood tests are normal, except for elevated C-reactive protein. Her antinuclear antibodies and antineutrophil cytoplasmic antibodies are also normal.

Question

Which of the listed diagnoses is most likely?

Answers

A Pulmonary tuberculosis
B Extrinsic allergic alveolitis
C Cryptogenic organising pneumonia
D Bronchiolitis obliterans
E Sarcoidosis

Question 5

Clinical scenario

A 44-year-old woman who is a lifelong non-smoker presents with a 5-month history of progressive exertional shortness of breath. Her GP diagnosed asthma, but she failed to respond to antiasthma medication, including a prolonged

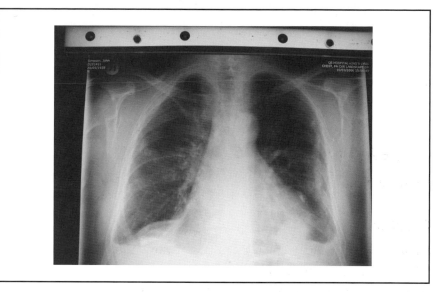

▲ **Fig. 44** Question 6.

trial of oral corticosteroids. Her CXR shows hyperinflated lung fields. Spirometry confirms irreversible airway obstruction. A CT chest scan shows no evidence of emphysema.

Question

Which diagnosis is most likely in her case?

Answers

A Pulmonary sarcoidosis
B Usual interstitial pneumonia
C Cryptogenic organising pneumonia
D Bronchiolitis obliterans
E Multiple pulmonary emboli

Question 6

Clinical scenario

A 68-year-old man, a retired RAF fireman, has developed symptoms of lower respiratory chest infection, which have left him with a hacking cough. His CXR is shown in Fig. 44.

Question

What would you arrange next to establish the diagnosis?

Answers

A A trial of inhaled corticosteroids
B Full lung function tests
C Fibreoptic bronchoscopy
D High-resolution CT chest scan
E Echocardiogram

Question 7

Clinical scenario

A 62-year-old man is referred to the chest clinic because of a productive cough, which has persisted for 6 weeks since his return from a holiday in India. He is an ex-smoker, having stopped 4 years ago. His physical examination is unremarkable. His CXR is shown in Fig. 45.

Question

What would you arrange next?

Answers

A Full lung function tests
B Fibreoptic bronchoscopy
C Mantoux test
D Sputum direct staining and culture for acid-fast bacilli
E Angiotensin-converting enzyme level

Question 8

Clinical scenario

A 65-year-woman, a lifelong non-smoker, has presented with an 8-month history of shortness of

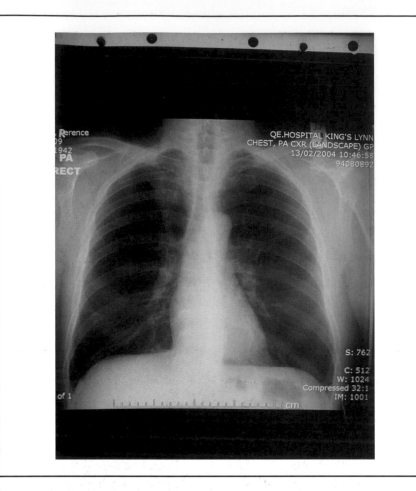

▲Fig. 45 Question 7.

breath and daily sputum production. Physical examination shows a left pleural effusion and yellow discoloration of nails. Diagnostic pleural aspiration shows exudate and no malignant cells.

Question

What would be the most appropriate action to take next?

Answers

A Bronchoscopy

B CT chest scan

C Pleural biopsy

D Simple pleural aspiration

E Pleural drainage with talc pleurodesis

Question 9

Clinical scenario

A 78-year-old woman with chronic obstructive pulmonary disease is planning to visit her daughter in the USA. Her forced expiratory volume in 1 second is 1.2 L (55% of predicted) and Sao_2 on air is 96%.

Question

What would you advise her to do?

Answers

A Say she should not fly

B Say she can fly but will need in-flight oxygen at a rate of 2 L/min

C Say she can fly but will need in-flight oxygen at a rate of 4 L/min

D Say there is no contraindication to air travel

E Say an altitude simulation test is required

Question 10

Clinical scenario

A 77-year-old man, a smoker of 20 cigarettes per day since the age of 18 years, is referred to a chest clinic with a 3-month history of progressive shortness of breath. There is no significant past medical history and he remains on no medications. On examination there are bilateral basal crackles. His CXR is shown in Fig. 46.

Question

What is the most likely diagnosis?

Answer

A Emphysema

B Left ventricular failure

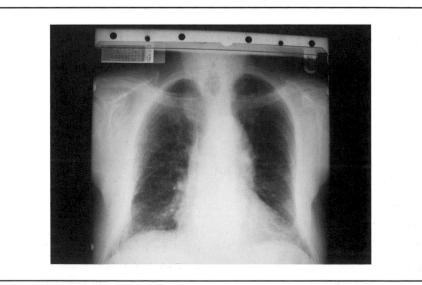

▲Fig. 46 Question 10.

C Usual interstitial pneumonia
D Sarcoidosis
E Asbestosis

Question 11

Clinical scenario

A 53-year-old man complains of increasing shortness of breath that limits his exercise tolerance to about 40–50 metres. His forced expiratory volume in 1 second (FEV_1) is 0.7 L (41% of predicted) and his forced vital capacity (FVC) is 1.4 L (67% of predicted), giving an FEV_1/FVC ratio of 50%. His CXR and CT chest scan are shown in Figs 47 and 48, respectively.

Question

What treatment should be considered?

Answers

A Simple pleural aspiration
B Pleural drainage
C Bullectomy
D Lung volume reduction surgery
E Lung transplantation

Question 12

Clinical scenario

A 52-year-old man, a lifelong non-smoker, complains of a productive cough that has persisted for the last 18 months. He denies shortness of breath. His past medical history is unremarkable, apart from the usual childhood infections. A physical examination is unremarkable. All routine blood tests as well as his CXR prove normal. His high-resolution CT chest scan shows distal bronchiectasis, most prominent in the lower lobes.

Question

Which of the following investigations would you arrange next?

Answers

A Bronchoscopy
B Serum immunoglobulin level

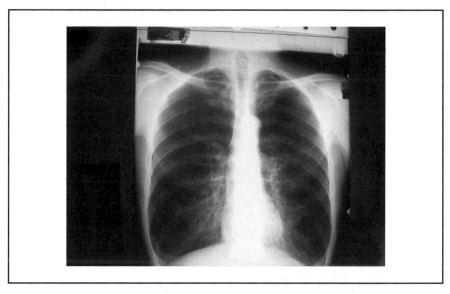

▲**Fig. 47** Question 11.

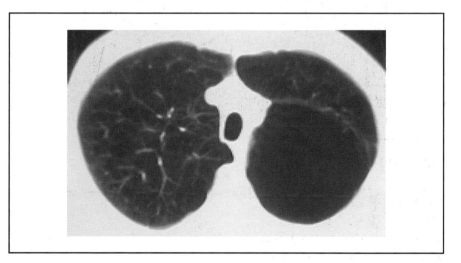

▲**Fig. 48** Question 11.

C Serum α_1-antitrypsin level
D C-reactive protein
E *Aspergillus fumigatus* precipitins

Question 13

Clinical scenario

A 38-year-old man is referred to the chest clinic as his GP is concerned that his asthma responds poorly to antiasthma therapy. Within the past few months he has required several courses of antibiotics and oral corticosteroid treatment. On examination there are few wheezes in his chest. His CXR is normal. Spirometry shows a moderately severe obstructive defect.

Question

Which of the listed investigations would be *least* relevant in further assessment?

Answers

A Antinuclear antibodies
B Antinuclear cytoplasmic antibodies
C Skin-prick test to *Aspergillus fumigatus*
D α_1-Antitrypsin deficiency
E High-resolution CT chest scan

Question 14

Clinical scenario

A 59-year-old retired plumber, smoker of 100 pack-years, has had a CXR as a part of a routine medical examination for insurance purposes. His past medical history is unremarkable and he remains on no medication. Apart from borderline hypertension, his physical examination is normal. His spirometry shows a mild obstructive defect. Oxygen saturation (on air) is 98%. His CXR shows interstitial shadowing, most prominent at both bases.

Question

Which of the following statements is *false*?

Answers

A Diffuse parenchymal lung disease (DPLD) is unlikely given the presence of an obstructive defect on spirometry

B DPLD is likely despite the presence of an obstructive defect on spirometry

C A high-resolution CT chest scan may reveal that the lower lobes of the lungs are 'squashed' by emphysematous upper lungs, giving the impression on a plain CXR of fibrotic changes at the bases

D An obstructive defect on spirometry could be the result of treatment with a beta-blocker for his hypertension

E A normal high-resolution CT chest scan virtually excludes the possibility of fibrosing alveolitis

Question 15

Clinical scenario

A 54-year-old man presents with a 6-month history of productive cough. His past medical history includes asthma, which lately has been poorly controlled, and perennial rhinitis. A physical

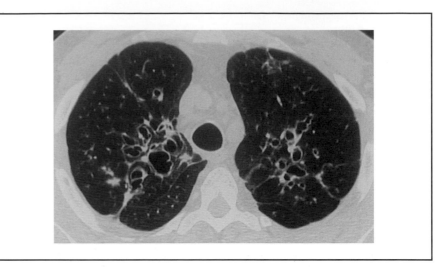

▲ **Fig. 49** Question 15.

examination shows widespread wheezes. His CXR is normal. A high-resolution CT chest scan is shown in Fig. 49.

Question

Which investigation would you request next in order to establish the aetiology of the radiological abnormalities?

Answers

A Rheumatoid factor

B Skin-prick test

C α_1-Antitrypsin

D Antinuclear antibodies

E Mantoux test

Question 16

Clinical scenario

A 78-year-old man has been found collapsed on the street and is brought to the Emergency Department. He is cold and clammy. His ECG shows an acute anterior myocardial infarction. His CXR is shown in Fig. 50.

Question

What is the most likely cause for this patient's radiological abnormality?

Answers

A Congenital absence of left upper lobe

B Pulmonary fibrosis secondary to tuberculosis

C Left pneumonectomy

D Left upper lobectomy

E Left thoracoplasty

Question 17

Clinical scenario

A 62-year-old woman, a lifelong non-smoker, is admitted for an elective laparoscopic cholecystectomy. A routine CXR taken prior to the procedure is shown in Fig. 51.

Question

What would be the most appropriate investigation to request next?

Answers

A Sputum direct staining for acid-fast bacilli

B Repeat CXR in 6 weeks' time

C Fibreoptic bronchoscopy

D Bone scan

E Mantoux test

Question 18

Clinical scenario

A 72-year-old man who has smoked 10–15 cigarettes per day since the age of 16 years complains of exertional shortness of breath

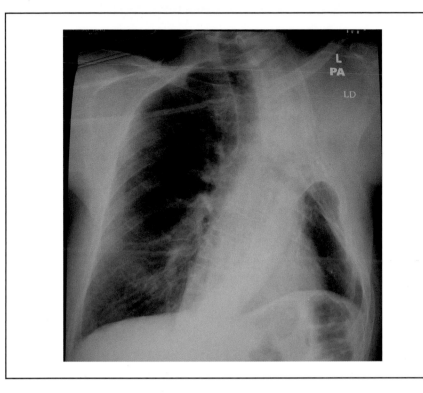

▲ **Fig. 50** Question 16.

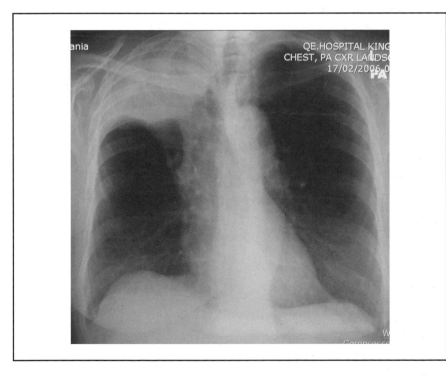

▲ **Fig. 51** Question 17.

and central chest tightness. A physical examination is unremarkable and his full lung function tests are normal. A CXR does prove abnormal, but as the cause of his symptoms remains unclear a high-resolution CT chest scan is carried out, which is shown in Fig. 52.

Question

What does the CT scan show?

Answers

A Emphysema

B Asbestosis

C Asbestos-related pleural plaques

D Pericardial effusion

E Asbestosis and asbestos-related pleural plaques

Question 19

Clinical scenario

A 62-year-old man has been referred to the chest clinic because he developed shortness of breath following accidental exposure to asbestos dust 4 months ago when his old fireplace was being replaced. Since then he has been complaining of shortness of breath on mild exertion and chest tightness. He also complains of feeling light-headed, having occasional sharp pains in his chest, and having pins and needles in both arms. His symptoms have been so troublesome that he has been off work for the last 3 weeks. He is a lifelong non-smoker. There is nothing on physical examination. His CXR, ECG, spirometry and oximetry are normal. He is very concerned that he is developing asbestosis.

Question

What would you tell him?

Answers

A Although his CXR is normal, a high-resolution CT chest scan is required to rule out the possibility of early asbestosis

B Although his ECG is normal, a treadmill test is needed to rule out angina

C A blood test will be arranged to rule out the possibility of clots in his lungs

D His symptoms are not due to asbestosis, which develops 20–30 years after exposure to asbestos, but he has most probably developed asthma and will be prescribed appropriate inhalers

317

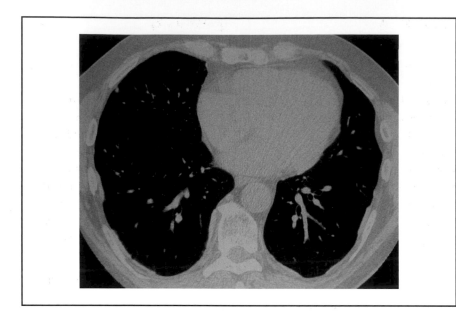

▲ **Fig. 52** Question 18.

E His symptoms are benign in
nature and should resolve
following breathing exercises

Question 20

Clinical scenario

A 62-year-old man, a smoker of
60 pack-years, is referred to the
chest clinic with a 6-month history
of progressive shortness of breath.
He is a keen golfer and is concerned
that he has recently had difficulty
in completing the game because
of dyspnoea, which is particularly
bad when the weather is cold or
windy. He gave up smoking 2 weeks
ago, which did not help. On direct
questioning he admits to having
had a 'smoker's cough' for years,
but denies any nocturnal symptoms.
His physical examination is normal.
Full lung function tests show a
forced expiratory volume in
1 second (FEV$_1$) of 1.4 L (63%
of predicted) and a forced vital
capacity (FVC) of 2.4 L (90% of
predicted), resulting in an FEV$_1$/
FVC ratio of 57%. His gas transfer
is 64%.

Question

What would you do next?

Answers

A Arrange a 2-week trial of oral
corticosteroid treatment and
repeat spirometry

B Start short-acting inhaled
bronchodilator

C Start long-acting oral
bronchodilator

D Arrange a bronchodilator
reversibility test to decide
whether inhaled corticosteroid
is indicated

E Start a combination of inhaled
corticosteroid and a long-acting
bronchodilator

Question 21

Clinical scenario

A 55-year-old woman attends the
chest clinic with a history of dry
nocturnal cough for over 6 months.
She has never smoked and is a
retired hotel receptionist. There is
no history of haemoptysis, wheeze
or weight loss. There are no nasal
symptoms. She suffers from

hypertension and is on perindopril
4 mg and bendroflumethiazide
2.5 mg daily. Examination is normal.

Question

Which of the following is most likely
to be responsible for her symptoms?

Answers

A Bronchogenic carcinoma

B Cryptogenic pulmonary fibrosis

C Drug-induced cough

D Late-onset asthma

E Bronchiectasis

Question 22

Clinical scenario

A 73-year-old woman known
to suffer from severe chronic
obstructive pulmonary disease is
admitted with a history of dyspnoea,
a cough with purulent phlegm and
wheeze. She is on home nebulisers,
long-term oxygen therapy and
maintenance prednisolone 15 mg
daily. She is house-bound and has
carers who help her daily. At the
time of admission arterial blood
gases on air reveal a pH of 7.30,
Paco$_2$ 8.9 kPa and Pao$_2$ 5.4 kPa; her
bicarbonate is normal. Her CXR
shows left mid-zone consolidation.

Question

Besides regular nebulisers, antibiotics
and oral prednisolone, which of the
following treatments is indicated?

Answers

A Endotracheal intubation and
ventilation in the intensive
care unit

B Intravenous aminophylline

C Controlled oxygen

D Bi-level positive airway pressure
ventilation

E Intravenous hydrocortisone

Question 23

Clinical scenario

A 67-year-old bus driver attends
the chest clinic with his wife.

He feels quite fine, but his wife says that he snores at night and has numerous daytime naps. He has hypertension despite taking atenolol 100 mg od, bendroflumethiazide 2.5 mg od and amlodipine 5 mg od. He has never smoked and his BMI is 39. His screening CXR and lung function tests are normal. On further questioning his wife mentions that he makes choking and gurgling sounds at night.

Question

Which of the following would be the best screening tool to apply to this man?

Answers

A Short form 36 questionnaire
B Hospital anxiety and depression score questionnaire
C Epworth Sleepiness Scale
D Medical Research Council dyspnoea scale questionnaire
E St George's respiratory questionnaire

Question 24

Clinical scenario

A 72-year-old man has been referred to the chest clinic by the cardiologists with a history of shortness of breath. He underwent an uneventful aortic valve repair 2 months ago. An echocardiogram is normal and a CXR shows a mildly elevated left hemidiaphragm. A CXR done prior to his surgery was normal.

Question

Which of the following investigations is most appropriate?

Answers

A High-resolution CT chest scan
B Regular peak expiratory flow rate monitoring
C Sitting and lying spirometry
D Arterial blood gases
E Bronchoscopy

Question 25

Clinical scenario

A 65-year-old woman attends the chest clinic with a history of dyspnoea on exertion and morning headaches. She also mentions daytime tiredness. On examination she is normal apart from pedal oedema and a BMI of 41. She has never smoked and is on no medications.

Question

What is the most likely diagnosis?

Answers

A Narcolepsy
B Obstructive sleep apnoea syndrome
C Chronic obstructive pulmonary disease
D Obesity hypoventilation syndrome
E Congestive cardiac failure

Question 26

Clinical scenario

A 73-year-old woman with a past history of thoracoplasty is admitted to hospital with a history of breathlessness on exertion for the last 4 months, morning headaches and mild ankle swelling. Her GP has started her on salbutamol inhalers without any improvement. There is no history of wheeze and she is a lifelong non-smoker. An examination shows chest wall deformity due to previous surgery and mild pitting ankle oedema. Arterial blood gases taken at 7 a.m. show pH 7.31, $Paco_2$ 8.8 kPa and Pao_2 6.9 kPa.

Question

What long-term treatment will she need?

Answers

A Antibiotics
B Oral steroids
C Nebulisers
D Oxygen
E Non-invasive positive-pressure ventilation

Question 27

Clinical scenario

A 68-year-old man with a history of obstructive sleep apnoea and who has been on nasal continuous positive airways pressure (nCPAP) for the last 3 years is referred to the sleep clinic with recurrence of daytime somnolence. He was previously well controlled on nCPAP and claims to use this treatment every night for at least 7 hours. He has recently gained 13 kg in weight.

Question

What is the best management plan?

Answers

A Try bi-level positive airway pressure
B Advice to lose weight
C Try a mandibular advancement device
D Start modafinil
E Consider tracheostomy

Question 28

Clinical scenario

A 40-year-old woman is admitted to the hospital with a parapneumonic effusion. A diagnostic pleural tap has been done.

Question

Which of the following is an indication for inserting a chest drain?

Answers

A Temperature above 39°C
B A rising white cell count and C-reactive protein
C Pleural pH <7.2
D Blood-stained pleural fluid
E Pleural fluid lactate dehydrogenase >200 U/L

Question 29

Clinical scenario

A 65-year-old retired builder is admitted with a left pleural effusion. He is an ex-smoker with a smoking history of 50 pack-years. As part of his employment he was exposed to asbestos 40 years ago. You suspect the underlying diagnosis to be mesothelioma.

Question

Which of the following is the investigation of choice?

Answers

A High-resolution CT scan of the lungs

B Bronchoscopy

C Pulmonary function test

D Video-assisted thoracoscopy and pleural biopsy

E Diagnostic pleural tap and insertion of a chest drain

Question 30

Clinical scenario

A 55-year-old man presents with a history of cough and haemoptysis of 2 weeks' duration. Six months ago he was diagnosed with sinusitis and started on some nasal drops. His CXR shows bilateral infiltrates and nodules with cavitations. He has never smoked and works in a zoo.

Question

What is the most likely diagnosis?

Answers

A Bronchogenic carcinoma

B Pulmonary tuberculosis

C Cryptogenic fibrosing alveolitis

D Sarcoidosis

E Wegener's granulomatosis

Question 31

Clinical scenario

A 44-year-old woman with steroid-dependent asthma attends the chest clinic. In her last visit, a leukotriene receptor antagonist was added and her oral steroid dose reduced. A series of CXRs over a period of 8 years has shown fleeting interstitial patchy shadowing. She has recently seen her GP as she has developed

subcutaneous nodules on the extensor surfaces of the arms. She has a mild normochromic normocytic anaemia, raised erythrocyte sedimentation rate, peripheral eosinophilia and a positive rheumatoid factor. In the past she was diagnosed with nasal polyps and sinusitis.

Question

What is the most likely diagnosis?

Answers

A Churg–Strauss syndrome

B Allergic bronchopulmonary aspergillosis

C Extrinsic allergic alveolitis

D Wegener's granulomatosis

E Rheumatoid lung disease

Question 32

Clinical scenario

A 48-year-old lorry driver has been referred to the sleep clinic with a history of snoring, daytime somnolence and nocturnal apnoeic spells. His score on the Epworth Sleepiness Scale is 14/24. You suspect obstructive sleep apnoea (OSA) and arrange for him to have a polysomnogram.

Question

Which of the following is true?

Answers

A OSA is usually more severe during rapid eye movement (REM) sleep

B OSA is worse in the prone sleeping position

C Alcohol increases REM sleep

D Normally REM sleep occurs during the first half of the night

E Benzodiazepines result in an increase in stages 3 and 4 (slow-wave sleep) of non-REM sleep

Question 33

Clinical scenario

A 28-year-old man is admitted to hospital with a suspected pulmonary embolism (PE).

Question

Which of the following is *not* suggestive of PE?

Answers

A Fever

B Haemoptysis

C Cough

D Wheeze

E Tachypnoea (respiratory rate >20/minute)

Question 34

Clinical scenario

A 27-year-old previously fit woman has been referred to the sleep clinic with excessive somnolence. There is no history of snoring. Her partner has noticed that on occasions when she is watching a comedy show on the television, she tends to drop whatever she is holding. A 2-week sleep diary shows that she sleeps for 8 hours every night and has numerous daytime naps.

Question

What is the most likely diagnosis?

Answers

A Sleep-disordered breathing

B Narcolepsy

C Insufficient sleep syndrome

D Restless leg syndrome

E Kleine–Levin syndrome

Question 35

Clinical scenario

A 33-year-old previously fit woman is admitted to the hospital with a 10-week history of progressive breathlessness and dry cough. She has never smoked and works in a supermarket. In the last 3 days she has developed painful dusky-coloured nodules on her shins. A CXR reveals bilateral hilar shadows.

Question

What is the most likely diagnosis?

Answers

A Bronchiectasis

B Tuberculosis

C Cryptogenic fibrosing alveolitis

D Lymphangioleiomyomatosis

E Sarcoidosis

Question 36

Clinical scenario

An 83-year-old man is admitted with a history of chronic obstructive pulmonary disease exacerbation. His forced expiratory volume in 1 second done 2 months ago, when he was well, was 1.1 L (36% of predicted). He has been treated with nebulisers, intravenous hydrocortisone, intravenous infusion of aminophylline and controlled oxygen. He has not improved despite this emergency treatment. You consider starting him on bi-level positive airways pressure (BiPAP).

Question

Which of the following arterial blood gas readings is an indication for BiPAP? (Normal values: pH 7.35–7.45, $Paco_2$ 4.7–6.0 kPa, Pao_2 >10.6 kPa, bicarbonate 22–28 mmol/L)

Answers

A pH 7.36, $Paco_2$ 7.3 kPa, Pao_2 6.6 kPa, bicarbonate 30 mmol/L

B pH 7.39, $Paco_2$ 5.0 kPa, Pao_2 7.1 kPa, bicarbonate 32 mmol/L

C pH 7.56, $Paco_2$ 3.7 kPa, Pao_2 8.9 kPa, bicarbonate 38 mmol/L

D pH 7.30, $Paco_2$ 4.0 kPa, Pao_2 6.9 kPa, bicarbonate 19 mmol/L

E pH 7.29, $Paco_2$ 8.9 kPa, Pao_2 6.1 kPa, bicarbonate 32 mmol/L

Question 37

Clinical scenario

A 56-year-old woman has a pleural effusion. The diagnostic tap shows a pleural fluid protein of 32 g/L.

Question

Which of the following is one of Light's criteria for differentiating pleural effusions into exudates and transudates?

Answers

A Pleural fluid protein divided by serum protein >0.5

B Pleural lactate dehydrogenase (LDH) divided by serum LDH >0.9

C Pleural fluid glucose divided by serum glucose >0.3

D Pleural fluid osmolality divided by serum osmolality >0.7

E Pleural fluid LDH less than two-thirds of the upper limit of normal serum LDH

Question 38

Clinical scenario

A 29-year-old woman is admitted with a 1-month history of increasing breathlessness and chest ache. The CXR shows a moderate-sized pleural effusion. As part of her diagnostic work-up a pleural tap is performed.

Question

Which of the following statements are true?

Answers

A Low pleural fluid glucose is highly suggestive of a pyogenic infection

B Normal pleural fluid pH is 7.6 due to an accumulation of bicarbonate ions

C Pleural involvement occurs in 50% of patients with rheumatoid arthritis and rheumatoid pleural effusions mainly occur in women

D Small pleural effusions occur in about 5% of patients with pulmonary embolism and about 20% are blood-stained

E In tuberculous pleurisy, pleural effusions are usually bilateral and smears for acid-fast bacilli are positive in 60% of tuberculous effusions

Question 39

Clinical scenario

A 19-year-old intravenous drug user is admitted febrile and with a loculated left-sided pleural effusion.

Question

Which of the following statements is *false*?

Answers

A In the management of empyema, nutrition is an important component of therapy

B 40% of infected pleural effusions are culture negative and so the measurement of pleural pH can be useful in establishing a diagnosis

C Patients who survive 6 months after an episode of pleural infection have a 4-year survival similar to that of healthy individuals

D The commonest cause of both community- and hospital-acquired pleural infection is the *Streptococcus milleri* group

E When empirically treating hospital-acquired pleural infection, the antibiotic regimen should cover Gram-positive aerobes (including methicillin-resistant *Staphylococcus aureus*), Gram-negative aerobes and anaerobes

Question 40

Clinical scenario

A 65-year-old smoker is referred to the clinic with haemoptysis of 2 weeks' duration. He is clubbed, has a palpable lymph node in the right supraclavicular fossa and has an oedematous right arm with superficial venous engorgement. The CXR shows a 3-cm spiculated mass extending from the right hilum.

Question

Which of the following is true?

Answers

A Over three-quarters of tumours can be seen and sampled at bronchoscopy

B About 50% of people with clubbing have carcinoma of the lung

C Hypercalcaemia is best treated by a low-calcium diet

D Patients over the age of 65 years with potentially resectable lung cancer, irrespective of comorbidity, will do badly after surgery

E Superior vena cava obstruction does not preclude a curative operative procedure

Question 41

Clinical scenario

A 69-year-old woman is admitted on an acute medical ward with severe breathlessness. Her past medical history is unremarkable, apart from an anterior myocardial infarction 6 months ago that was complicated by a ventricular tachycardia arrest. According to her daughter she has become progressively short of breath over the past 6 weeks. She is cyanosed and there are bilateral crackles in her lower and mid

zones. Her arterial blood gases on air reveal pH 7.34, P_{CO_2} 5.0 kPa and P_{O_2} 5.2 kPa. Routine blood tests are all normal apart from eosinophilia. Her CXR is shown in Fig. 53.

Question

What are the two most likely diagnoses?

Answers

A Left ventricular failure

B Bilateral bronchopneumonia

C Amiodarone-induced pneumonia

D Angiotensin-converting enzyme-induced pneumonia

E Aortic dissection

F Pericardial effusion

G Pulmonary embolism

H Usual interstitial pneumonia

I Bronchiolitis obliterans

J Cryptogenic organising pneumonia

Question 42

Clinical scenario

A 67-year-old retired builder with a smoking history of 45 pack-years is admitted with breathlessness. This started 2 months ago and has gradually worsened. A CXR shows

a large right pleural effusion, which a pleural tap confirms to be an exudate. In the past he is known to have had paroxysmal atrial fibrillation and has been on amiodarone for over 3 years.

Question

Which two of the following are true?

Answers

A Malignant effusions have a high glucose level

B Pleural effusions due to rheumatoid arthritis have low glucose levels

C Benign pleural effusions due to asbestos exposure are usually transudates

D Amiodarone can cause pleural effusions

E Pleural effusions occur in over 90% of patients with pulmonary embolism

F In parapneumonic pleural effusions, intrapleural streptokinase reduces duration of hospital stay

G Pleural transudates are never blood-stained

H Benign pleural effusions due to asbestos exposure are never blood-stained

I Pleural effusions in acute pancreatitis are mainly right-sided

J Pleural effusions in mesothelioma are usually transudates

Question 43

Clinical scenario

A 23-year-old previously fit man is admitted with a spontaneous left pneumothorax. He smokes 20 cigarettes per day and works as a labourer.

Question

Which two of the following are true?

Answers

A He should be treated with a chest drain irrespective of the size of the pneumothorax

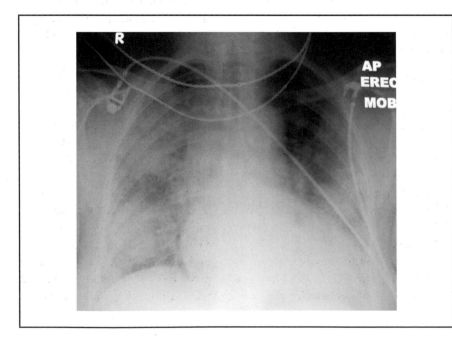

▲Fig. 53 Question 41.

B There is a direct relationship between physical activity and the pneumothorax

C Smoking has no relation to recurrence of pneumothorax

D Re-expansion pulmonary oedema does not occur with reinflation of the lung in the context of pneumothorax

E In a patient with pneumothorax admitted for observation, high-flow oxygen (10 L/min) will increase the rate of resolution of the pneumothorax

F Simple aspiration is the treatment of choice in a large pneumothorax in a patient with severe chronic obstructive pulmonary disease

G Large (20–24F) chest drains are better than small (10–14F) drains for drainage of the pneumothorax or a pleural effusion

H If suction is applied to the chest drain, a high volume and low pressure (10–20 cmH$_2$O) should be used

I Patients can be allowed to go deep-sea diving 8 weeks after successful treatment of a pneumothorax

J All patients with a primary spontaneous pneumothorax should undergo talc pleurodesis

Question 44

Clinical scenario

A 56-year-old woman is admitted with a right-sided pleural effusion. She is asymptomatic apart from breathlessness on exertion of 3 months' duration. She has a smoking history of 35 pack-years and is known to suffer from rheumatoid arthritis (RA) for which she is on prednisolone 10 mg daily and weekly methotrexate.

Question

Which two of the following are true?

Answers

A Pleural effusions associated with RA are usually transudates

B Pleural effusions associated with RA have high glucose level

C Pleural effusions in RA typically develop in young women

D Pleural effusions in RA have a high pH (>7.50)

E The treatment of choice is talc pleurodesis

F Pleural effusions in RA have a high triglyceride level (>110 mg/dL)

G Pleural effusions in RA have high levels of cholesterol

H The treatment of choice is to increase the dose of methotrexate

I Pleural effusions in RA develop in patients with subcutaneous nodules

J Pleural effusions in RA have very high C4 complement levels

Question 45

Clinical scenario

A 55 year-old retired coal miner with rheumatoid arthritis complains of breathlessness of 4 months' duration. He has never smoked and at present is on prednisolone 20 mg daily and methotrexate 15 mg every week.

Question

Which two of the following are *not* lung problems associated with rheumatoid arthritis?

Answers

A Pulmonary embolism

B Bronchiolitis obliterans

C Bronchiectasis

D Pulmonary nodules

E Pleural effusion

F Elevated hemidiaphragm

G Pneumothorax

H Interstitial pulmonary fibrosis

I Caplan's syndrome

J Apical fibrobullous disease

Question 46

Clinical scenario

A 59-year-old male asylum seeker is admitted with weight loss, nocturnal sweats and a productive cough. The CXR shows bilateral upper lobe infiltrates.

Question

Which two of the following statements are *false*?

Answers

A Erythrocyte sedimentation rate is an unreliable indicator of disease activity in patients with suspected pulmonary tuberculosis (TB)

B Inactivity of tuberculous disease can be inferred from the CXR

C A depressed (anergic) response following a BCG is found in sarcoidosis and lymphoma

D TB enteritis can occur as a result of swallowed sputum

E Ethambutol is useful in preventing the emergence of resistance to other drugs

F If sputum smears are negative for alcohol and acid-fast bacilli in this patient, then a bronchoscopy may increase diagnostic yield

G Rifampicin can cause thrombocytopenic purpura, and if this occurs it should never be given again

H Corticosteroids should be given in addition to antituberculous chemotherapy in patients who have ureteric obstruction

I A previous BCG usually causes a Heaf grade 1 or 2 reaction (ie Mantoux test: 5–14 mm)

J Pyrazinamide is bacteriostatic and has poor cerebrospinal fluid penetration: it therefore has limited use in tuberculous meningitis

4.2 Self-assessment answers

Answer to Question 1

D

This patient is too old for either bilateral lung transplantation or heart–lung transplantation. Single lung transplantation is highly unlikely because of the shortage of donors. He should be considered for lung volume reduction surgery (LVRS). The goal of LVRS is to reduce lung volume by 20–30%, which probably improves pulmonary and chest wall mechanics at rest and during exercise. Several randomised trials have compared LVRS with optimal medical treatment and have shown that patients with upper lobe-predominant emphysema and a low exercise capacity benefit the most from LVRS. Contraindications include forced expiratory volume in 1 second <20% of predicted, diffusing capacity of the lungs for carbon monoxide <20% of predicted and homogeneous changes on CT chest scan, because this group of patients is at high risk of death after surgery and is also unlikely to benefit from LVRS. (See Sections 1.2.5 and 2.3.)

Answer to Question 2

E

Emphysema due to α_1-antitrypsin deficiency predominantly involves lower lobes. Most patients are between 30 and 45 years of age at the time of presentation. In contrast, emphysema due to smoking has upper lobe predominance and usually does not cause severe airflow obstruction until patients are in their mid-sixties. (See Sections 1.2.5 and 2.3.)

Answer to Question 3

E

Inhaled corticosteroids should be prescribed for patients with a forced expiratory volume in 1 second less than or equal to 50% of predicted, and who have had two or more exacerbations of chronic obstructive pulmonary disease (COPD) requiring treatment with antibiotics or oral corticosteroids in a 12-month period. The aim of treatment is to reduce exacerbation rates and slow the decline in health status, not to improve lung function *per se*. Maintenance use of oral corticosteroid therapy in COPD is not normally recommended. (See Sections 1.2.5 and 2.3.)

Answer to Question 4

C

Pulmonary tuberculosis, extrinsic allergic alveolitis and sarcoidosis are unlikely as in these conditions upper lobe predominance would be expected. Consolidation is not a feature of bronchiolitis obliterans, which usually presents either with a normal CXR or with signs of hyperinflation. Bilateral airspace radiological changes not responding to an antibiotic may suggest cryptogenic organising pneumonia (COP). A tissue diagnosis (video-assisted thoracoscopic lung biopsy) should be obtained, as COP requires long-term oral corticosteroid treatment, initially in high dose. (See Section 2.7.2.)

Answer to Question 5

D

The absence of emphysema on the CT chest scan of a patient who has severe airway limitation and no clinical manifestation of asthma may suggest bronchiolitis obliterans. Mosaic pattern is usually seen on high-resolution CT chest scans carried out during expiration. Lung biopsy may be required to establish a diagnosis. (See Section 2.7.2.)

Answer to Question 6

C

The CXR shows a rounded mass behind the heart that is highly suspicious of a lung cancer, bilateral calcified pleural plaques consistent with previous asbestos exposure, an enlarged heart and bilateral small pleural effusions. The risk of developing lung cancer amongst those who have been exposed to asbestos is significantly greater in smokers than in non-smokers. The relative risk of lung cancer for cigarette smokers with a history of asbestos exposure is 59-fold, compared with a 6-fold relative risk for non-smokers with a history of asbestos exposure. Cigarette smoking without a history of asbestos exposure is associated with an 11-fold increase in the risk of lung cancer. (See Sections 2.6.1 and 2.9.1.)

Answer to Question 7

B

The CXR shows signs of early collapse and consolidation in the right apex. An endobronchial lesion must be excluded. (See Section 3.6.4.)

Answer to Question 8

E

Yellow nails and pleural effusion suggest yellow nail syndrome. She most probably also has bronchiectasis, which is part of the syndrome. This would explain her daily sputum production. No further investigations are required. As pleural effusion is likely to recur, pleural drainage with talc pleurodesis is recommended. (See Section 1.2.4.)

Answer to Question 9

D

There are no contraindications to air travel if Sao_2 is over 95%, or if it is between 92 and 95% and there are no risk factors. In-flight oxygen is indicated if Sao_2 is below 92%. If Sao_2 is between 92 and 95% and risk factors are present, then hypoxic challenge should be carried out. Risk factors include severe chronic obstructive pulmonary disease/asthma, severe restrictive disease, cystic fibrosis, pulmonary tuberculosis, comorbidity with other conditions worsened by hypoxaemia (cerebrovascular accident, ischaemic heart disease and congestive cardiac failure), risk of or previous venous thrombosis, recent pneumothorax, pre-existing requirement of oxygen or ventilatory support, history of travel intolerance with respiratory symptoms and any travelling planned within 6 weeks of discharge from hospital for acute respiratory illness. (See Section 2.12.1.)

Answer to Question 10

C

This CXR shows bilateral peripheral interstitial reticular shadowing, predominantly in lower and mid lobes. This is characteristic of usual interstitial pneumonia. (See Sections 1.2.2 and 2.7.1.)

Answer to Question 11

C

The CXR shows hyperinflated lungs with areas of arterial deficiency and hypoattenuation. The CT chest scan shows a large left upper lobe bulla. The most common indication for a bullectomy is severe dyspnoea in the setting of a large bulla, occupying

at least 30% of the hemithorax. Another indication is history of a pneumothorax. (See Section 2.3.)

Answer to Question 12

B

Acquired hypogammaglobulinaemia should be excluded, as it requires specific treatment with regular immunoglobulin infusion. In allergic bronchopulmonary aspergillosis, proximal bronchiectasis would be expected. (See Sections 1.1.3 and 2.4.)

Answer to Question 13

A

The following should be excluded: vasculitis (antineutrophil cytoplasmic antibody), allergic bronchopulmonary aspergillosis (skin-prick test is the best screening), emphysema secondary to α_1-antitrypsin deficiency as well as the possibility of bronchiolitis obliterans (if other investigations prove normal). (See Section 2.2.2.)

Answer to Question 14

B

Patients with diffuse parenchymal lung disease (DPLD) usually have a restrictive defect in spirometry. However, in the early stages of DPLD, spirometry may be normal. An obstructive defect may be seen in some patients with DPLD, eg in those who have sarcoidosis. A mixed defect can be seen if chronic obstructive pulmonary disease coexists. (See Section 2.7.)

Answer to Question 15

B

The high-resolution CT chest scan shows extensive bilateral cystic bronchiectasis of proximal distribution, most likely secondary

to allergic bronchopulmonary aspergillosis (ABPA). A skin-prick test to *Aspergillus fumigatus* should be the first step in screening for ABPA. If the skin-prick test is positive, serum total IgE and serum precipitins to *A. fumigatus* should be requested next. ABPA is excluded if the serum total IgE level is less than 1000 ng/mL or if serum precipitins to *A. fumigatus* are negative. (See Sections 1.1.3 and 2.4.)

Answer to Question 16

E

The CXR shows left thoracoplasty. Before streptomycin and then isoniazid became available, apical pulmonary tuberculosis was sometimes treated with thoracoplasty. This involved the removal of several ribs from the chest wall in order to collapse a lung and to close open tuberculous cavities. The average patient required the removal of seven to eight ribs. (See Section 1.2.7.)

Answer to Question 17

C

The CXR shows right upper lobe collapse. An endobronchial lesion must be excluded. Some lung cancers (adenocarcinoma and carcinoid) are not smoking-related. (See Section 3.6.4.)

Answer to Question 18

C

Multiple pleural plaques are present, which suggests previous asbestos exposure. There is no evidence of pleural fibrosis or emphysema. The patient's shortness of breath and chest tightness are unlikely to be respiratory in nature. The possibility of angina should be excluded by further appropriate investigations. (See Section 2.6.1.)

Answer to Question 19

E

This man presents with symptoms typical of chronic hyperventilation syndrome. A referral for physiotherapy should be made for breathing retraining. (See Section 1.1.8.)

Answer to Question 20

B

There is nothing to suggest asthma. A mild obstructive defect with reduced corrected gas transfer is compatible with emphysema. Neither oral corticosteroid reversibility nor single bronchodilator reversibility are recommended as these do not predict a response to inhaled corticosteroids. If he remains symptomatic on an inhaled short-acting bronchodilator, then long-acting inhaled bronchodilators should be prescribed. (See Section 1.2.5.)

Answer to Question 21

C

A chronic cough is defined as one persisting for at least 8 weeks. In approximately 90% of cases presenting to secondary care the cause is one of asthma, rhinitis/sinusitis or gastro-oesophageal reflux disease. However, in this group of patients the GP has usually considered any drug-related causes prior to referral; in this woman it is likely that the angiotensin-converting enzyme inhibitor is responsible, and should be stopped. (See Section 1.1.5.)

Answer to Question 22

D

This woman has type II respiratory failure, which needs treatment with bi-level positive airways pressure (BiPAP). If her oxygenation does not improve with this alone, controlled oxygen therapy may be used in conjunction. An early decision needs to be made with the patient about whether she wants, and is suitable for, intubation and ventilation should the BiPAP fail. Some texts quote radiographic consolidation as a relative contraindication to non-invasive ventilation, due to worries about sputum impaction and difficulties expectorating. In fact, positive airways pressure facilitates sputum clearance (it is used by some physiotherapists in bronchiectasis for this purpose) and a nasal mask can be used where there is copious sputum production. (See Sections 1.2.5 and 2.3.)

Answer to Question 23

C

The Epworth Sleepiness Scale is a validated tool for screening for obstructive sleep apnoea syndrome. It comprises seven questions scoring a maximum of 3 points each. A total score of over 11 in an appropriate clinical scenario is highly supportive of the diagnosis. (See Sections 1.1.6 and 2.1.1.)

Answer to Question 24

C

The diaphragm has to work harder to inflate the lungs when lying down, because there is no assistance from gravity. Normally no functional effect is seen, but in diaphragmatic weakness there will be a relative reduction in forced inspiratory flow (and pressure, which is more difficult to measure) when lying down compared with standing or sitting. (See Section 2.1.1.)

Answer to Question 25

D

Obesity hypoventilation eventually leads to chronic type II respiratory failure and cor pulmonale. Patients often have coexisting obstructive sleep apnoea syndrome. (See Section 2.10.)

Answer to Question 26

E

This woman has developed type II respiratory failure and cor pulmonale secondary to her chest wall deformity. Even though this deformity may have pre-existed for many years, advancing age and comorbidities (chronic, such as kyphosis or chronic obstructive pulmonary disease, or acute, such as pneumonia) often accumulate to produce chronic respiratory failure. This woman has chronic symptoms, and in the absence of any reversible factors will require home ventilation. (See Section 2.12.3.)

Answer to Question 27

B

Weight loss is central in the management of obstructive sleep apnoea syndrome. This is often initially difficult to achieve with severe daytime somnolence, but many patients are able to lose weight after successful initiation of treatment. This man needs input from the physiotherapist and dietitian so that his previous symptomatic improvement can be regained. (See Section 2.1.1.)

Answer to Question 28

C

Indications for the urgent insertion of a chest drain for a pleural effusion include empyema (pus in the pleural cavity), haemothorax (not the same as blood-stained fluid) or a pH <7.3, which indicates a highly metabolically active collection (almost always due to infection or malignancy). In all cases, the fluid is likely to form locules with thick fibrous septa, and hence early intervention to prevent this is required. (See Section 1.4.4.)

Answer to Question 29

D

It is important to make an accurate diagnosis, and to treat the effusion. Pleural tap has about a 60% sensitivity for pleural malignancy, whereas thoracoscopic biopsy will make the diagnosis in 98% of cases. In addition, the fluid can be drained and pleurodesis performed in the same procedure. If mesothelioma is confirmed, the patient will need to have radiotherapy to the site to prevent extension of tumour along the tract. (See Sections 1.2.4 and 2.9.2.)

Answer to Question 30

E

Wegener's granulomatosis affects the upper and lower respiratory tract and kidneys. Further investigation includes urgent measurement of serum antineutrophil cytoplasmic antibodies and mucosal biopsy (nasal is the easiest), preferably prior to commencement of immunosuppression. (See Section 2.8.4.)

Answer to Question 31

A

The use of leukotriene receptor antagonists has been associated with the development of Churg–Strauss syndrome in asthma, although almost always in the context of a reduction in oral steroid use, which is the more

likely precipitant. It should be considered in all patients with deteriorating asthma, especially where there is blood eosinophilia and interstitial shadows on the CXR. Systemic vasculitis with skin, cardiac and renal involvement may follow. (See Section 2.8.5.)

Answer to Question 32

A

Obstructive sleep apnoea (OSA) is usually worse in the supine position and during rapid eye movement (REM) sleep. Alcohol worsens OSA as a result of its sedative effect (although it does not increase REM sleep) and by relaxing the pharyngeal muscles. (See Sections 1.1.6 and 2.1.1.)

Answer to Question 33

D

The most common symptoms in acute pulmonary embolism (PE) are dyspnoea (73%), tachypnoea (70%), pleuritic chest pain (66%), cough (37%) and haemoptysis (13%). Although wheeze may occur in pulmonary hypertension (perhaps secondary to bronchial compression by adjacent enlarged pulmonary arteries), it is very rare in acute PE and points towards an alternative diagnosis (eg asthma).

Answer to Question 34

B

Narcolepsy is characterised by excessive daytime somnolence (can be measured by the Epworth Sleepiness Scale), cataplexy (sudden onset of muscle weakness, which may be focal or generalised), hypnagogic hallucinations (vivid hallucinations occurring at the onset of sleep) and sleep paralysis (inability to move on falling asleep or wakening, often

accompanied by hallucinations). (See Section 2.1.1.)

Answer to Question 35

E

Bilateral hilar lymphadenopathy and erythema nodosum is a typical presentation of sarcoidosis. The diagnosis should be confirmed by tissue biopsy, and the other main differential, tuberculosis, excluded. (See Section 2.8.2.)

Answer to Question 36

E

Bi-level positive airways pressure is indicated for acute type II respiratory failure with a pH <7.35, although there is less evidence for benefit if pH <7.25. (See Section 2.12.3.)

Answer to Question 37

A

Light's criteria for differentiating an exudative from transudative pleural effusion are the presence of one or more of fluid protein/serum protein >0.5, fluid LDH/serum LDH >0.6 and fluid LDH more than two-thirds over the upper limit of serum normal. (See Sections 1.2.4 and 1.4.4.)

Answer to Question 38

B

The fluid pH should always be recorded: a low pH is associated with highly cellular/metabolically active effusions, commonly caused by infection or malignancy. (See Sections 1.2.4 and 1.4.4.)

Answer to Question 39

D

Although *Streptococcus milleri* is the most commonly isolated organism from community-acquired empyema (although only isolated in 16% of cases; 34% are culture negative), in nosocomial infections methicillin-resistant *Staphylococcus aureus*, Gram-negative organisms and anaerobes are more common. (See Section 1.4.4.)

Answer to Question 40

A

Hypercalcaemia in malignancy needs to be managed aggressively with intravenous fluids and bisphosphonates. Superior vena cava obstruction may be caused by extrinsic but non-invasive compression or by thrombosis, and so must always be investigated by CT with or without venogram. (See Section 2.9.1.)

Answer to Question 41

A and C

The CXR shows extensive bilateral interstitial infiltrates. Causes include oedema, pneumonia and pneumonia: the history and particularly the subacute

onset favours the former two. (See Section 2.8.6.)

Answer to Question 42

B and D

Benign asbestos-related pleural disease usually causes a blood-stained exudate. It usually occurs shortly after the exposure period (as opposed to mesothelioma, which occurs 20–40 years later). Traumatic blood-staining of a transudative effusion may also occur during thoracocentesis. Nevertheless, bloody pleural effusions always need investigating thoroughly, in particular to exclude malignancy and pulmonary embolus. (See Section 2.8.6.)

Answer to Question 43

E and H

Continued smoking significantly increases the risk of recurrence of spontaneous pneumothorax, even in the absence of chronic obstructive pulmonary disease. Diving should be permanently avoided, unless the patient has

had bilateral successful pleurodeses. (See http://www.britthoracic.org.uk/c2/uploads/PleuralDiseaseSpontaneous.pdf)

Answer to Question 44

G and I

Pleural effusion is one of the many pulmonary complications of rheumatoid arthritis and its treatment. (See Section 2.8.3.)

Answer to Question 45

A and F

The pulmonary complications/associations of rheumatoid arthritis are many. (See Section 2.8.3.)

Answer to Question 46

B and J

Certain radiographic features, such as apical fibrosis and interstitial granulomas, imply previous tuberculosis, but do not exclude the presence of active disease. (See Section 1.2.8.)

THE MEDICAL MASTERCLASS SERIES

329

Haematology and Oncology

HAEMATOLOGY

Cardiology and Respiratory Medicine

CARDIOLOGY

Gastroenterology and Hepatology

GASTROENTEROLOGY AND HEPATOLOGY

Neurology, Ophthalmology and Psychiatry

NEUROLOGY

PACES Stations and Acute Scenarios 3

Endocrinology

ENDOCRINOLOGY

Nephrology

NEPHROLOGY

Rheumatology and Clinical Immunology

RHEUMATOLOGY AND CLINICAL IMMUNOLOGY

Note: page numbers in *italics* refer to figures, those in **bold** refer to tables.